Training Your Brain To Adopt Healthful Habits:

Mastering The Five Brain Challenges

Fourth Edition
2024

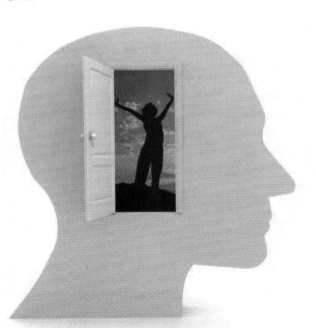

By:
Jodie A. Trafton, Ph.D.
William P. Gordon, Ph.D.
& Supriya Misra, Sc.D.

Published by:
Institute for Brain Potential (IBP)

Library of Congress Cataloging-in-Publication Data
Training Your Brain To Adopt Healthful Habits: Mastering The Five Brain Challenges, Fourth Edition
ISBN: 978-0-9832465-8-9

Copyright © 2024 by Institute for Disease Management, a division of Institute for Brain Potential (IBP).

Institute for Brain Potential (IBP) is a non-profit organization dedicated to providing advances in Behavioral Medicine through publications and conferences. IBP is a 501(c)(3) organization (tax identification number 77-0026830) founded in 1984 as Institute for Cortext Research and Development. Over four million health professionals have completed our live, online, and recorded programs or text-based continuing education available at ibpceu.com. Over 30,000 health professionals have purchased prior editions of Training Your Brain to Adopt Healthful Habits. Updated in 2024, this text can also provide 24 hours of continuing education for most health professionals.

Printed in the United States of America

Table of Contents

- Smiling

Brain Challenge #3: Enhancing Resiliency to New Threats and Chronic Stressors

Challenge 5: Creating an executive system that supports problem-solving to optimize health benefits for health care enrollees **302**
- Ensuring clinical practices optimize patients long-term health
- Managing health care finances

Appendices **308**

References Cited **341**

PREFACE

One of the most difficult challenges in life is learning to make healthful decisions, whether it is about how we eat, exercise, take prescribed drugs and illicit drugs, drink, smoke or manage our emotions. Most people know what they should be doing but fail to heed the recommendations of their physicians and other caregivers.

Why is it so hard to maintain healthful habits? This book, updated in this fourth edition, will explain successful processes to initiate and maintain change from a neuroscience perspective. Specifically, we will examine five key brain challenges that underlie many of the most effective cognitive, behavioral, and pharmacological strategies for changing health behaviors and maintaining healthful practices. The neuroscience is presented simply and focused on the practical. While advances in optogenetics, neuroimaging techniques, behavioral economic modeling, and other scientific methods are rapidly increasing our understanding of how brains make decisions and control behavior, one does not need to understand the methods or fine-grained details to make use of the findings. Here, we filter down complex science into simple applicable concepts that you can use in your everyday life and clinical practice. Each of the brain challenges is followed by exercises to target the brain processes, encouraging you to change your brain responses as you learn about them. Research has consistently shown that behavior change requires active participation rather than just passively learning concepts. As such, this text will walk you through activities as you learn how and why they work.

It is remarkable that the same brain circuits that participate in self-destructive drug dependence and substance misuse, including nicotine, alcohol, cocaine, amphetamines, and heroin, can also encourage self-benefiting practices that we will call healthy pleasures (e.g., eating healthy foods, engaging in stimulating physical activity, thinking calming thoughts, fostering genuine friendships and collaborations, and doing productive activities). Just as use of addictive substances can become automatic and compulsive, positive behaviors can be acquired and become habit-forming. Once learned and supported in your everyday life, both negative and positive habits can be performed without much conscious effort. However, acquiring a health-promoting habit takes a good deal of effort and focused attention. We will show you how.

Many books purport to enable their readers to make changes that are quick and easy. The overwhelming evidence is that changing habits is neither quick nor easy. Making real change requires making thoughtful decisions every day and deferring immediate gratification even when you are stressed or in a hurry. Moreover, making real change normally involves the need to reinstate the behavior multiple times. Lapses and relapses are a normal part of the process of achieving positive health habits, just as they are part of the process of overcoming self-destructive behaviors such as drug dependence. Read the chapters, participate in the exercises, and put them into practice, and you will have an excellent chance to create meaningful and lasting change. We challenge you to try and try again to continually come closer to realizing your optimal health. Your goal should be to continue to work on optimizing your health rather than to attain a specific weight or level of fitness. Health is a process, a state of being, and an ongoing activity rather than a specific outcome or marker of achievement.

Your odds of adding years to your life and life to your years are greatly increased if you avoid tobacco cannabis, excessive alcohol use, and illicit drugs, maintain a healthy weight, eat healthful foods, and avoid infections, toxic agents, risky sexual behaviors, unsafe use of firearms, and reckless driving. You already know this. However, what is less understood is that an estimated half of all deaths in the United States and the industrialized world are related to self-destructive behaviors and habits (Mocdad et al., 2004; McGinnis 2013). As of 2020, the top four causes of U.S. deaths were poor diet, tobacco use, obesity, and alcohol and drug use. Inactivity, motor vehicle crashes, firearm accidents and incidents, and unsafe sexual behaviors, are also large contributors to mortality. However, it is very difficult to stop smoking, drinking, over-eating, under-exercising, emotionally over-reacting, and other seemingly intractable habits. The table below provides some statistics demonstrating the impact of these risks.

<u>Top Causes of Mortality in the United States</u>

(CDC, Data Brief 427: Mortality in the United States, 2020)

Disease Associated with Death		**Behavioral Causes of Death**	
Heart Disease	659,000	Diet	>525,000
Cancer	602,000	Tobacco	~500,000
COVID-19	351,000	Obesity	>375,000
Accidents	201,000	Alcohol and drug use	~175,000
Stroke	160,000	Inactivity	~100,000
Lung Disease	153,000	Unsafe Sex	~20,000
Alzheimer's disease	134,000		
Diabetes	102,000		
Pneumonia/Influenza	54,000		
Kidney Disease	53,000		

<u>Legend:</u> This table provides the number of people per year who died in the United States based on (1) the top diseases that contributed to their death in 2020 or (2) the leading behavioral risk factors that contributed to their death in 2016.

Conclusions About Changing Health-Related Habits
* *Information alone is rarely sufficient to meaningfully alter behavior.* Information about why to change a behavior may be necessary to motivate change, but practice and support for new behaviors are needed to create enduring health-related habits.
* *Learning "how" to change a behavior is of much greater value than learning "why" a*

behavior should be changed. We offer more than a lecture about why you should change and what behaviors you should adopt. We help you take positive steps to discover what works for you and to make these new behaviors an ongoing part of your life. We show you how to initiate action, learn from mistakes, and refine healthful behavior.

* *Chronic interventions are more effective than acute interventions.* Learning to convert a health behavior into a habit often requires chronic interventions from health professionals and coaches. Chronic interventions to promote behavioral change work best for chronic conditions but most interventions provided by physicians and allied health professionals are provided in acute care settings. We will show you how to build an environment and support structure that will help you achieve chronic health, using tools such as automatic reminders, scheduling, environmental modification, networking, and revaluation of health-related choices.

* *Relapse is the norm rather than the exception. Therefore, it is very helpful to build in back-up strategies at the start.* We show you how to reinstate healthful behaviors by identifying what worked previously and evaluating what went wrong.

* *Daily or frequent self-monitoring is immensely valuable in helping you focus on what you are trying to achieve, the obstacles to change, and everyday problem-solving.* We show you several ways to institute self-monitoring. We also provide you with forms and tools so that you can easily review your progress.

* *A support system is extremely helpful for maintaining changes.* We will show you how to recruit family, friends and health professionals who can encourage, remind, or participate in what you seek to change. We will also show you how to recognize when family or friends unwittingly sabotage your efforts to institute and maintain change.

* *Defer immediate gratification.* We will explain why your brain is biased toward seeking short-term pleasure at the expense of long-term health. We go into substantial detail to describe how the part of the brain that drives automatic behavior to get immediate rewards (the limbic reward system) can overwhelm other higher brain centers (the prefrontal executive system) that facilitate the ability to delay gratification.

* *Make healthful habits automatic through practice and reinforcement.* A habit requires little conscious effort whereas a conscious behavior requires short-term memory and initiating or reminding events. We will show you how to convert healthful conscious behaviors into habits, this time focusing on the basal ganglia, the part of the brain that learns and retains new habits even when your short-term memory does not function well.

* *It is possible to acquire more than one health-related habit at a time. If you want to try this program, be bold as you work for meaningful results.*

What Is New About This Book
1. To our knowledge, this is the first book to break health behavior change into specific neural processes, describing first the underlying brain activity that needs to be changed and then providing exercises to help you alter these processes. You will learn how to reprogram your reward circuits and prefrontal cortex to achieve your health objectives.
2. We draw our recommendations based on the totality of evidence from our extensive catalog of continuing medical education seminars and books (ibpceu.com), where leading experts have curated the latest research into actionable behavioral health information for health professionals.
3. We explain how the addiction-related reward circuits of the brain can be reprogrammed

to help people acquire and maintain healthful habits. Emphasis is placed on the four health-related habits of greatest interest to health professionals:

- Changing preference for healthful food to achieve a healthy weight;
- Changing a sedentary lifestyle to include regular and rewarding physical activity;
- Changing the way emotions and emotion-driven thoughts are managed;
- Addressing pain safely and effectively to support function and wellness.

4. We provide interactive exercises for the learning components of this book. We invite the readers who have completed the exercises to contact the authors to help us update the exercises based on what works, what is confusing, and what is unhelpful. We seek to improve the book on a regular basis. We invite you to participate.

5. We provide suggestions regarding effective strategies for not only changing health habits in individuals, but also for changing clinical practices in health care systems to support behavioral health care delivery that is safe and effective for both patients and providers.

About The Authors

Jodie Anne Trafton, Ph.D., William P. Gordon, Ph.D., and Supriya Misra, Sc.D. are behavioral neuroscientists and health service delivery experts deeply interested in the neural mechanisms underlying change, the psychological processes that facilitate meaningful health-related change, and health care practices that support patients and providers in making change. They are committed to creating a clear, practical resource for health professionals, clients and anyone who seeks to change health-related behaviors.

Both Drs. Trafton and Gordon are actively involved in innovation of methods to create meaningful, enduring change in health behaviors, and development of trainings, books, and programs to help others achieve these objectives. Their goal is to not only spur initial attempts to reach a health objective, but also to encourage reinstatement of the behavior until it becomes an enjoyable lifelong habit. They link basic science findings and clinical trials evidence to not only share the most evidence-based clinical practices with clinicians, but also explain the neurobiology and learning mechanisms that underlie their effectiveness. Here, we highlight practices culled from comprehensive review of long-term clinical trials of behavioral health interventions (e.g., as we curated in the four-volume series, *Best Practices in the Behavioral Management of Chronic Disease*, a 52-chapter series where experts in management of chronic health conditions systematically reviewed clinical trials research on behavioral health interventions for each condition) and in collaboration with leading academic and clinical experts to develop continuing medical education for health professionals over 4 decades.

Disclaimer To Neuroscientists

For us to explain many of the neurobiological processes important for encouraging healthful behavior change in a clear, concise manner, we are forced to oversimplify systems and underlying cell biology to isolate the process of interest. Neuronal systems rarely do only one thing and have layers and layers of modifiers, regulatory processes and feedback loops that keep behavior both flexible and stable. Trying to discuss all that we know about these systems, their detailed and changing connections, and the chemical interactions that modify cellular activity over short and longer time scales, would take an encyclopedia, confuse all but the most dedicated neurobiologists, be extremely dull in many places, and, most importantly, not help clinicians or patients understand the key elements of how to change health behaviors. There are places in this text where we oversimplify the neurobiology to the point that the details are not precisely accurate: a few neurons in a circuit are missing, effects are ascribed to a single neurotransmitter or receptor system when many are involved with much more intricate interactions and regulatory effects, or we leave out the effects and processes occurring in whole brain regions. Although the broader literature is exciting and may contribute greatly to our understanding, there is just too much to discuss. So please forgive us in places where the details are fudged for the sake of simplicity. We have purposely chosen to focus on the broader concepts and processes that guide these neurobiological systems. Apologies to the neurobiologists whose decades of work are summarized in a sentence, have been stripped of their subtleties or are ignored all together. We have sacrificed the detail of your work to make it accessible to those with a day rather than a decade to understand it.

INTRODUCTION

Imagine how vastly we could improve the health of people in the industrialized world simply by changing their habits. The top contributors to disease in these countries are all unhealthful behaviors. With effective behavior change, no new medications, medical devices, diagnostic tests and machines, or surgical techniques are needed to eliminate the biggest contributors to disease and death in our population. But then why have most people not altered their health behaviors? Education cannot be the main problem. Who does not know that smoking, drinking, taking drugs, eating unhealthful food, not exercising, playing with guns, driving too fast or when intoxicated, and having unprotected sex are bad for you? So why do so many of us do these things anyway? Why is it so hard to make healthful choices and act on them consistently?

Immediate Gratification: The Deadly Trade-Off

One major problem is that these unhealthful behaviors can seem fun and rewarding at the time. While cookies and a soda might make a lousy lunch in terms of nutrition, they still taste good, and the sugar and caffeine are highly rewarding to our brains. In the moment, risky sex, fast driving, substance use, gun play, or laying around watching TV can all seem exciting, relaxing, thrilling, or enjoyable, even if they make us feel bad, get sick, or risk injury later. To behave healthfully, we need to control our actions and keep ourselves safe when these quick pleasures present themselves. That can be a very difficult thing to do.

To make good choices that lead to long-term wellness, we need to be able to forgo immediate gratification at least some of the time. Shortsighted decisions keep us from reaching our health potential. In this book, we explore the brain circuits that influence our search for immediate gratification. We discuss how we learn bad habits and why we favor bad habits over more objectively rewarding behaviors. We describe how feeling helpless, stressed, and out of control can make it difficult to make good choices. We demonstrate why not recognizing opportunities in your life can make you impulsive. We explain how unrealistic expectations, stigma, social pressure, and media exposure can lead our brain to overvalue quick fixes. Most importantly, by revealing how these systems work, we provide techniques for shaping these circuits to support your quest for long-term health and happiness. Lastly, we offer exercises to help you practice these important psychological techniques.

To focus our exploration of the neurobiological and psychological basis of good health choices, we have broken the process of health behavior change into five steps or challenges. These steps map onto a simplified brain circuit that processes information to guide your behavior. These steps are as follows:

Challenge #1: Learning to highly value behaviors that promote wellness and devalue behaviors that lead to poor health.

When we make decisions, our brains weigh options and consider the expected benefits, including immediate gratification, of one action versus another. If you expect big benefits from behaviors that lead to poor health, then you will make self-destructive choices. If you expect healthful behaviors to be boring, painful, or unpleasant, then you probably will not do them. For example, if I think of a big five-scoop ice cream sundae as a delicious reward then I will probably want to eat it. If I instead think of the stomachache that it will likely produce shortly after, I probably will not. If I think of how much my legs will hurt while I go running, I probably will not go running. If I think of the warm glow I will experience after I run, I probably will. Altering our expectations about the benefits of behaviors can lead to big changes in health.

Challenge #2: Enriching your life to tame the need for immediate gratification.
Our brains keep track of opportunities in which we know how to do things to obtain quick benefits. When opportunities are rare, our brains will drive us to habitually take advantage of these rare opportunities, even when the benefits may be short-lived and the negative consequences may be relatively great. If you spend your days feeling neglected and deprived, you will find it hard to turn down the quick pleasure presented by the cookies at the convenience store. Conversely, when our brains recognize that we have many opportunities, they slow down and consider options more thoughtfully and deliberately. If you have a rich life with lots of positive interactions with people and choices about what to eat and how to spend your time, you will find it easier to turn down a quick reward and stick to your long-term goals. Learning to recognize and take advantage of more opportunities in your life can help you make decisions with greater long-term benefits. Learning to recognize problems, negative emotions, and connections with people as opportunities to make your life better can be a helpful step.

Challenge #3: Enhancing resiliency to new threats and chronic stressors.
Threats to our well-being cause us to favor quick fixes over potentially better or more durable solutions. When we feel threatened, it feels so important to do something to make things better immediately, that we may not even consider other options that would provide much greater long-term benefits. Feeling endangered brings out bad habits, and inhibits careful, purposeful problem-solving. When we reduce stress in our lives and feel in control of our fate, we are more likely to be able to make good choices that lead to excellent health. As we will show, by increasing the predictability of unpleasant events and increasing your sense of control over them, you will become resilient both emotionally and physically. Eating, smoking, and drinking are common responses to feeling unsafe and are well-known health-related risks. By learning ways to keep your physiology in balance and change your response to threatening situations, you can avert self-destructive choices in trying times. The key is to create life patterns and responses that promote safety and confidence.

Challenge #4: Training your addiction circuits to make health behaviors habitual.
It is much easier to do behaviors regularly when they become habits. But to make a behavior habitual, we must first learn it and then practice it a lot. Finding ways of learning new behaviors, encouraging practice, and rewarding good behavior is key to learning new habits that will keep us healthful as we age. We will show you first how to efficiently learn a new behavior. We will then teach you how to convert behaviors into habits by introducing monitors and rewards for your attempts. For example, if you want to consistently walk half an hour a day, it is very helpful to keep a log of your daily physical activity and find a buddy to check your log and praise your successful efforts.

Challenge #5: Empower your brain to make healthful, flexible choices.

Even with the best health habits, life provides us with challenges that we cannot resolve with quick, easy answers. In these situations, you need to be able to imagine new responses, think through the long-term consequences of your choices, and plan novel and potentially complex solutions. For example, it is very helpful to think out ways of handling problems you are apt to encounter before you try something, rather than waiting until an emergency arises. Pre-planning solutions to problems you are likely to encounter can help you avoid relying on quick fixes that save you in the moment but generate more problems later. We show you techniques for making creative, flexible, future-focused plans and generating more adaptive long-term solutions to obstacles.

What You Will Take Away

In sum, you will learn to reduce the tendency to make impulsive and self-destructive actions while acquiring strategies to help you progress towards your long-term goals. At the end of each challenge, we include exercises to help you practice what you learn. Feel free to modify or adapt these to meet your needs. In chapter 6, we combine the five challenges into an individual case study entitled "The Example of Achieving a Healthful Diet and Body Weight". We walk back through each of the sections of the book and provide suggestions to apply what we have learned to the specific health behavior goal of achieving a healthful weight and diet. This understanding goes beyond eating healthfully and exercising consistently to tackle the underlying behaviors we need to undertake to value health, enrich our lives, develop stress resilience, train good habits, and improve problem-solving to reach and maintain weight or other health behavior goals.

Lastly, we provide a guide to addressing these challenges in health care delivery. The effectiveness of health care depends on clinicians having the supports and structure necessary to provide advice and treatments that enhance patients' long-term health and well-being. Clinicians' must develop practice habits that bring safe and effective health care interventions to patients in a manner that patients can access. But, as humans, clinicians are vulnerable to incentives and stressful or opportunity-poor environments that can favor quick fixes over effective health care. Without attention to the five challenges, health care systems can unintentionally encourage and reinforce clinical practices that worsen long-term wellness of patients and providers alike. We explore evidence-based methods to improve health care outcomes through health care system interventions that support providers in effective practice habits.

In this book, we present these processes from a brain-based perspective. We will discuss findings from neuroscience, but these are presented to help you understand why specific behavior change processes work. We have attempted to keep the concepts simple and understandable for readers without a detailed knowledge of neuroscience – it is not crucial that you know and remember the neuroanatomical structures or understand the detailed cellular mechanisms, as long as you grasp the behavior change processes. Nevertheless, we expect that some readers will want to understand the neurobiology more explicitly, so we have included appendices that provide more information about the brain structures we mention (Appendix 1), and more information about the cellular processes involved in learning (Appendix 2). Additionally, Appendix 3 contains an alternative conceptualization of three different circuits of the brain that have to do with the acquisition, retrieval, or modification of habits. If you find the sections on neurobiology difficult to conceptualize, we suggest starting with the Appendices 1 and 2 first. These are not necessary reading, but we hope they will be helpful to those more curious about the neurobiological mechanisms of the health-related processes we describe.

To make best use of this book, it is helpful to take an honest inventory of your own health behaviors before proceeding. With your own risks and habits in mind it will be easier to relate the processes to your life and make effective use of the included exercises. On the next page, complete the checklist of risk factors. You can refer back to it as you work through the book and identify your specific health goals for the various exercises.

What Are My Health Risks?

Risk Factor	Check if you have this risk	Personal Notes
High Level of Stress		
Low Level of Life Satisfaction		
Chronic Anxiety or Depression		
Easily Angry or Upset		
High Cholesterol		
High Blood Pressure		
Exercise <30 Minutes Daily		
Body Mass Index over 27.5		
Smoke Tobacco or Cannabis		
Harmful Alcohol Use*		
Illicit Drug Use		
Failure to Use Safety Belts		
Unsecured Gun in the Home		
Have Unprotected Sex		
Excessive Recreational Screen Time**		
Take Too Much or Too Little Prescribed Medication		
Sleep <6 hours Nightly		
Work >50 hours Weekly		
Excessive Sitting		
Absenteeism		
Other (specify):		
Other (specify):		

*For men: greater than 14 standard drinks per week or more than 4 in a sitting; for women: greater than 7 standard drinks per week or more than 3 in a sitting.

**For our purposes, defined as more than 2 hours of recreational screen viewing a day.

With these risks in mind, we encourage you to explore the key neurobiological challenges to reshaping your lifestyle and decisions and begin and repeat the exercises and practices that will make healthful choices and actions habitual.

Brain Challenge #1
Learning to Highly Value Behaviors that Promote Wellness and Devalue Behaviors that Lead to Poor Health

Challenge Introduction

You are dining with friends and are served an extra-large piece of hot apple pie with a huge scoop of vanilla ice cream. You know this is not good for you, but ah, the aroma, the sight of it, the encouragement of the host; it's her special recipe and you do want to please, right? How can you possibly stick to your diet when everything and everyone is encouraging you otherwise?

Your health-related decisions depend upon your brain's perception of the value of your options. When you make a decision to do something, you are inevitably choosing not to do something else. In deciding between two or more actions, you want to pick the choice that improves your life the most. To do this, you must estimate how much each of the possible actions will help you. Should you eat the apple pie and ice cream or finish your meal with a cup of tea instead? The answer depends on what you expect eating the pie or drinking the tea will do for you. Will the apple pie or tea taste better? Will the people around you approve of you more or make you feel a part of the group if you choose the pie versus the tea? Will your host be upset if you turn down her pie? Your brain carefully calculates and keeps track of estimates and expectations about the outcomes of your possible actions based upon your past experiences and observations about each option. Using a well-developed system, you automatically assign a value to every behavior you know how to do in a given situation. You then use these estimates to choose between options available at any given time. Thus, your expectations about the value or results of a behavior are hugely important in determining what you choose to do over time. If you highly value or expect greater benefits from healthful behaviors, you will generally choose healthful behaviors over other options. If you have strong expectations that doing unhealthful behaviors will better your life, improve your social status, or make you feel good, then you will tend to do those unhealthful behaviors rather than make more healthful choices. This can lead you down a path towards chronic health problems.

Your brain will consider many factors when estimating the benefits of an action. Your previous experiences will shape your estimations. Your perception of how others close to you will react to the behavior will strongly color your estimates. If doing a behavior gains you immediate approval from people important to you, you will learn to expect social rewards for that behavior in the future. Your own expectations about the results of the action, objectively accurate or not, will strongly influence your estimates. Your expectations may be strongly influenced by cultural stories about the meaning or results of a behavior. You may have learned to associate the behavior with other good or bad things through advertising, entertainment, or interactions you have seen. Your current emotional or physiological state may drastically affect your judgments about the value of an action. For example, you will probably expect the benefits of eating apple pie to be greater when you are hungry than when you are not. The impact of the action on your long-term goals may change your estimates. If you use addictive substances, you will overestimate the benefits of using these substances because of the pharmacological effects of the substances on your brain. On the next page is a checklist of possible factors that may lead you to over- or undervalue options when you are making a decision.

Factors that can influence our evaluation of the benefits of health options
- Previous experiences
- Beliefs and expectations
- Social norms
- Social approval
- Cues we associate with the behavior
- Physiological states
- Current thoughts
- Directed attention
- Emotional states
- Long-term goals
- Substance use
- Novelty
- Stress
- How quickly we will receive the benefit

In Challenge #1, we will examine each of these influences on your estimates of the benefits of your potential actions. In Chapter 1.1, we discuss how your brain, and specifically your dopamine neurons, generates value estimates so your brain can weigh options when making health-related decisions. In Chapter 1.2, we reveal how opportunities for reward can get overvalued through social pressure, expectations, and advertising. In Chapter 1.3, we explain additional social factors that contribute to this overvaluation and how that can sabotage your health. In Chapter 1.4, we specifically address how addictive substances can hijack the brain's reward system. In Chapter 1.5, we suggest ways in which you can learn to correct your value estimates and assess the true value of a reward.

Because there are so many factors that contribute to your judgment of the value of doing a behavior, there are many ways in which your estimates can become harmfully inaccurate. Beliefs, social pressures, learned associations, and unpleasant emotional states can lead you to overvalue unhealthful behaviors and undervalue healthful ones. Correcting these inaccurate estimates can help you make more healthful choices.

Chapter 1.1: How Your Brain Weighs Options When Making Health-Related Decisions

In this chapter, we discuss how the brain calculates and keeps track of expectations of the outcomes of our health choices. We will provide examples of ways in which actions can become over or undervalued. We then discuss effective psychological techniques for changing our expectations. Throughout, we provide exercises to encourage these changes in ourselves and in others.

What parts of your brain calculate the value of an opportunity?
Our brains contain an intricate network of neurons that provide ongoing assessment of opportunities in the environment. These neurons generally contain the chemical messenger dopamine, a neurotransmitter that has been associated with disorders of habit and impulsivity. Firing of these neurons encodes the expected value of an opportunity: the greater your expectations about the benefits afforded by an opportunity, the faster these neurons fire. This firing encourages you to repeat the behavior, regardless of how you feel when you are doing it. These dopamine neurons are important for understanding why we make self-destructive versus healthful choices, particularly when tempted by the promise of quick pleasures.

It is important to note that our reward system is not a pleasure system, although many things that are rewarding are also pleasurable in the moment. The reward system motivates behavior, rather than setting mood. While feelings of pleasure may occur around the same time as firing of these neurons, they are neither the cause nor the outcome of it. A reward is something that 1) improves your immediate, if not your long-term, well-being, and 2) encourages learning such that you try to repeat the experience whenever an opportunity presents itself. You will gravitate toward and attend to situations, thoughts, and behaviors that previously led to activation of your reward system regardless of whether the situations, thoughts or behaviors provided benefits, happiness, and health, or hassles, stress, and disease over the long-term. Thus, the dopamine neurons do not signal pleasure but identify immediate opportunities and estimate their potential value.

Neurobiologists have found that these dopamine neurons fire both tonicly and phasicly (Paladini & Roeper, 2014). In the languages of the brain, tonic refers to an ordinary, stable rate of neuron firing and phasic refers to quick bursts of neuron firing that occur at the time of an event. In this system, dopamine neurons fire slowly and consistently (tonically) in the absence of an opportunity. When your brain has not identified any particular prospects for making life better, your dopamine neurons calmly plod away, firing slowly and steadily. However, when your brain detects a chance to improve on your current state, dopamine neurons come to attention, firing a burst of neuronal impulses (phasic firing) to indicate the presence and value of that opportunity. The intensity of firing during these brief bursts tells our brain systems our expectations about the benefits of the present opportunity. Encoded in that burst of dopamine neuron firing is our anticipation of benefits awaiting us if only we take action to claim them. How big of an incentive is that apple pie? The intensity of that burst of dopamine neuron firing when your host offers you the apple pie will determine how strongly you are driven to take it. The more you find the pie enticing, the more rapidly your dopamine neurons will fire. If you are having trouble visualizing how these dopamine neurons work, think of them like a Geiger counter for radiation or a metal detector for metal objects. Your dopamine neurons beep slowly (fire tonicly) until you come near a known opportunity for immediate gratification or relief. When you come near an opportunity, they start to beep faster, with the speed of the beeps indicating how big an opportunity you have just encountered (phasic firing).

Because brains are adaptive, your dopamine neurons do not just relay signals about your expectations; they also constantly learn and update expectations based on the near-term outcomes of your chosen actions (Berke, 2018). This learning happens within a single experience, as part of the process. The brain estimates, makes a decision, and then adjusts its estimations for next time, after it experiences the near-term result of the decision. Perhaps you just took a bite of pie, driven to action by the anticipatory burst of phasic dopamine neurons firing generated by your hosts offer. Was it what you expected? If so, your dopamine neurons are done. Their predictions were great, and their work is finished. But if they were wrong, they will send feedback about their mistakes. How big was the error? Was the pie much better than you anticipated? Was it worse?

In the case that the outcome was worse than expected, tonic firing becomes important. Because these dopamine neurons still fire when no opportunities are present, they are able to slow down below their normal, tonic firing rate to indicate when they made a mistake, such as when an opportunity that they predicted would be present does not pan out. For example, suppose your host was not such a good cook after all, and her beautiful looking pie tasted terrible. Your brain would need some way of warning you not to get so excited about *her* apple pie in the future. Because your dopamine neurons can both speed up or slow down from their resting state, they can provide both positive and negative feedback about your expectations, in terms of dopamine concentration in a brain region called the nucleus accumbens (Hart et al., 2014). This slow, constant firing allows these neurons to dampen their expectations when they overestimated the benefits at the outset. This signals the brain to decrease its expectation of reward in the future, reducing behaviors to seek reward given that same opportunity (Chang et al., 2016). Thus, the rate at which dopamine neurons fire provides two pieces of information for every decision: (1) they make a prediction about the benefits to be had before the choice is made, and (2) they provide feedback about the accuracy of their prediction after the choice occurs.

How do our dopamine neurons come up with their estimates?
Our dopamine neurons get information from all over the brain. These other brain regions provide information about what we are currently observing, what we have experienced in the past, and what our goals are for the future. Each of the brain regions that talk to the dopamine neurons can slow down or speed up the rate at which the dopamine neurons fire. Thus, the information they provide shapes the firing patterns of the dopamine neurons to provide an estimate of the value of a given behavioral choice.

To get a sense of all the things that shape our expectations about our options, it may be helpful to briefly explore some of the neuroanatomy that underlies the predictions made by our dopamine neurons. The dopamine neurons that make these predictions originate in part of our reward circuit, in a brain region called the ventral tegmental area (VTA) (see the Figure on page 23 and Appendix 1 for further details). These reward circuits are a highly conserved and ancient computational system, similar throughout mammalian and reptilian species, and are crucially important for long-term survival. These dopamine neurons receive input from a number of other brain regions that strongly influence their firing patterns, each of which can alter estimations of the value of an opportunity. So what are some of these brain inputs and what do they contribute to our expectations? We need to know what is going on if we are going to create expectations about possibilities in our immediate future. First, we need sensory information. But information about our environment is not enough. We need this information in a personal context. We need to know about our current environment in terms of our past experiences and current goals. Let's go back to that apple pie example. There are a wide variety of sensory cues being observed by various parts of the brain, including the smell and sight of the pie and the sound of the pie being removed from the oven. If this is not your first exposure to apple pie, your memories of these smells, sights and sounds, and things you have learned in eating apple pie previously, will influence how you interpret these sensory experiences.

Additionally, we need information about your current state and goals. For example, if you are hungry and looking for something to eat, that will change how you perceive the pie. Conversely, if you have eaten your fill already, your dopamine neurons will consider your satiated state in their estimates (Papgeorgiou et al., 2016). The prefrontal cortex keeps track of our goals and our intentions, and inputs from this region can also influence the amount these dopamine neurons fire (Del Arco & Mora, 2008). From these prefrontal cortex inputs, information about long-term goals and expectations contribute to the influences on the dopamine neuron firing patterns and thus our valuation of an option.

This is a lot of complicated information, but fortunately, a part of our brain with the virtually unpronounceable name of pedunculopontine tegmentum (PPTg) pulls all of it together to send to our dopamine neurons. The PPTg integrates sensory information from the auditory, visual, and somatosensory (sound, sight, touch and other forms of body-awareness) systems with information from the limbic system (including our emotional memory and reward circuits) and prefrontal cortex (conscious problem-solving and decision-making), and can then change dopamine neuron firing (Grace et al., 2007; Vitay & Hamker, 2014). This allows the PPTg to combine information about what we are hearing, seeing, and feeling with information about our emotional state and long-term goals. The PPTg uses this combined information to guide our dopamine neurons as they estimate the value of opportunities, like a piece of pie, that we encounter. All of this happens while you are sitting at the table, perhaps even before you realize that you are making decisions about whether to eat the pie.

Moreover, a part of your brain called the hippocampus helps recall conscious memories and provides information to dopamine neurons about the novelty of a situation. Our brain finds new options more exciting and motivating. Instead of the usual apple pie, if you are served French apple pie, the hippocampus will help amplify dopamine neuron firing to let you know that this is a new option (Grace et al, 2007). When an opportunity is novel, your brain will inflate its estimates of the benefits to be gained through these circuits, encouraging you to test out a situation that you have not experienced before (Lak et al., 2016). Dopamine neurons are also sensitive to delays in receipt of rewards, even on the order of seconds, and they value delayed rewards less than prompt rewards (Kobayashi and Shultz, 2008). This shapes choices to favor quick rewards over those that require a wait.

Together, the inputs to your dopamine neurons provide information about what we are encountering, our knowledge or experience with similar situations in the past, our current state and goals for the future, the novelty of the experience, and the speed at which the reward will arrive. Thus, all these elements will color your valuation of a choice.

<u>FIGURE: Projections of the dopamine reward neurons</u>

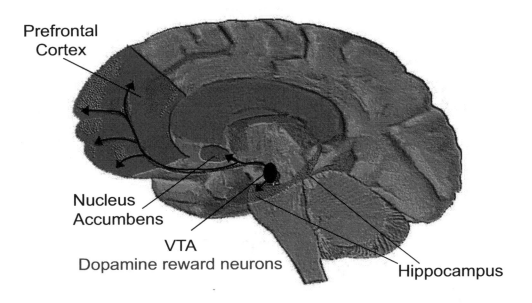

Legend: Reward circuit dopamine neurons originate in the VTA (black oval). They receive inputs from and project back to regions throughout the brain (black arrows). In particular, inputs to the VTA are consolidated in a region of the brain known as the PPTg (not shown). This combines information from the limbic reward system, including the hippocampus, and the prefrontal cortex. The hippocampus provides memories of what we experienced in the past and helps alert us when we encounter something new. The neurons use this consolidated information to predict – based on our previous experience, current states, and future goals – how much we might gain from doing a behavior in our current setting. The dopamine neurons then send outputs back to the limbic reward system and the prefrontal cortex. The prefrontal cortex can modify these predictions based upon additional information about our long-term goals.

What does your brain do with the value estimates that the dopamine neurons provide?

Some of the same regions that provide inputs to the dopamine neurons also receive the outputs. The main targets of these dopamine neurons are the limbic reward circuit and the prefrontal cortex, which use this information to make decisions about how to respond to opportunities. Dopamine neurons provide both brain regions with similar information. In both brain regions, the phasic firing of these neurons represents the expected value of the reward that will be obtained by doing a behavior. The faster the dopamine neurons fire, the greater the expected value of the reward. This firing rate is used to guide the choice of habitual behaviors. This has been observed directly in the nucleus accumbens, part of the limbic reward system (Abler et al., 2006), and in the orbitofrontal cortex, a part of the prefrontal cortex (Roesch & Olson, 2004).

For both short and long-term decisions, the brain must compare between the expected benefits of one choice versus another. Both the limbic reward circuit and the prefrontal cortex must make these choices based on the firing rate of the dopamine neurons.

The limbic reward circuit uses this information to decide whether to carry out well-learned, habitual behaviors to meet an immediate need or desire. It focuses on habits and the NOW. The limbic reward circuit uses the estimates from dopamine neurons to ask, "Can I make my life better this very moment by doing a well-practiced behavior to get something nice or get rid of something unpleasant?"

The prefrontal cortex uses the estimates from dopamine neurons to make broader decisions about behavior. It focuses on new behaviors and the LATER. It asks, "Will this opportunity help me reach a long-term goal? Do I need to do a new or less trained behavior to get the most out of this opportunity? Do I need to do something special because of the unique social or environmental context of this opportunity? Can I solve a complex, multi-part problem with this opportunity?"

Thus, dopamine neuron information is used simultaneously to answer two questions to plan behavior: (1) The limbic system determines if this opportunity can provide immediate gratification—the NOW. Will it provide immediate pleasure or relief? (2) The prefrontal cortex determines if this opportunity can lead to longer-term benefits or goals—the LATER. Will it make life better in the future?

The battle between the "here and now" of the limbic reward circuit and the "what could be" of the prefrontal cortex
To a substantial extent, these two brain regions make their decisions in parallel rather than collaboratively. They can be considered to compete for control over your behavior. When the limbic reward circuit predominates, you will tend to favor behaviors that benefit you right now, the hot apple pie moments of life, regardless of their effect on your future. When the prefrontal cortex predominates, you will tend to favor behaviors that benefit you in the future, even if they involve delay of immediate gratification in the moment or denial of pleasure for the foreseeable future.

The competition between these two brain circuits for control over behavior is influenced by the speed at which they make their choices. The limbic reward circuit tends to make faster decisions than the prefrontal cortex. This reflects the more complex processing that the prefrontal cortex carries out. The limbic reward circuit tends to follow a pretty standard calculation for picking between options whereas the prefrontal cortex can use a variety of logic or decision-making rules in making its choices. This flexibility is crucial for making wise long-term decisions. However, not having clearly set decision-making rules like the limbic reward circuit can slow down choices (Saling & Phillips, 2007). This means that the limbic reward circuit can beat out the prefrontal cortex in controlling behavior, simply by choice. Once this limbic-driven behavior is started, other better choices that the prefrontal cortex was planning may no longer be possible. For example, if your limbic system already directed you to eat the pie, you can no longer choose to search for a more healthful dessert. To keep the limbic system from constantly preempting decisions, the prefrontal cortex has connections with the limbic reward circuit that can inhibit limbic decisions from being carried out. Overall, the prefrontal cortex has some ability to stall or override limbic decisions both while it completes its analysis and if it comes up with a better behavioral plan. However, when you strongly overvalue a habit or have a powerful drive for immediate gratification, your prefrontal cortex will find it difficult to delay behaviors, and your limbic decisions will start to win out over your more careful long-term plans.

EXAMPLE: How do you develop expectations about the value of an opportunity? How much is pie worth to you?

At an early age, one of the author's (W.G.) dopamine neurons linked the smell, taste, and sight of apple pie with positive memories of sweet, satisfying food and a caring family. My overindulgent grandmother loved to bake tasty apple pies. From that point on, I have been compelled to attend to suggestions of apple pie. The smell of pie reorients my attention, distracts me from what I am doing and sends me searching for the source. I have learned to highly value apple pie, and these learned cues get my dopamine neurons firing rapidly. How did I become so driven by the smell of apple pie? How did my experiences shape the firing patterns of my dopamine neurons? Scientists have worked out how our expectations about the benefits of a choice are calculated and modified over time. We will walk through this process step by step to help illustrate how the reward system works.

As we have stated, dopamine neurons use a feedback system to learn and update estimates of the value of an opportunity. Dopamine neurons use this feedback system to guide learning of cues that predict opportunities in the environment. My wonderful experience eating grandma's apple pie induced learning, so that on my next visit to grandma's house, my dopamine neurons were happily firing awaiting the next opportunity. Once cues that predict an opportunity are learned, our brains pay more attention to and alert us to their presence. These cues become emotionally important to us. Apple pie becomes linked with love, caring, and grandma. We notice these cues among the myriad of other things in our environment, and consider changing our behavior in response. For each of these cues, our dopamine neurons learn and update an estimate of the value of responding to the cue or opportunity. Whining about how hungry I am is apt to produce bigger rewards if I whine during my visit with grandma, rather than on the car ride over. My dopamine neurons recognize this and their anticipatory firing at grandma's house encourages my brain to begin doing things that might get me pie when I arrive. The estimates provided by our dopamine neurons help our brain to decide whether an opportunity is worth responding to in comparison to other possibilities. To help clarify how our dopamine neurons develop this estimate, let's walk through an example of this feedback system in action.

<u>EXAMPLE: How do dopamine neurons learn to identify opportunities?</u>
Another author (J.T.) recalls how dopamine neurons can even train behavior in graduate students studying dopamine neurons. Specifically, I describe the example of training neurobiologists to attend science seminars. Let's consider how my graduate program trained my classmates and me to regularly attend optional seminars from invited guest speakers using cookies as bait. At each point in the learning process, I will illustrate how dopamine neurons fire to guide decision-making and learning.

When starting graduate school, I had no expectations for seminars beyond the seminar itself. My dopamine neurons fired only to indicate my expectations of the benefit I would receive from hearing the speaker. For simplicity's sake, reflecting my burned out and overwhelmed state as a graduate student, let's assume I didn't consider it much of an opportunity at all and pretend my dopamine neurons didn't change their firing rates at all. Nevertheless, I followed orders and compliantly went to the seminar. Once there, I was quick to notice the free cookies and juice offered at the back of the room. This offer of free sugar was quickly detected by my dopamine neurons, which increased their firing rate to signal that I could head to the back of the room for a snack should I so desire.

Thus, at my first seminar experience, my dopamine neurons fired as in line A (see diagram below). There was no dopamine neuron firing at the time I saw the seminar announcement. But when I entered the seminar and got a cookie, my dopamine neurons increased their firing by one cookie's worth. My dopamine neuron firing after I entered the seminar signaled my brain to try to find and learn cues that predicted the availability of cookies in a room. Putting my expensively trained intellect to work, it didn't take long for me to guess that the free cookies were part of the seminar series.

The next time I saw a posting for a neuroscience seminar, my dopamine neurons predicted that this indicated an opportunity for free cookies. The posting elicited a cookie's worth of dopamine firing, alerting of my brain of this nutritional resource. Having made this prediction, my dopamine neurons then expected the cookies when I got there. When the cookies were there as predicted, my dopamine neurons didn't respond any further. They had already let me know of the opportunity and done so accurately, therefor the presence of the cookies didn't elicit anything new. There was nothing else to learn, and no corrections to make. My dopamine neurons fired as in line B.

Thinking I had figured out the seminar/cookie connection, I started noticing flyers for other seminars around campus. Feeling particularly hungry one day, I saw a flyer for a seminar for medical doctors put on by a well-known drug company. My dopamine neurons dutifully increased their firing by a couple of cookies' worth to let me know of the opportunity presented by this seminar. To my surprise and delight, this seminar was stocked not only with cookies, but also with freshly made sandwiches and salad. My dopamine neurons had underestimated the opportunity this seminar provided, and quickly started firing again (a sandwich and salad's worth of firing to be exact) to indicate the additional opportunity that this presented. This notified my brain of the original error in my prediction and told me that there was more to learn. I guessed that pharmaceutical company seminars are better funded, and my brain quickly learned to distinguish between pharmaceutical-related

27

seminar flyers, worth a full meal plus dessert, and neuroscience-program-related seminar flyers, worth only cookies. Thus, I increased my dopamine neuron firing more when pharmaceutical-related seminar flyers were identified. In this situation, my dopamine neurons fired as in line C.

I began to favor seminars about new pharmaceuticals. When I saw a flyer for a seminar targeting pharmacy students, my dopamine neurons fired a full meal's worth and I headed expectantly to the talk. I entered and, to my shock, there was no food at all at the back of the room. My dopamine neurons slowed their firing well below their stable rate and fired as in line D. They had made a mistake. There was no meal, no cookies. Something was wrong with the prediction, and I needed to learn new cues to stop me from making that mistake again. I had confused pharmaceutical-related with pharmaceutical company-related. The pharmacy school was even poorer than the neuroscience graduate department. Not only did they not provide lunch, they did not even provide cookies. My brain quickly noted this contingency and from then on was very careful to distinguish between pharmaceutical company-funded seminars (a meal's worth of dopamine neuron firing) and pharmacy school seminars (no change in dopamine neuron firing).

FIGURE: Dopamine neuron firing rate

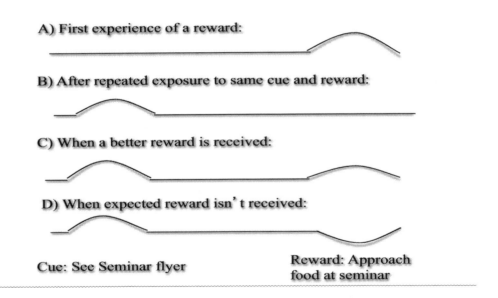

A) First experience of a reward:

B) After repeated exposure to same cue and reward:

C) When a better reward is received:

D) When expected reward isn't received:

Cue: See Seminar flyer   Reward: Approach food at seminar

Legend: A) The rate of dopamine neuron firing following the first unexpected experience of a reward in the form of cookies, B) After repeated exposure, considering going to a seminar that should have cookies brings about dopamine neuron firing even before the cookies are encountered, C) Attending a seminar with sandwiches and salads instead of cookies provides an even better reward than expected, leading to increase in dopamine neuron firing, and D) attending a seminar with no cookies – the expected reward is not received – results in a decrease in the rate of dopamine neuron firing.

What this set of lines signifies is the process by which the brain develops predictions about rewards it could seek. The technical name for this form of learning is called an "error signal learning model". Specifically, learning is guided by a process of prediction and correction based on the accuracy of the prediction. In other words, the error signal is the difference between the prediction and the actual occurrence at the time the predicted reward is expected to materialize. The rate at which dopamine neurons fire during the prediction encodes the predicted reward value. The actual value of the encountered reward is the combination of (1) the firing during the prediction and (2) the error signal firing at the time of the predicted reward. Errors in the original prediction trigger learning of new cues and contingencies. In other words, dopamine neuron firing at time the reward should be encountered encourages new habit learning. Scientists have observed this process in both monkeys using intercellular recording (Schultz, 1998; Tobler et al., 2005), and humans using fMRI during learning exercises (e.g., Rodriquez et al., 2006).

The concept of the predicted "value" of a reward might seem a bit abstract, particularly when we are talking about the value of relief from a bad mood or the solution to a distressing problem. It may help to think of it in more concrete terms like the "value" of a specific purchase. Our brain uses the same process to make fast decisions in the realm of personal economics, and dopamine neurons guide our shopping decisions. The quick choices that we make regarding what to purchase – our impulse buying – depend on the value predictions of the dopamine neurons that provide input to our nucleus accumbens.

For example, a study examined how we make decisions about what to purchase by having people shop while being monitored in an fMRI machine, a device capable of recording images of ongoing brain activity (Knutson et al., 2007). People were shown items, then a price, then given 4 seconds to choose whether to purchase the product. The investigators found that the amount of activity in the nucleus accumbens during the time that people were shown the items predicted whether or not they would choose to buy them. This was a better predictor of whether they would purchase the product than what they *said* was their preference for the product. As we mentioned earlier, dopamine neurons that indicate predicted reward value are the major input to the nucleus accumbens, so this study shows that the brain uses these reward predictions to guide rapid decisions about the worth of an opportunity, even when someone may not realize it. In this case, the decision was about whether it was worthwhile to spend money, a form of stored work, on an opportunity. In everyday life, we buy things based on our dopamine neurons' estimates of the reward value of objects all the time. In fact, recent studies have shown that reward value estimates in the nucleus accumbens of pilot testers considering crowd-funding proposals were better predictors of the future success of the crowd-funding proposal on Internet sites than the actual funding choices that the pilot testers made (Genevsky et al., 2017), highlighting the power of these neuronal reward value estimates on human choices regarding how to spend our money, time and energy. If we overvalue certain products, because of advertising, perceptions that the product will improve social status, the addictive nature of the product, or stress (see Challenge #3), our shopping cart may get filled with these immediate-gratification items.

Chapter 1.2: Great Expectations: How Do Opportunities for Reward Get Overvalued?

When reward appraisal works optimally, we create realistic expectations about our options and our limbic reward circuit and prefrontal cortex work together to ensure that we are both taken care of in the moment and on-track to achieve our long-term goals. However, there are many ways in which our estimates can become biased and cause us to favor behaviors that do not objectively help us, or more ominously, are self-destructive (e.g., addictions of all kinds).

Social factors, artificially associated rewards, and drugs of abuse are just a few of the things that can fool these brain regions into overvaluing unhealthful behaviors. We will discuss some of the most common and well-understood ways in which the process of learning reward value can get manipulated to favor thoughts and behaviors that make us unwell. Dopamine neurons that talk to a brain region known as the nucleus accumbens play an important role in this process by relaying our expectations about the immediate benefits of doing habit behaviors. Notably, you do not need to understand the neurobiology of dopamine neurons to effectively shape behavior. In fact, external parties such as social groups and advertisers often use these techniques to their advantage to manipulate the behavior of those around them. Being aware of these influences is a first step towards preventing others from manipulating your expectations to the detriment of your health.

Social reinforcement and peer pressure

What we hear from others about the effects or importance of a health-related choice can greatly influence our calculation of reward value, even changing how we respond to the opportunity when we encounter it. We learn a lot about how certain behaviors, products or experiences are supposed to make us feel by watching or talking to others, or seeing them in the media. Our brains use these social observations and rumors to set up expectations about the value or effect of various behaviors, often long before we have ever experienced their effects ourselves. Our observations of the effects and rewards of a behavior on other people get factored into our estimates of reward value. In other words, our interpretations of other peoples' experiences influence our value estimates just like our own experiences do.

Rumors can change peoples' behaviors by altering their expectations about the risks and benefits of a health-related choice, even when they are not true. Because we cannot always have our own experiences ahead of time, we often rely on information from others without always knowing or confirming its validity. For example, an uproar over purported risk of autism resulting from vaccines containing trace amounts of mercury unduly scared parents from vaccinating their children. Media-driven fears reduced the expected value of the vaccines, thus making them a less appealing option. This had a significant effect on vaccination rates, even though the vaccines had proven beneficial effects on health and the single report suggesting a risk was shown to be incorrect. Similarly, the social buzz around fad diets, though not evidence-based, often drives people to alter choices about what to eat, demonizing hamburgers one month and then buns the next. What we hear about certain foods can change our predictions about how good they are for us, and change what we eat.

Because of this, the human brain is more likely to base choices on social norms than objective realities. Because our expectations are so vulnerable to suggestion, our choices often reflect opinion more than true experience. Objectively, vaccination has overwhelmingly positive benefits, reducing suffering related to infectious disease. But our brains have no way of knowing this ahead of time, so we rely on what we hear from others, though it may be highly evidence-based or complete fabrication. By altering our expectations about the value of specific health choices, what we hear and observe can change how we react to things, even when we have not experienced them ourselves.

This process can lead whole groups or cultures of people to harbor beliefs about the effects of a certain behavior that may have no objective basis in fact. Are dogs a tasty treat or a disgusting horrible thing to eat? It depends on what those around you tell you and how they react when offered dog meat. Will crystals prevent you from picking up other people's bad moods or negative energy? It depends on what you have been told, how others react when you wear the crystals, and how you interpret your own behavior while you are wearing them. The stories we create around behaviors and objects will shape our expectations about their effects, color our observations and interpretations of their actual effects, and even change our responses to experiences. We tend to act the way we think we are supposed to in response to opportunities even if there is no real objective reason to do so. Someone of European heritage may throw up their dinner after learning that they just ate dog, even though the dinner was in no way poisonous or less healthful than their common dinner of pig. They are responding to their expectations about eating dog rather than the actual effects of eating dog on their physiology. In other cultures, a dinner of dog is considered a luxury. It is not uncommon for cultures or groups to develop expectations about behaviors or objects that lead to unhealthful or even dangerous behaviors. Recognizing these expectations and working to correct these false beliefs can be very helpful for changing behavior in a more healthful direction.

EXAMPLE: The impact of expectation on behavior

To illustrate the impact of expectation on behavior (in this case dietary choice), one of us (J.T.) will share another story from her graduate school years. Having both a horrendous family history of heart disease, and migraines triggered by meat and dairy products, I followed a vegan diet (no meat, eggs, and dairy products), more than two decades before anyone mainstream thought this was a kind, green, or remotely cool way to eat. My lab-mates were all very aware of my diet, as it provided endless opportunity for mocking, taunting, and teasing during lab outings and meals. So, when I was assigned the duty of picking up bagels for our 7:00 am lab meetings, I felt perfectly justified in buying the soy-based imitation cream cheese that they sold at the bagel shop. Because few other people bought the fake cream cheese by the container, the store had to repackage their giant container of soy-cheese into smaller plastic containers that didn't have any labels. So I brought soy cream cheese in unmarked containers to lab meetings.

I never explicitly announced that I was purchasing soy cream cheese for the meetings, but I also never hid the fact that I was smearing large quantities of the stuff all over my bagels, and assumed that anyone who gave it a thought would know it was not really cream cheese.

No one ever complained and everyone in the lab ate lots and lots of soy cream cheese with their bagels each week. So, all was fine and I was very happy breakfasting vegan for a full year and a half. But then the bagel shop decided they were selling enough packaged soy cream cheese to keep smaller containers on hand. Now, the soy cream cheese package boldly announced the fact that it was imitation, non-dairy, vegan cream cheese. But, no worries, I thought, everyone has been happily eating the stuff for 18 months.

Boy, was I wrong. The minute I put the soy cream cheese package on the table, there were complaints; vocal, outraged, angry complaints. There was no way the rest of the lab was going to eat weird soy-products on their bagels, and how dare I bring this to the lab meeting. When I pointed out that this was exactly what I had been bringing for the last year and a half, just without the fancy lid, and everyone liked it before, I completely infuriated one of our senior scientists. She scowled, saying that she knew that there was something wrong with the cream cheese all that time, and that it was disgusting and horrible. I noted that she had nevertheless put it on and ate it with at least two bagels each Monday morning for the last 78 weeks, without ever once mentioning her concerns. But that was the end of her experience with soy. She never again ate a bit of the soy cream cheese, and I was forced to buy additional tubs of real cream cheese to appease my lab-mates who had distaste for things that say "soy" on the cover.

In exchange for having the senior scientist hate me for a few days and suspiciously examine the cream cheese during lab-meetings for the next few weeks, I got a great demonstration of the power of expectation. While she thought the soy cream cheese was real cream cheese, our senior scientist ate it with gusto. If she didn't like it, she didn't show it, and ate it whenever offered and without complaint. When she thought it was soy, her expectations changed completely. She would no longer even taste the stuff, refused to eat it, and told anyone who asked how nasty it was. Her expectations completely changed her thoughts and behaviors about soy cream cheese, and never once did it get valued highly enough for her to eat it knowingly, at least at any of our lab-meetings.

To counter scientific illiteracy promoted by the commercial media and unreliable online sources, we urge you to draw inferences directly from evidence-based sources when making health-related decisions. For example, if you want to review research on safety of vaccines, go to the publicly available National Library of Medicine through PubMed at www.ncbi.nlm.nih.gov/pubmed/ and enter key terms, read the abstracts, perhaps review articles or read reviews of scientific studies. We shamelessly promote our *Institute for Brain Potential* seminars and distance learning as but one source of worthy information about changing health-related behavior at www.ibpceu.com.

Our ability to learn from others' experiences relates to the fact that our dopamine neurons respond to and learn from not only rewards that we receive personally, but also from rewards that we observe other people receive. Neuroimaging has shown that watching others receive rewards activates reward-learning circuits in the nucleus accumbens (Morelli et al., 2018), although the amount of activation varies for different people. This brain response to watching others benefit was unrelated to how much one responds to personally receiving rewards, but was related to prosocial behaviors such as self-described excitement at seeing others benefit, personal tendencies to help others in everyday situations, and giving to charity and others. Being sensitive to the rewards received by those around us can have big benefits in terms of building supportive communities, even while making us vulnerable to the biases of others. It is possible to remain sensitive to the gains of those around us while also learning to test assumptions made while observing them. This can help us build prosocial communities without falling victim to expectations of our peers that may or may not be grounded in truth.

The power of suggestion: Placebo and nocebo effects

Expectations about an experience or treatment can have a huge effect on the perceived outcome. The effect of expectations can be positive, in which case they may produce a placebo effect or benefits beyond those produced by pharmacological or objective actions alone. But expectations of bad outcomes can be negative, in which case they produce harmful effects such as worsening of symptoms, medication inefficacy, or side effects. These are called nocebo effects.

Scientists interested in pain have studied placebo and nocebo effects in depth. Suggestion has large effects on the feelings, thoughts, and behaviors produced by a potentially painful stimulus. When people fear something or expect it to be particularly painful, they find it to be particularly painful. Often, peoples' expectation about how painful something will be is a better predictor of reported pain following the experience than the actual intensity of the painful stimulus itself.

These expectations work in the opposite direction as well. When people expect something to hurt less, it will. This was shown in a brain imaging study that used a fake "analgesic cream" (Wager et al., 2004). The researchers caused a painful sensation by heating up volunteers' forearms, then told the volunteers they were applying an analgesic cream that would reduce but not eliminate pain. The researchers then repeated the study with the same cream but told the volunteers it was just the base for the analgesic medication. In both cases, the heat stimulus was the same and the cream had no medication in it. All that differed was what they were told was in the cream. However, when told that they had received an analgesic cream, clients reported less pain and brain imaging showed less brain activity in regions that represent emotion and regions that transmit information about potentially damaging stimuli (i.e., things that might cause pain). Their expectations had changed how they experienced the heat sensation, and how their brains responded.

Another brain imaging study observed people when they were expecting a painful stimulus rather than during the painful stimulus itself (Koyama et al., 2005). They showed that expectation alone altered brain activity in the cortical brain regions involved in the experience of pain (anterior cingulate cortex, insula cortex), judgment of the value of responding to potential rewards or punishments (prefrontal cortex), and the gating or filtering of sensory information to cortical brain regions (thalamus). Expecting that a painful stimulus was coming set up the brain to respond to the pain, including starting to feel the experience in advance, preparing itself for the possible need to escape, and activating pain control regions to either amplify or dampen the impending painful signal. In other words, guessing how much an upcoming stimulus would hurt changed activity in brain regions that generate behavioral and emotional responses. This guess set up the brain to respond to the expectation when the stimulus actually arrived.

Lastly, a brain imaging study observed how a certain region of the brain that receives information from dopamine neurons (the nucleus accumbens) responded when people were given a placebo painkiller (Scott et al., 2007). Using positron emission tomography (PET) to view changes in the amount of dopamine released (by seeing how many D2 dopamine receptors were dopamine-free), they showed that being told you were given a painkiller increased dopamine release in the nucleus accumbens when people were anticipating a painful stimulus. In other words, if you knew a painful experience was coming, just thinking you had been given a painkiller made your reward circuits expect a reward (e.g., relief from pain). The amount of dopamine release was related to how much pain relief the individuals expected to experience when they were given the placebo "drug"; greater expected pain relief was associated with greater dopamine release.

Moreover, expectations and the amount of dopamine release during anticipation of the pain stimulus predicted how much pain relief participants experienced when the painful stimulus was actually applied. The researchers also looked at activity in the nucleus accumbens of these same participants when they anticipated receiving a monetary reward. They found that the people who expected larger pain relief and released more dopamine in anticipation of the painkiller also showed greater dopamine release when anticipating a monetary reward. Thus, placebo expectations and responses may be related to how much your reward system anticipates rewards in general. This study clearly demonstrates that the dopamine-based process of reward learning in the nucleus accumbens is involved in generating our expectations and responses to opportunities both when we can get something nice or escape something unpleasant. It also shows that expectations, rather than true reality, change how our brain responds and thus shape our behavior. Lastly, it shows that individual differences in the brain's responsiveness to rewards have meaningful effects on how people react to opportunities and expectations.

While the effects of expectation have been studied extensively as they relate to the experience of pain, the clinical impact of expectation-driven placebo and nocebo effects are much broader. As Fabrizio Benedetti describes in detail in his book, *Placebo Effects: Understanding the Mechanisms in Health and Disease* (2021), expectations of clinical improvement can have a substantial effect on symptoms for a wide variety of disorders. For insomnia, placebos can induce behavioral and electroencephalographic (a measure of neuronal firing patterns) changes. In depression, the rate of improvement in placebo groups is high and has increased over the past years, presumably because of advertising touting the virtues of antidepressant medications. In addiction, tobacco smoking and nicotine intake reveal large placebo effects, perhaps because expecting a drug of abuse may make using it more pleasurable. Sexual function may improve after placebo and worsen after nocebo. Cough is powerfully reduced by placebo treatments, as is bronchial hyper-reactivity in asthma. Reduction of gastrointestinal symptoms is common in clients who receive placebos for gastrointestinal and genitourinary disorders including irritable bowel syndrome. Reduction of subjective lower urinary tract symptoms is greater than objective symptoms in placebo groups. Placebo surgery is associated with clinical improvement at high rates, even in those who incorrectly believe they have received organ transplantation.

Expectation may also induce unpleasant side effects in clients receiving inert medications. Such nocebo effects are common in control groups in cardiovascular trials. Nocebos can even mimic the depressant effects of narcotics on breathing rate in respiratory disorders. As the above series of studies show, our expectations about the effects of treatments modify the reward estimates of our dopamine neurons. These differences in dopamine neuron firing influence activity in the nucleus accumbens and alter our body's choice of habit responses – thereby changing the physiological effects of the treatment. Our expectations influence not only our outward behaviors and emotions, but also our internal responses to situations.

To practice creating positive expectations and examples of how to make use of placebo in clinical practice, see Exercise 1A (page 66).

TIPS FOR HEALTH PROFESSIONALS:

Using expectation to improve pain management and treatment effects

1. *Talk about wellness, not pain.* Clients' pain intensity ratings are consistently and significantly lower after verbally reinforcing "well talk" in contrast to verbally reinforcing pain talk (White & Sanders, 1986); therefore, a focus on wellness and recovery more meaningfully reduces pain than a focus on the pain itself. When treating clients with pain or mood disorders, focus on what will lead to wellness, not the pain. Focusing directly on the pain itself can heighten the pain; focusing on recovery may reduce it. For example, in response to concerns over untreated pain, the Joint Commission encouraged assessing pain severity on a 0-10 scale at all clinical visits as a vital sign. Primary care physicians who had implemented pain as a vital sign screening for years, described the negative consequences of this approach, highlighting that it often caused patients who did not come in with concerns about pain to reflect on pain they did experience and start to think of themselves as disabled or broken (Ahluwalia et al., 2018). The primary care physicians recommended an alternative approach of asking patients about their health goals and how they tried to manage their symptoms, bringing up pain challenges from the frame of empowering the patient to take control of their health, rather than encouraging reflection on ways their conditions hurt or limit them.

2. *Model positive outcomes.* Clients can learn a placebo effect by social observation. For example, when people observed someone else not respond in pain to a procedure they expected would be painful, they found it less painful (Colloca & Benedetti, 2009). Help your clients learn positive outcomes by watching other clients. Expose your clients who are too scared to try activities like exercise and physical therapy to your clients who have used these methods with good results. Seeing that these clients weren't hurt by these activities may reduce their expectations of pain and increase pain tolerance. Seeing that these clients benefited from treatment may help them to believe that they will benefit too.

3. *Provide hope.* Helping clients feel hopeful about their life and treatment can improve mood and amplify the effects of analgesics, antidepressants and other treatments that target emotions and emotional behavior. Even simple exposure to a sunny day can reduce the

need for pain management. For example, clients recovering from spinal surgery who stayed on the on the sunny side of a hospital unit used 22% less analgesic medication per hour and had lower perceived stress (Walch et al., 2005).

4. *Take time to demonstrate competence and warmth in your interactions with patients.* A patient's perception of the competency (e.g., skills, knowledge, experience) and warmth (e.g., understanding of the patient and their goals as a person, empathy, rapport) of their provider can alter their response to treatment by moderating their placebo response (Howe et al., 2019). Across multiple studies, when providers followed protocols designed to demonstrate their competency and warmth, the patient experienced more relief from the pain, irritable bowel syndrome, or allergic reactions that the treatment was meant to address. Protocols for demonstrating competency and warmth included establishing the clinician's experience with the problem, focusing carefully during an evaluation, making empathic statements, and asking the patient about their understanding of the treatment and/or effects of the condition on their lifestyle.

Expectancy and alcohol: Thinking you are drinking when you are not

Many research studies have examined the effects of having both strong positive and negative expectations about the effects of alcohol. The most famous and creative versions of these studies asked people about their expectations about the effects of alcohol and then observed them in a simulated bar environment while they drank "alcoholic" beverages. The bar was actually a lab staffed by researchers and equipped with cameras and two-way mirrors. Some participants were given true alcoholic drinks; others were given placebo non-alcoholic drinks that were made to smell and taste like typical cocktails. Additionally, some participants were told they were drinking alcohol and some were told they were not. These studies allowed researchers to separate the effects of drinking alcohol from the effects of thinking you are drinking alcohol.

Not surprisingly, this type of study showed that drinking alcohol had effects on both physiology and behavior. For example, drinking alcohol impaired motor performance and information processing, and improved mood (Hull & Bond, 1986). However, these studies also showed that thinking that you are drinking alcohol had significant effects on social behaviors. For example, people who thought they were drinking alcohol but actually were not still showed significantly increased sexual arousal to erotic stimuli, drank more "alcoholic" beverages, and showed mildly reduced aggression (note: true alcohol actually tends to increase aggression) (Hull & Bond, 1986). Thinking they were drinking alcohol changed how participants behaved after drinking. Presumably, social beliefs that drinking alcohol disinhibits sexual behavior, makes it hard to stop drinking, and makes people more relaxed and mellow made people more likely to act this way when they thought they were drinking. Peoples' expectations about how they would behave when they drank alcohol changed how they actually behaved after they drank a beverage. Presumably, people felt that it was more socially acceptable to act in these ways when they were drinking. By changing behavior to match preconceived beliefs about alcohol's effects, expectations not only increase the expected value of an opportunity but also alter one's experience to reinforce the original beliefs.

Advertising, observation, and cultural mores can shape expectations about alcohol and other substances. Expectations about alcohol can have profound and prolonged effects upon health starting at an early age, as they predict how much, when, and why one drinks both now and in the future. For example, it has been demonstrated that expectations about the effects of alcohol were associated with how teenagers drank alcohol (Christiansen et al., 1983). Teenagers who believed alcohol would make them more social tended to drink frequently with friends. Teenagers who believed alcohol would improve their cognitive and motor functioning were more likely to report having alcohol-related problems. To demonstrate that these beliefs also influenced future behavior, researchers asked seventh and eighth graders what they thought the effect of drinking alcohol would be on their feelings, behaviors, and social interactions. When they assessed actual alcohol drinking behavior in these same adolescents a year later, the researchers found that the adolescents' beliefs about the effects of drinking one year earlier predicted how much, how often and how problematically they were drinking now (Christiansen et al., 1989). More recent studies have confirmed that positive expectations in early adolescence predict greater drinking and alcohol purchases in subsequent years (e.g., Chen et al., 2018). Our beliefs about the effects of a behavior directly impact the decisions we make about when, where, and how often to do that behavior.

How to challenge alcohol-related expectancies

A few studies have tested interventions that challenge alcohol expectancies by having groups of people experience alcohol use in a situation where people do not know whether they or others are drinking alcoholic or non-alcoholic drinks. Following this experience, the group members discuss who they thought was drinking alcohol and how they came to that conclusion. They are then told who really was or was not drinking alcohol. Inevitably, many of the guesses about whether individuals were drinking alcohol are wrong, thus providing a direct example and opportunity for discussion about the errors in their assumptions. This intervention has been tried with groups of college-age students in single or multiple sessions, and with content tailored towards typical male versus female expectations about the effects of alcohol. Meta-analysis of trials suggests that that it can change expectations about the effects of alcohol in young adults and lead to reductions in alcohol use and heavy drinking over the subsequent weeks to months (Scott-Sheldon et al., 2012; Darkes & Goldman, 1993; Darkes & Goldman, 1998; Lau-Barraco & Dunn, 2008). The intervention demonstrated to young adults that their beliefs about the effects of alcohol were not accurate and many of the effects of alcohol depended on what people thought they were drinking rather than what they were really drinking. This simple demonstration produced changes in their beliefs about the effects of alcohol and the changes in beliefs were associated with reductions in actual drinking behavior in the next month. These studies provide experimental evidence that our beliefs about the effects of our behaviors, in this case alcohol use, have a direct impact on whether we choose to do the behavior. It also shows that changing our beliefs changes our behavior. When we have exaggerated expectations of the positive effects that an unhealthful behavior will produce or underestimate the immediate negative effects of an unhealthful behavior, we are apt to develop unhealthful patterns of behavior. However, it is possible to train ourselves to develop more realistic expectations of the effects of certain behaviors. To translate these findings into practical results, we urge parents and health professionals to avoid unwittingly promoting positive expectations related to alcohol, nicotine, or cannabis use or other unhealthful behaviors. It may be useful to ask a child or teenager what he or she thinks it would be like to smoke, vape, or drink and guide him or her to more accurate information about the objective effects of these substances.

Challenging our beliefs about the effects of our behaviors can help us develop more accurate expectations about the outcomes of our behaviors and potentially improve our health. We may challenge our beliefs by directly observing outcomes on ourselves, by asking other people to report their observations about the outcomes of a behavior, or even by learning more about the objective effects of a behavior, perhaps by reading medical reports or scientific studies. When our brains make decisions using more accurate information about the outcomes of our choices, we tend to make decisions that provide greater benefit for our health and happiness. We will discuss techniques and exercises to encourage this process at the end of this chapter.

How do advertisers seduce us into buying their products?
Random cues, items, behaviors or feeling states can become overvalued and overused when they become paired with unexpected rewards. Such pairings are created intentionally all the time by advertisers intent on training you to favor their product. By linking immediate gratification – a pretty face, the suggestion of sex, the promise of money or power – with a commercial product, advertisers create an association between their product and these unexpected rewards in your limbic system. Whether the product is a can of soda, a car, or a financial service, your brain will now relate that product with the opportunity for reward, most commonly in the form of approval from the opposite sex or a position of status among peers. These associations, whether or not you are aware of them, can alter your estimates of the value of a behavior or thing, and bias your choices.

In an elegant study, researchers mimicked the advertising process by showing volunteers arbitrary cues (pictures of unrelated things) along with pictures of attractive female faces and measuring their brain activity using fMRI (Bray & O'Doherty, 2007). Viewing the attractive faces activated reward circuits, indicated by an increase in blood flow to the nucleus accumbens. This suggests that seeing attractive faces is rewarding and might train the volunteers' brains to seek out cues that were associated with the faces. As it turns out, the volunteers had developed behavioral preferences for the arbitrary cues, liking cues that had been linked with attractive faces more than cues that had not been linked with attractive faces. *In other words, they overvalued things that had been associated with people they found attractive.* The study showed that the amount of nucleus accumbens activity predicted how much the person learned to prefer the cue associated with the attractive face. This suggests that the more rewarding the dopamine neurons in the reward circuits found the attractive faces, the more the person learned to value the cue. In other words, the value that the pretty face added to the product cue predicted how much the person would favor the product cue in the future.

Another study demonstrated that activation of the nucleus accumbens was related to behavioral measures of preference for an attractive face (i.e., how much you would press a button to see the face), but not your stated assessment of how attractive the face appeared

(Aharon et al., 2001). This suggests that learning directed by the reward circuits controls your tendency to do a behavior, but not necessarily your conscious assessment of the value of doing that behavior. Pairing rewards and cues might train you to actively seek a cue and do more work to get the cue, even if you were not aware that you liked or wanted the cue more. In other words, you may not even be aware that your brain values a behavior and causes you to repeat it. For example, a commercial that showed an attractive person drinking a specific soda might train you to drink more of that soda even if you still thought and told people that you did not really like that beverage.

This same reward learning process may also overvalue cues when they are paired with rewards by chance rather than capitalist intention. For example, your new jeans might become your favorite when the queen bee of your middle school compliments you on them; your smelly gym socks may become crucially important to your participation in future athletic competitions when you win the biggest competition of your life while wearing them; you may decide pears are the most amazing fruit in the world when the person you've had a crush on for the last two years bakes you pear tarts for your birthday. The cue takes on the value of the outcome with which it was associated, even if those associations were completely arbitrary or random. Regardless of whether these associations stem from advertising or coincidence, they can lead to irrational and sometimes impulsive behaviors.

Social influence can also moderate both expectations and actual responses to a product or cue. Having another person confirm or deny an expected experience of a product can not only alter someone's beliefs about the product, but also their physiological, psychological, and behavioral responses to it. For example, Crum and colleagues (2016) labeled plain water as containing 200 mg of caffeine, and randomized participants to consume it alone, with another person who denied effects on alertness, or with another person who endorsed effects on alertness. Those randomized to consume it with someone who endorsed effects on alertness showed not only greater self-reported alertness, but also greater changes in systolic blood pressure, improved performance on a Stroop Task assessing cognitive interference, and greater endorsement of the product, as compared to those who drank the water with someone who denied effects on alertness. Observing someone else obtain benefit from a product or experience can alter not only one's own perceptions of the product, but also their physiological, cognitive, and behavioral responses to it. Social influencers use this technique to encourage viewers to purchase products. But this same effect can significantly shape health behaviors and treatment responses of peer groups or patients in group treatments. Being aware of these effects can help providers correct expectations to motivate behavior change or enhance the benefits of treatments.

Marketing your own expectations and rewards
In short, our beliefs about the effects of behaviors or things have an enormous impact on how we value opportunities to do these behaviors or gain these things. In addition, external advertising or coincidental associations may lead us to develop incorrect believes that inaccurately associate certain cues and behaviors with reward.

These beliefs can lead us to make choices that are bad for our health. We may ignore our doctors' warnings to cut back on cholesterol by substituting soy products for animal products because we think soy will taste bad or be disgusting. We may avoid getting screened for breast or colon cancer because we fear it will be a painful, terrible experience. We may drink large quantities of alcohol on the weekends because we think it will make us more attractive and social and will help us have more fun. Objectively, we may not even notice the difference in taste between soy and animal products, the injury and discomfort from the screening tests may be far less than that we experience playing our favorite sport, and alcohol may make us act in embarrassing ways, smell funny, and make us feel terrible the next day. But we may never experience or notice these realities while our beliefs contradict them. Changing your beliefs about the effects of behaviors can have a huge impact on your health choices. Correcting such beliefs is a large component of many psychosocial interventions that improve health behaviors.

Try to create your own "commercials" or associations between the behaviors you want to do and cues that attract you. For example, if I ruminate on how much I love getting together with family at Thanksgiving and how my aunt's green bean and pearl onion dish is so delicious, I may be able to trigger warm positive feelings and overeating responses to green beans. To help reinforce this more, I might post some pictures of my favorite people eating green beans on my refrigerator. If I gorge myself on green beans, I will likely eat less of other less healthful options. If I want to start running regularly, and I know I enjoy spending time with my friends, then I can plan an outing with a friend each time I complete a run. If I let my friends know this is my plan, they can also ask me about my running behavior when they are planning something with me. Some of my friends may want to start running with me to achieve similar goals, creating external reminders of the associated cue between running and time spent with friends. If I run regularly, I will be less likely to sit in front of the TV and stay inside all day. The best way to discourage or reduce a behavior with "commercials" and cues is to encourage another one, such as eating green beans to prevent yourself from eating three servings of pie and running to avoid spending the entire day on the couch.

To help identify cues that trigger your healthful or unhealthful behaviors, see Exercise 1B (page 69). To practice creating "cues you can use" to encourage healthful behaviors, see Exercise 1C (page 70).

Chapter 1.3: Social Factors that Can Overvalue Habits and Sabotage Our Health

Our beliefs about what other people do and consider normal will also shape our evaluation of an opportunity and change our behavior. People are socially influenced and do not like to do behaviors that are different from their peers. Moreover, people tend to surround themselves with people who act like they do. For example, a person who smokes is much more likely to know other smokers than is a non-smoker (Christakis & Fowler, 2008). Smokers will spend more time in places with high numbers of smokers; smokers necessarily cluster in smoking areas and frequent places where cigarettes are purchased. While they are smoking, smokers will tend to receive more positive feedback from other smokers, and thus may prefer to be around them. Thus, people tend to create social networks where the people they see act like they do. Based on their experience, they tend to overestimate how common or normal it is to do a behavior. Because of their desire to act like others, they will favor doing behaviors that are similar to those around them, overvaluing reward opportunities that make them seem more like their peers.

Habits are contagious

Interestingly, this tendency to overvalue conformity can lead to the spread of behaviors in patterns like the spread of a disease. Behaviors and thus their health consequences appear to be contagious. For example, obesity appears to spread through social ties. Drs. Christakis and Fowler (2007) examined how weight gain spread through a social network of over 12,000 people during a 32-year period. People with close social ties were more likely to have a similar body mass index, showing that obesity tended to cluster in social networks. Moreover, when one person gained weight the chance that their friends and relatives gained weight in the near future increased substantially. If a friend became obese, a person's risk of becoming obese subsequently increased 57%. If a sibling or spouse became obese, their risk increased 40% and 37% respectively. Weight gain in neighbors did not increase risk of obesity. Thus, spread of obesity was not due to location, but to social interactions. A very similar pattern was observed for spread of smoking and smoking cessation behaviors in these same networks (Christakis & Fowler, 2008). Our desire to be like those around us even shapes the emotions we feel from day to day. Examination of these networks showed that even emotional responses, specifically feeling happy, spread socially through groups based upon the closeness of their ties (Fowler & Christakis, 2008). People who reported being happy tended to have close relationships with other people who reported being happy. These studies highlight the importance of social norms and reinforcement of behaviors in close networks of family and friends in modifying health risk. We tend to mimic the behaviors of people close to us. Making friends that behave the way we want to behave can help us develop their desirable behaviors. If friends and family behave in ways that increase health risk, we are at risk of sharing their illnesses. But if family and friends make healthful choices, we may just "catch" their health.

Why do those we love sabotage our attempts at self-improvement?

Notably, part of the reason that social norms are so contagious is that people regularly punish others for violating social norms. People express satisfaction with and are willing to continue punishing others for breaking social norms even when it costs them substantially to carry out the punishment. In an elegant study, researchers demonstrated that punishing others for purposely not following expected social behavior activates brain reward circuits (de Quervain et al., 2004). *In other words, punishing others for breaking social norms is personally rewarding.* This study involved a game in which two players were given money. If the first player chose to give some of that money to the second player, the money that was shared would be quadrupled. The second player was then given the opportunity to give some of that money back to the first player. Thus, the expected best strategy would be for the first to give all of money to the second, and the second to give half of the quadrupled money back. But if the second chose to not follow expected social norms and kept all the money, the first would lose all the money from that round. Following such an unfair interaction, the first player was given the option of punishing the second player. In the real punishment condition, the first player could pay $1 for every $2 that would be taken away from the second player. In the symbolic punishment condition, the first player could assign as many "punishment units" as they desired to the second player, but it had no effect on either player's money.

To compare the effects of the second player's intentional desire to keep the money versus simply being a passive recipient of it, the researchers looked at a few scenarios while the first player was in a positron emission tomography (PET) scanner. Sometimes, a study team member played the second player and purposely kept the money. At other times, the first player was told that a computer would decide how much money the second player kept, so that he or she was not really responsible if any money was kept. The researchers were interested in the brain activity during the time when the first player was deciding whether to punish the second player's decision.

The researchers discovered that real punishment, but not symbolic punishment, activated the reward circuits of the first player. In other words, the first player's reward circuits were activated when the second player experienced real punishment for his or her decision not to return half of the money to the first player. The greater the activation of the reward circuits while deciding whether to punish, the more a person was willing to spend to punish second player for breaking expectations. Additionally, the first player chose to punish the second player more and their reward circuits were activated more when they believed the second player made the decision to keep the money than when the computer made the decision to keep the money. In other words, the participants only found it rewarding to punish people who had purposely treated them unfairly even though they were just as hurt by the response in both cases. Human brains are wired to encourage us to punish others for breaking social norms, even if it costs us to enforce the punishment. However, if the person who treated us unfairly had done so accidentally, then we do not find it rewarding to punish them. *These studies tell us that revenge for being intentionally hurt by another person is rewarding, and likely an automatic response in our brains.*

This tendency to punish intentional norm breaking can make it difficult to change our unhealthful habits if those around us share our unhealthful behaviors. Refusing to do something that everyone else in the group is doing, even if it is harmful or unhealthy, is breaking the social norms of the group. Group members are apt to go out of their way to punish you for your attempts at new healthful behavior. Tell your drinking buddies that you have decided not to drink any more and, at a minimum, it is unlikely that they will be particularly helpful and supportive of your new habit. It is much more likely that you get mocked and insulted. Likewise, tell your friends with whom you used to discuss your favorite TV show that you have decided to take a yoga class at that time instead, and they probably will not congratulate you on your healthy decision and encourage you to keep going. This is one of the reasons why mutual help groups consisting of those dedicated to meeting a shared health goal, such as Alcoholic Anonymous for those attempting to remaining sober, can be especially helpful by creating a supportive peer group that encourages change.

This helps to explain why people who associate with groups with extreme behaviors tend to follow those behaviors despite the potential harms from conforming. Not only do people receive social approval for acting like those around them, they are also likely to be punished by their peers when they act differently. Thus, it can be very helpful for people in social groups with extreme behaviors to begin associating with people from social groups with different norms. Making people in these extreme social groups aware that other peers outside the social group do not follow these norms can be a substantial step in that direction. Thus, some effective interventions focus on making people aware of more healthful social norms in the broader population or encourage people to associate more with people with more healthful social norms. Without changing these social influences, it can be extremely difficult for a person to stop engaging in the dangerous behaviors of their friends and family. Why would you continue to do a new healthful behavior when those around you punish you every time you try to do it?

The fact that punishing others is rewarding if they have hurt you, highlights another useful concept for supporting behavior change. Provocation can encourage revenge, triggering reflexive, aggressive, punishing behaviors from those that you insult, prod, or anger. When you hurt or take something away from someone else, you provide the person you hurt with a reward opportunity. Specifically, he can now benefit from getting revenge on you. Your taunt will encourage the other person's reward circuits to do habitual, aggressive behaviors to get you back, with insults, physical attacks, or other unpleasantness.

Using a competition between players whose brains were being imaged by fMRI, Chester and Dewall (2016) watched such an interaction in action. They showed that provocations from the other player, specifically blasting his competitor with a loud noise after he won a trial, activated the insulted player's nucleus accumbens. The larger the taunted player's nucleus accumbens activation, the more likely the taunted player was to aggressively retaliate by doing the same back to his competitor on the next trial. When prefrontal cortex activity was paired with the nucleus accumbens activity, the likelihood of retaliation was reduced. Essentially, taunting another puts you at the mercy of their reward circuits. If they have good control over their habit behaviors (e.g., via prefrontal cortex circuits), you might get away with the harm you inflicted; otherwise, you can expect habitual aggressive revenge-seeking responses in return.

This finding not only helps to explain aggressive behavior, but also highlights a common pitfall of early behavior change. Part of the behavior change process often involves recognizing the negative aspects of your own behavior and the reasons why you might want to change. Learning to recognize the parts of your own behavior that are undesirable tends to make those same behaviors in others around you obvious and potentially upsetting. It is not rare for someone trying to make a personal behavior change to become outwardly critical of that same behavior when they observe it in others. As you improve your own health, it is natural for you to want to share your newly found knowledge and behaviors with those you care about. Problematically, that can often come out as criticism, and criticism can act as a provocation for revenge from those it is directed towards.

EXAMPLE: Becoming a missionary for a vegan diet

At age 11, my father's first triple bypass caused me to become acutely aware of the dangers of cholesterol and thus meat consumption. I not only stopped eating meat, but I felt obliged to share my new knowledge with everyone I encountered who was eating meat. I didn't want them to go through what my Dad had experienced. "That steak is going to clog your arteries and kill you!", I helpfully informed my dining relatives and peers. But was I thanked by my dining-partners for my well-intentioned knowledge-sharing, while they traded in their meat for more salad, broccoli, and grain? Not exactly. Instead, my criticism provoked them. I had, in essence, just taken an anticipated reward right out from under their nose. My outburst just turned the juicy steak that they had been drooling over into a poison that would slowly sicken and incapacitate them. I might as well have taken a cookie right out of a toddler's hand. At the time, I was horrified by the reactions I triggered. Some told me my vegetarian meal was disgusting, and at least they would enjoy their shortened life. Others told me I would go to hell for my dietary deviance from prevailing culture. Some tried to sneak meat into my food. A few even tried to physically force feed me meat. In my enthusiastic proselytizing towards healthful food choices, my negative comments stole anticipated food rewards from others and triggered revenge responses in many forms. After some years of struggling with a horrified sense of betrayal by a self-destructive humanity (I was a young adolescent after all.), I learned to not judge other people's choices, to share information in less charged contexts (e.g., without food present), and to explain my behavioral decisions in terms of my personal context. I note that I didn't stop trying to shape the health behavior of people I cared about. I just stopped antagonizing people about their health choices in an attempt to save them and worked on shaping their environments instead. I offered to cook dinners and do the grocery shopping, modeled healthful eating, praised people for their healthful food choices, commented on how delicious the healthy food options looked, and so forth. This not only reduced conflict, but actually reduced meat consumption in those around me.

Behavioral Couples Therapy incorporates this behavioral truism into treatment, including loved ones in therapy for substance use disorders and training them to avoid criticizing and berating their partner for drug use (other beneficial components of Behavioral Couples Therapy will be discussed in Chapter 4.3). Not only does this avoid triggering drug use as a revenge for the insult, but also it reduces relationship conflict. Less conflict reduces stress, another common driver of short-sighted reward-seeking behaviors (as we will discuss in Chapter 3). When you learn to avoid provoking those around you, you make your life more enjoyable, limit others' attempts to sabotage your behavior change, and more successfully encourage others to adopt your new health behaviors.

To research ways to become more aware of the norms surrounding your target health behavior, see Exercise 1D (page 72).

When helping is hurtful: Rescuing, doting, and enabling

From the time we are toddlers, we are taught the importance of being nice to other people. It seems like a simple concept. Anything we do to help people and make them feel better is a good thing, right? If someone were having a hard time with something, then presumably helping him or her would be a particularly nice thing to do. But unfortunately, behavior is not that simple. In certain situations, helping people can make them worse and even train them to be chronically sick or miserable.

Being too nice to someone when they feel bad, are anxious, do something wrong, or are hesitant to try something can reinforce unpleasant feelings or bad behaviors. While these responses to other people's distress or discomfort are generally well intentioned, they can have extremely negative effects on others health, mood, and life functioning. If unpleasant feelings, thoughts, or behaviors are rewarded, the brain will encourage them to be repeated, attracting people to situations and encouraging responses that recreate the unpleasant experience. Over time, having their bad feelings, thoughts or behaviors rewarded can lead people to chronically feel bad, think bad things, or misbehave. *Thus, for some chronic behavioral and mood disorders, such as chronic pain, substance use disorders, and conduct disorders, having an important person in your life who rescues you, dotes upon you, or enables your misbehavior when you feel bad has been shown to be a major risk factor for development of or poor recovery from these disorders.*

To demonstrate how this process occurs, we present an example of how children can be trained to misbehave and not pay attention at school. In the extreme, such training could potentially win them a diagnosis of conduct disorder or ADHD. More commonly, it may lead to isolated problems with classroom discipline and learning.

As we can likely remember from our own childhood experiences, everyone feels bored or restless every now and again at school. Moreover, most children crave attention and acknowledgement. Some children may feel bored and restless more often than others to start, and some children may be more starved for attention than others. Such variation may make some children more vulnerable to learning bad behavior. But what provides the training? Consider (1) an over-crowded classroom where the teacher has no hope of providing regular individual attention to each student, and (2) a teacher with a low tolerance for disorganization or a strong need to feel her students are focused directly on her. To keep her classroom in line, the teacher quickly responds to any perceived misbehavior. "Johnny, stop fiddling with your pencil." "Sue, stop whispering to your friend." "Aiden, don't call out answers without raising your hand." The problem with this technique is that it assumes that because the teacher's attention is negative and critical, it is a punishment and not a reward. This may be true for some of the children, particularly those who are shy, get plenty of positive attention and are very sensitive to criticism. But for other children, any attention from adults is rewarding. First, the child got a busy teacher to focus on them. Second, they just figured out a way to get a reaction out of an authority figure. They managed to gain at least temporary control over a big powerful person, which is surely some sign of power and status. If the child finds this response from the teacher rewarding, even if it only remains rewarding briefly before becoming a hassle, the behavior *and the feeling that preceded it will be reinforced.* Thus, the child will be more likely to misbehave again and feel bored and restless more often.

As evidence that this technique does contribute to conduct problems in children, there are programs that effectively reduce conduct problems in children by teaching parents and teachers to avoid unintentionally rewarding bad behaviors, thoughts, and feelings. These programs focus primarily on getting teachers or parents to stop attending to bad behavior and start explicitly rewarding good behavior instead. For example, a program called "Peace Builders" has been shown to reduce conduct problems in schools where bad and even violent behavior had become a problem (Flannery et al., 2003; Krug et al., 1997; Embry et al., 1996). This program uses mediation to resolve disputes and trains teachers to ignore non-dangerous misbehavior and provide praise to children they catch acting appropriately. Thus, this program helps teachers stop reinforcing bad behaviors with attention. In parallel, it encourages teachers to reinforce good behavior with attention. This concept is also a primary focus of other evidence-based treatments for conduct disorder and ADHD, including "The Incredible Years Program" (Larsson et al., 2009; Jones et al., 2008; Webster-Stratton et al., 2008; Jones et al., 2007), "Parent-Child Interaction Therapy" (Thomas & Zimmer-Gembeck, 2007; Nixon et al., 2004; Nixon et al., 2003; Eyberg et al., 1995), and "Problem-solving skills training with parent management training" (Kazdin et al., 1992). *When bad behaviors and the feelings that lead to them are ignored and not rewarded, they lose their value and are no longer worth doing.*

WARNING: Extinction bursts

Ending rewards for a bad behavior, whether or not those rewards were intentionally provided, is crucial to getting rid of the bad behavior. However, the bad behavior will not disappear immediately when the rewards are stopped. In fact, the *bad behavior will tend to escalate the first few times the reward is not received, even in adults.* Behavioral scientists refer to this increase in the behavior when the reward is withheld as an "extinction burst". Only later, after the behavior has consistently stopped eliciting a reward, will the behavior go away. When you are trying to get rid of bad behaviors by eliminating rewards, the behavior will temporarily get worse before it gets better.

To understand "extinction bursts" without straying too far from the rat models where it was first described, think of a soda machine. Most of us have been trained that when we put money in the machine and press the button of our choice, a soda will fall out of the slot in the bottom. Think of a time when a soda machine did not work when someone put money in and pressed the button. Did the person immediately decide that the machine did not work or was empty and walk away? Probably not. Chances are they pressed the button repeatedly, perhaps pushing harder and more angrily with each try. Maybe they pressed all the other buttons including the change return, shook the machine, yelled at the machine,

---

tried reaching up the soda delivery slot, or went looking for the machine's owner to complain. Maybe they tried adding more money and pressing the button again. In other words, they escalated the behavior that normally provides the soda reward, making it bigger and more dramatic. The first response to a missing reward is to make the typically rewarded behavior more extreme, perhaps just to make sure that the lack of a reward was not because the behavior was not noticed.

One broken soda machine is probably not enough to lead someone to give up on soda machines and never use them again. However, if someone put money in ten soda machines in a row and none of them delivered a soda when a button was pressed, then they might give up on soda machines, stop noticing them, and stop trying to make them work. But, when you are trying to get someone to stop a behavior, you should expect to go through a period when that person throws temper tantrums before you achieve your goal.

The problem with extinction bursts is that they can be extremely unpleasant to endure, and very discouraging to the person withholding the reward. Withholding a reward may cause screaming, crying, begging, anger, frustration, sadness, and other unpleasant reactions from the person used to getting the reward. It will almost certainly be easier for the person withholding the reward to give in and provide the reward than it will be to bear witnessing the person's response. It may also be difficult to realize that the process may eventually achieve your goal of eliminating the undesirable behavior. This fact has resulted in hoards of toddlers getting cookies that surely ruined their appetite for dinner, young children staying up past their bedtime, and adults being given just one more drink even though everyone else knows they have had too much already. Extinction bursts are extremely effective for ending people's well-intentioned attempts to stop enabling bad behaviors in those close to them.

Understanding and expecting extinction bursts can make it a bit easier to stop rewarding bad behaviors in others. If you are expecting and are prepared for an outburst, you have a better chance of persevering through the reaction. When the person withholding the reward knows the reaction is only temporary and will eventually go away after the reward is withheld consistently, they may be better able to stick to their intentions. For example, providing warnings before encouraging parents to stop rewarding a bad behavior in their children may greatly increase the chance that they successfully eliminate the reward because they will know that a previously rewarded bad behavior will get worse before it is eliminated.

Behavioral training not only encourages behavioral problems in children, but also can lead to chronic emotional problems in adults. For example, studies of the mechanisms that encourage development of chronic pain problems and factors associated with poor recovery have identified "solicitous spouses" as a contributor to long-term experience of pain following an injury (e.g., see Romano et al., 1995; Sorbi et al., 2006). A "solicitous spouse" refers to someone close to a person with an injury or pain problem who immediately pampers or rescues their loved one whenever they experience or complain of pain. A "solicitous spouse" could be the wife who encourages her husband to rest when his back hurts, gets him his pain meds, and then fluffs his pillows before making him dinner.

Alternatively, it could be the father who lets his son who hates school stay home, watch movies, and eat ice cream whenever his stomach hurts. In these cases, the "solicitous" family member rewards their loved one every time they feel bad. While this may help a genuinely hurting person feel better, because reward encourages your brain to repeat the state that preceded getting the reward, this reward will train the loved one to feel bad more often. The husband's back will start hurting more and more often. The son may develop chronic stomachaches. Typically, the best way to get rid of such pain is to have the solicitous family member stop being so nice when their loved one feels sick.

How verbal reinforcement can alter sensory and emotional experience
Positive reinforcement, relief and other rewards can rapidly alter how one feels, even if the reinforced feelings are unpleasant or punishing themselves. For example, positive reinforcement can quickly train people to experience more pain. Jolliffe and Nicholas (2004) provided simple verbal reinforcement, saying things like "that's right," or "very good," when volunteers reported that having their arm squeezed with a blood pressure cuff was marginally more painful than they did the time before. This verbal reinforcement led volunteers to report an increase in the amount of pain produced by the blood pressure cuff stimulus an hour later. The increase in pain associated with just one hour of verbal encouragement was more than 1 point on a 0-10 pain scale from "no pain" to "worst pain imaginable." To put the magnitude of this change in pain in context, this one-point change in pain produced solely by an hour of verbal encouragement is greater than that produced by medical marijuana or opioid analgesics (i.e., narcotic painkillers) in trials in chronic pain clients (Martín-Sánchez et al., 2009; Martell et al., 2007). When volunteers were encouraged to experience more pain when their arm was squeezed, they reported more pain in response to the same amount of squeezing. A group of volunteers who experienced the same pressure stimuli without the verbal reinforcement did not show this increase in pain level. Hölzl and colleagues (2005) did a similar study but changed the intensity of the pain stimulus in response to pain perception. Specifically, they rewarded increases in perceived temperature from a painful heat stimulus with reductions in the temperature of the heat stimulus. In other words, when participants reported that a stimulus was hotter, they were rewarded by having the painful heat reduced on the next exposure. They found that rewarding participants with this reduction in heat intensity led to changes in heat perception within an hour of testing. By the end of the hour, rewarded participants reported thinking that a given temperature stimulus was hotter than they did at the start of the study. They had also changed their perception of temperature compared to non-rewarded participants. The reward provided by the reduction in heat made them more sensitive to potentially painful heat.

Flor and colleagues (2002) directly studied the impact of a solicitous spouse on pain experience and brain activation in clients with chronic back pain. They brought in participants with chronic lower back pain who had a solicitous spouse. These spouses were known to pamper and attend to the client whenever they experienced or complained about back pain. They exposed these participants to a painful shock to their lower back or finger (i.e., a site where they had not been rewarded for experiencing pain) while recording brain activity in the limbic cortex by EEG. They repeated this process in two different ways: 1) when the spouse was not present, and 2) when the spouse was present. They found that while the solicitous spouses were out of the room, the back pain clients reported similar moderate levels of pain and had similar brain activity in response to the painful shock whether it was applied to the back or the finger. However, when the spouses were in the room, the clients reported a near doubling of the amount of pain that the shock to their back elicited, and activity in their limbic cortex was similarly elevated. There was no change in response to the stimulus to the finger. This suggests that the solicitous spouses had trained an increase in back pain experience in their loved ones. A stimulus to the back now caused more pain when the spouse was present. The spouses well-meaning attempts to save their loved one from feeling pain had trained the loved one to experience more intense back pain when the spouses were around.

In essence, when someone receives rewards when he feels or acts badly, he will be encouraged to feel or act badly again, even if those feelings or behaviors hurt him severely over the longer-term. The rewards may be simple and unintended: attention from others, the power to change a situation or get a reaction out of someone, sympathetic comments or responses, encouragement, special treats, favors or expressions of love or affection. It can be difficult to stop others from providing maladaptive rewards, and sometimes the best solution is to remove oneself from those interactions. These social rewards can greatly inflate estimates of the value of an unhealthful behavior, even so far as to drive one to do or feel things that would normally be punishing (e.g., criticism or pain).

TIPS FOR HEALTH PROFESSIONALS: What helps, what hurts.

The above sections have described how over-solicitous spouses or health professionals can increase the perception of pain. As the "Tips for Health Professionals" on page 34 recommend: 1. Talk about wellness, not pain, 2. Model positive outcomes, and 3. Provide hope.

One elaboration of these recommendations is to monitor functional or recovery outcomes (e.g., whether the client is doing things in life that matter to them, like work, interacting with family, engaging in valued activities) rather than monitoring pain level. Using these outcomes to gauge treatment success and guide pain treatment planning can improve outcomes and is a major recommendation of recent pain management guidelines. Family members could benefit from shifting their focus here as well – help by supporting one's engagement in life rather than trying to ease their pain, distress, or negative mood.

To assess social influences that may hurt or help your efforts to improve a health behavior, see Exercise 1E (page 73) and Exercise 1F (page 75).

Chapter 1.4: Hijacking The Brain's Reward System: The Attraction of Addictive Substances

Drugs of abuse, specifically alcohol, tobacco, cannabis (i.e., marijuana), opioids (e.g., heroin, narcotic pain-killers), stimulants (e.g., cocaine, amphetamines (meth)), benzodiazepines, barbiturates, and even caffeine, have special effects on our dopamine neurons. Drugs of abuse differ from other drugs specifically in their ability to trick the brain into over-valuing them over other opportunities. This ability to trick the brain into over-valuing them has something to do with the fact that these substances increase firing from the dopamine neurons that code reward value.

These addictive substances cause many different effects on the brain and body, but they all share one common effect: they all pharmacologically cause the dopamine neurons to fire and/or induce release of dopamine in the nucleus accumbens (Wise & Bozarth, 1985; Bardo, 1998; for discussion of cannabis specifically, see Bloomfield et al., 2016). Because of the direct actions of these drugs, these dopamine neurons will fire even if the signals they receive from other neurons would not normally encourage dopamine neuron firing. *In other words, drugs of abuse hijack the reward system, making the brain's reward circuits react as though the drugs are highly rewarding and valuable, even when the rest of the brain recognizes that drugs are objectively causing harm or worsening well-being.*

Dopamine neuron firing after taking drugs of abuse depends on the pharmacological properties of the drug rather than the social, environmental, or physiological effects of taking the drug. Regardless of what you have previously learned, your expectations, or what you experience when you take the drug, these chemicals will make your dopamine neurons release dopamine into your nucleus accumbens. This pharmacological property disrupts and confuses your brain's natural system for judging the value of various opportunities.

Spiraling out of control: The stepwise increase in overvaluation of drug reward
Models of how this pharmacological property of drugs of abuse influence reward prediction error learning and estimates of reward value can help to explain some of the cardinal features of drug addiction (Redish, 2004; Shultz, 2011), so we will walk through a simplified version here. The first time a person uses drugs of abuse, the effect on the user's dopamine neurons are about the same as the effects of any other unexpected reward. Dopamine neurons fire at their normal (tonic) baseline rate until the drug is taken. Then the drug causes those neurons to increase their firing and release dopamine. Thus, the drug produces a signal that a new, unexpected opportunity for life improvement has been identified and the brain should do its best to learn to repeat this opportunity.

The next time there is an opportunity to use drugs, our dopamine neurons recognize this, and increase their firing to indicate the expected value of this opportunity based upon the amount of dopamine released the last time when you used the substance. If this were a normal reward, there would be no further increase in dopamine neuron firing when you actually took the drug because your brain had already perfectly predicted the effect of the drug. If this were a normal reward, it would produce changes in the environment or your physiology that are detected by your sensory systems and then interpreted by your reward system to trigger dopamine release. However, because these drugs act directly on receptors or proteins on reward system neurons to pharmacologically increase dopamine release, your dopamine neurons will fire again when you take the drug regardless of what you experience or sense through other brain systems. This indicates to your brain that this time the same drug reward was even better than predicted. Thus, your brain looks for more cues to predict the availability of drug reward and increases its estimation of how good taking drugs will be. This process will continue each time you use a drug of abuse until eventually your reward circuitry has so greatly overvalued the drug reward that your dopamine neurons cannot fire any faster. To keep comparisons between natural rewards and drug rewards to scale, your brain is forced to start reducing dopamine neuron firing in response to natural rewards.

FIGURE: Dopamine neuron firing rate in addiction

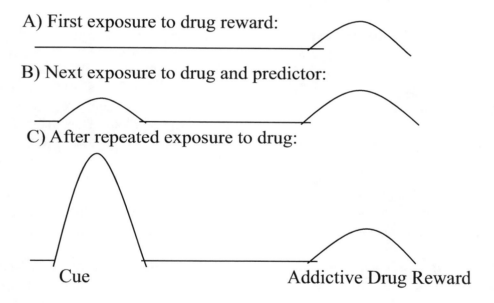

A) First exposure to drug reward:

B) Next exposure to drug and predictor:

C) After repeated exposure to drug:

Cue   Addictive Drug Reward

Legend: A) The rate of dopamine neuron firing following the first use of the drug (the same as unexpected cookies at a seminar), B) The next exposure to the drug leads to an increase in dopamine neuron firing in anticipation of the reward (just like the expectation of cookies at a seminar) but then the neurons fire again when the drug is used (unlike when the expected cookies are received, and because of the direct pharmacological effects of the drug on dopamine neurons rather than the brain's perception of rewarding effects of drug use), C) After repeated exposure to the drug, the anticipation of the drug leads to a high rate of dopamine firing that continually increases with each exposure, because the firing when drug itself is used causes the neurons to recalculate their expectation of the reward (even though the benefits from the drug remain unchanged, and may be low or non-existent).

Therefore, as you continue to take drugs of abuse three things happen: First, your limbic reward circuit predicts enormous rewards for taking drugs. Objectively, the drug may not improve well-being much if at all, but your limbic reward circuit will always think that you lucked out and got even more than the jackpot you expected. Second, because the drug causes additional dopamine release every time it is taken, your limbic reward circuit will start to learn that every possible feeling, object, person, or place that is present while you use drugs indicates an opportunity to use drugs. Drug cues will become ubiquitous—they will be everywhere. Every liquor store, every association with a person with whom you have been drinking, every mood and thought that preceded the drinking, will remind you of the drug reward. And these cues will induce cravings to take drugs when they are around. You will start craving drugs more and more frequently. Lastly, at least to your limbic reward circuit, everyday rewards will seem miniscule and worthless in comparison to the opportunities provided by drugs (Kalivas & Volkow, 2005). Gaining social approval will not seem very important. Doing well in school or work will become much less important than using drugs. Taking good care of yourself will get moved down the list of priorities. Drugs become so overvalued that the things that truly improve well-being become ignored. Natural true rewards will no longer drive automatic behaviors, and your body will lose part of its ability to maintain its well-being.

Typically, when this process is explained to health professionals there are several reactions. First, people say, "Well that sounds grim. Does that mean drug-users are doomed to slowly die as their lives are taken over by drug use?" Second, they say, "Wait a minute. That doesn't make sense. I know lots of people who drink a little bit of alcohol every night or take drugs occasionally, and they still prioritize other things in their lives." Luckily, that second viewpoint is correct and this is not just a doom and gloom story. Happily, we do have other parts of our brain, particularly our prefrontal cortex, that can over-ride the suggestions and estimates of our limbic reward circuit. We will discuss this in detail in Brain Challenge #5. Additionally, beliefs and expectations about the effects of drugs, as we discussed in Chapter 1.2, still modulate the dopamine response to drugs. This occurs despite the pharmacological effects of the drug on dopaminergic reward circuits. For example, Gu and colleagues (2015) used fMRI to monitor activity in the reward circuits of smokers when the smokers were given cigarettes with and without nicotine and were variably told the truth about the nicotine content of what they were smoking. They found that being told that the cigarette did not contain nicotine reduced both the expected reward value signal and the reward prediction error signal from the dopamine neurons, even when the cigarette did contain nicotine that certainly pharmacologically activated the dopamine neurons. This emphasizes the complexity of the inputs and computations that go into estimates of reward value about natural and addictive drug rewards, even in the limbic reward circuit alone. Each component that influences perceived value, including beliefs and expectations, social reinforcement, prior experience, and pharmacological effects on dopamine neurons, contributes to the estimated reward value signal. Modifying any of these will reshape priorities and decisions about habit behaviors.

Speed and intensity of drug absorption separate addiction from recreation
It is also important to consider what pharmacologists call the "pharmacokinetics" of a drug of abuse. The limbic response to drugs of abuse depends not only on what chemical is

ingested, but also how much hits the brain and how fast the drug is absorbed. Remember that your limbic brain only pays attention to immediate effects, say ten minutes into the future. It learns best when a drug of abuse hits the brain quickly and all at once – when blood concentrations go from low to high almost immediately. The slower and more gradually the drug concentrations in your blood change, the less dramatic is the learning, and the less your limbic brain will overvalue the drug.

Thus, how someone takes a drug of abuse will have a big effect on whether the drug becomes overvalued and starts to take over his or her life. Directly injecting a drug of abuse into one's blood stream will almost instantaneously increase drug concentrations in the brain and thus dopamine release in the nucleus accumbens. This intravenous use will rapidly lead to over-valuation of drug reward and its associated consequences. Smoking a drug of abuse delivers the drug to the brain nearly as rapidly. One's lungs take up the drug rapidly from the air and deliver it straight to the brain. Thus, this method of use is also extremely addictive. Snorting a drug of abuse is a bit slower, but still a pretty quick way of increasing drug concentrations in the brain. Swallowing a drug of abuse takes longer to increase drug concentrations in the brain than these other methods. It may or may not deliver the drug to the brain quickly enough to powerfully and swiftly release dopamine in the nucleus accumbens.

Filling an empty stomach with a ready-to-absorb drug will still increase blood levels of drug rapidly. However, slowly consuming a drug over an hour or two in combination with a large, high-fiber meal will increase drug concentrations in the blood more slowly; perhaps slowly enough that the nucleus accumbens barely notices. For example, downing two glasses of wine in two minutes on an empty stomach will lead to greater over-valuation of alcohol reward than will drinking the same two glasses of wine over the course of a three-hour five-course meal. From the perspective of your nucleus accumbens, the first case would cause a clear spike in dopamine neuron firing after chugging the wine. Here, it would not be too hard for your brain to guess that this big increase is related to the drinking and to attribute that bump in dopamine to the alcohol. In the second case, there would be a long, slow drift towards increased dopamine neuron firing over the course of dinner. Not only does this make it less likely that the dopamine neurons notice the increase, but it also decreases the chance that the nucleus accumbens correctly attributes the increase in dopamine neuron firing to the wine. Maybe it is the restaurant that is slowly making your life seem better. Maybe it is the wonderful food. Maybe it is the charming person with whom you are dining, the way she is looking at you, or the fascinating conversation in which you are engaged. The slow uptake of the alcohol makes it both less likely that your nucleus accumbens notices the increase in dopamine release and more likely that it associates the increase with something other than alcohol use. Thus, chugging wine is likely to lead you to overvalue wine and encourage you to drink more. Slowly drinking wine with fine dinners may lead you to overvalue fine-dining or your dinner companion and encourage you to spend a disproportionate amount of money on fancy meals and your dinner date.

Why treating triggers does not reduce substance use

When trying to stop typical habit behaviors, it can be helpful to work on reducing exposure to cues that trigger reward seeking. For example, many people over-eat when they watch television, and reducing television viewing can help reduce over-eating (e.g., Jason & O'Donnell Jr., 2008). Reducing television viewing does not make food less rewarding, but it does prevent the television advertising cues from initiating a food-seeking behavior. Clinical researchers have tried to apply that logic to developing treatments for substance use disorders but failed repeatedly in their attempts. For example, drug withdrawal symptoms are known to be triggers for drug seeking. Withdrawal symptoms signal to a dependent substance user that using a drug will make them feel better, by relieving the unpleasant withdrawal symptoms. Numerous clinical trials have treated withdrawal symptoms with medications, expecting that this should reduce drug seeking and substance use. But trial after trial has shown that reducing withdrawal symptoms, while providing medical stabilization for the patient, does nothing to reduce the likelihood or frequency of drug use. Likewise, "using to cope" is one of the strongest predictors of development of substance addiction, as people learn to "self-medicate" negative mood with addictive drugs. Here, undesired feelings (e.g., depression, anxiety, sadness, stress, loneliness) trigger drug-seeking behaviors. Recognizing this connection, numerous clinical trials have also tried to reduce substance use by treating negative mood states; for example, by using antidepressant medications. But these, too, were unsuccessful, with antidepressants having no more effect on substance use than placebo (e.g., Ipset et al., 2015; Torrens et al., 2005). People regularly report using drugs in response to withdrawal symptoms and negative feelings. And these interventions were able to successfully reduce withdrawal symptoms and depression and anxiety symptoms. So why do these treatments fail at reducing drug seeking and use? Why does reducing exposure to common triggers work for over-eating but not for substance use?

This lack of effectiveness can be blamed on the fact that addictive drugs, unlike natural rewards, pharmacologically trigger dopamine release each time they are used. Remember, the dopamine signal at the time of the reward tells the brain to learn to new cues to trigger drug-seeking with each experience. Normally, cues that correctly predict opportunity for reward will not produce an error learning signal at the time of the reward, and the brain will not learn additional new associations with the reward. So, the first cue that correctly triggers reward-seeking is the only cue that triggers the reward-seeking behavior. But addictive drugs release dopamine, generating an error learning signal that drives the brain to learn additional cues to trigger drug use. For example, this can include any extraneous information at the time of drug use, such as where you were or whom you were with. So even though withdrawal symptoms are one trigger, the substance user will learn all sorts of additional associations that also trigger substance use. Medicating the withdrawal symptoms does not remove all the other learned cues, which will continue to trigger drug-seeking. Because of the ubiquity of these learned cues for drug-seeking, removing one trigger, even the most salient cue of withdrawal symptoms, does not have a meaningful impact on substance use. The pharmacological release of dopamine that occurs every time addictive drugs are taken creates so many learned cues that addressing common triggers for drug use does not appear to be an effective strategy for reducing substance use.

How medications for substance use disorders normalize reward learning

So, what does work for reducing drug-seeking? Here again, clinical research has confirmed what the error signal learning model would predict. If you prevent drug use from causing dopamine release, then the drug use stops being reinforced and drug-seeking is minimized. Treatments that eliminate or minimize the dopamine release at the time of drug use effectively reduce drug seeking and substance use. Many of the most effective treatments for substance use disorders take this approach; medications that prevent drug use from triggering dopamine release in reward circuits have been very effective for reducing opioid, nicotine, and alcohol use.

Unfortunately, misperceptions by the public about how these medications work has limited our ability to provide this effective care for people suffering from substance use disorders. A major reason for this is that these medications have the same receptor targets as drugs of abuse, even though their impact on reward learning is completely different. Though the medications interact with the same receptors as the addictive drugs, the timing of their interaction with these targets is different, leading to completely different effects on habit learning. To address these misperceptions, we will walk through each of these treatments and how they work to correct the broken reward learning process caused by addictive drugs.

To understand these medications, first consider how addictive drugs break the reward learning process. Here, reward circuits are listening for immediate changes in internal or external environment as feedback about the results of the drug-seeking behavior. Changes in blood levels of the addictive drug are detected by receptors in the reward circuits; these quick changes in drug level trigger the phasic firing of dopamine neurons in the reward learning circuits. The brain recognizes this phasic firing as a sign of having experienced a reward. Note that here the reward learning circuit is responding to the *detected change* in blood level of the addictive drug. If we want to stop the reward learning circuits from experiencing drug use as rewarding, we need to stop these circuits from detecting a change in blood levels of the addictive drug.

Functionally, there are two ways of stopping reward learning circuits from detecting a change in bloods level of the addictive drug. You can jam the receptors that detect blood level of the drug either in their ON state or in their OFF state. Since the receptors have to change from OFF to ON to detect a change, getting them stuck in either the ON or OFF position will prevent them from noticing the change when addictive drugs are used. Medications have been developed that take both approaches at the relevant receptors for the addictive drug being treated. While these two approaches have opposite actions, where one turns on the relevant receptors (i.e., agonist therapy) and the other turns them off (i.e. antagonist therapy), functionally they both do the same thing to the reward learning process: They stop the addictive drug from registering as a reward in the reward learning circuits, training the brain that the drug-seeking habit is no longer of benefit.

What are these medications and how are they used? Two agonist therapies are used for opioid use disorders, the medications methadone and buprenorphine, which turn on opioid receptors. One antagonist therapy is also used for opioid use disorders, the medication naltrexone, which turns off opioid receptors. For tobacco use disorders, two agonist therapies are used, nicotine replacement therapy and varenicline, which turn on nicotinic acetylcholine receptors. Lastly, for alcohol use disorders, naltrexone is also used as an antagonist therapy, as the effect of alcohol on dopamine neuron firing involves activation of opioid receptors. In all cases, these medications are provided to patients in formulations or with dosing schedules designed to keep the targeted receptors completely saturated with the medication at all times. With the medication filling all of the targeted receptors, use of the addictive drug cannot be detected by the receptors. Either all of the targeted receptors are already on (i.e., with agonist therapy) or they are all blocked from being turned on (i.e., with antagonist therapy).

Where does the public misperception come from? In the case of agonist treatments for opioid and tobacco use disorders, the effect of the addictive drug and the medication on the targeted receptor is the same. For example, heroin, fentanyl, methadone, and buprenorphine all turn ON opioid receptors. Considering just the drug target, it sounds like the addictive drug and the medications do the same thing! This has led misinformed people to suggest that these agonist treatments are simply doctors taking over the role of a drug dealer, supplying patients with a different version of the drug to which they are addicted, and continuing the addiction. But when you consider the effects of the addictive drug versus the agonist treatment on the reward learning process, you realize that the addictive drug and the medication have completely different effects. The addictive drugs trigger dopamine release at the time of drug use, reinforcing the drug use behavior that just occurred and encouraging its repetition. The agonist therapy keeps the target receptor stably stuck in the ON position, preventing the addictive drug use from triggering dopamine release, and preventing the perception that drug use was rewarding. The addictive drug hijacks the reward learning circuits to reward drug use that is not actually beneficial. The agonist therapy forces the reward learning circuit to stop listening to the addictive drug, so that drug use no longer shapes habit decisions and predominates behavior driven by the brain's autopilot. The addictive drug warps the brain's autopilot to favor drug-seeking over all else. The agonist therapy makes the brain's autopilot insensitive to the addictive drug, allowing it to readjust its learned habits to favor ones with real benefit.

The misunderstanding of how agonist therapy works has also led to ineffective use of this treatment in some health care clinics. Belief that agonist therapy was just substituting for the patient's more dangerous illicit drug habit led some clinicians to try to minimize the amount of medication that they gave the patient. But with a minimal dose, the target receptors are not saturated; some receptors still remain empty to respond to use of the addictive drug. While the medication might dampen the dopamine neuron firing in response to the addictive drug, drug use would still trigger some reward signal and continue to promote drug-seeking. This on-going drug use reinforced those clinicians' belief that agonist treatment did not work and that patients receiving it were still addicted. Without a dose sufficient to block the dopamine response to drug use, the medication does not stop drug-seeking and normalize habit learning the way it is intended.

Recognizing that agonist and antagonist therapies do the same thing to help address substance use disorders, why would you choose to use one over another? When it comes to clinical effectiveness, the key difference between agonist and antagonist therapies comes down to medication adherence. To work, these treatments require that the target receptors are consistently stuck ON or OFF. If the medication wears off, then the addictive drug will be rewarding again, and drug-seeking behaviors will return. Here, agonist therapy has an advantage. Because the receptors are constantly turned on, the brain starts to adapt to having the receptors constantly on, reaching a new normal with the medication present but becoming disrupted when the medication goes away. In other words, the brain becomes physically dependent on the medication, and the patient will have withdrawal symptoms when they forget to take their medication. These withdrawal symptoms provide a helpful, though unpleasant, reminder to the patient to take their medication. With methadone, for example, a patient would have to endure about a week's worth of miserable flu-like withdrawal symptoms before taking the addictive drug would become rewarding again. Not surprisingly, patients on methadone rarely forget to take their medication. But with antagonist therapy, there is no signal for the brain to adapt to, and patients do not become physically dependent on their medication. For example, if a patient forgets to take their oral naltrexone, they will feel perfectly normal. Later that day, if they take the addictive drug, the drug use will be rewarded and drug-seeking starts again. This leads to big differences in adherence to these treatments, which is why oral treatment with methadone has historically been much more effective than treatment with oral naltrexone. To address the adherence problem with naltrexone, a new medication formulation that keeps naltrexone levels stable for a full month after an injection was recently developed. This has greatly improved the effectiveness of antagonist treatment for opioid use disorders, as the patient only needs to remember to get their medication once per month rather than every day.

A second serious consideration in choosing between agonist and antagonist therapies stems from the difference in physical dependence. Part of development of physical dependence is development of tolerance to the effects of the drug. When tolerant or physically dependent on a drug, a person will experience less of a physiological effect to a given dose of a drug. In a tolerant state, taking relatively large quantities of a drug may not produce an overdose, even though the dose consumed would be sufficient to cause dangerous and even life-threatening effects in a person without tolerance. Because patients on agonist therapies will maintain a physically dependent and tolerant state, in the case that they do use the drug for which they are being treated, they will have minimal response to that drug and are unlikely to overdose. But patients on antagonist treatments will lose their tolerance to the drug over time, and in the case that they use the drug for which they are being treated while their naltrexone levels are low, they will experience the effects of the dose consumed. If patients on antagonist therapy use the quantity of drug that they regularly used when tolerant (e.g., before treatment), they are at significant risk of overdose if they miss their medication. This difference between agonist and antagonist treatment is a specific concern for treatment of opioid use disorders, as opioid use causes respiratory depression that can lead to death. Because oral naltrexone effects wear off quickly, doses can be missed without noticeable consequences to the patient. As patients lose tolerance to the effects of opioids, oral naltrexone is both not effective and puts patients at risk of overdose. Thus, it is not a recommended treatment for opioid use disorders (The ASAM National Practice Guideline for the Treatment of Opioid Use Disorder, 2020). Extended-release naltrexone, which provides stable dosing for a month with a single injection, reduces risk somewhat, as the naltrexone should help block the effects of opioid use and minimize its effects. But practically, patient adherence to treatment isn't perfect, and clinical trials comparing risk of overdose during treatment with extended-release naltrexone versus extended-release buprenorphine suggest that patients on the antagonist treatment naltrexone had 3.8 times greater risk of overdose than those on the agonist treatment buprenorphine (Ajazi et al., 2022). For these reasons, agonist treatments are favored over antagonist treatments for opioid use disorder, despite similar impact of the treatments on reward learning processes.

Chapter 1.5: Getting What You Pay For: How to Assess the True Value of a Reward

As we have reviewed in the last chapters, there are many ways in which our brains can be tricked to overvalue specific rewards. When this happens, we will tend to work hard to get these rewards, even though the benefits we obtain from them may be low or the harms may be great. In essence, we are being bamboozled by our culture and experience. We have been trained to pay more, in effort, for rewards that simply are not as beneficial as we expect. How can we fix this training, so that we only pay for what we truly get?

How can we correct our value estimates?

A number of effective therapies have been developed that include a focus on changing expectations about the relative value of healthful or unhealthful behaviors. Cognitive Behavioral Therapies and Motivational Interviewing are two effective treatments for treating addictive and mood disorders and encouraging more healthful habits.

Part of generating accurate value estimates is identifying what already has value estimates associated with them. In addition to requiring knowledge about the consequences of thoughts and behaviors, we also need to be aware of our own habits. Often, we do things so automatically that we do not even know we are doing them. People close to us may be more aware of our tendencies and behaviors. Thus, it can be helpful to ask others to point out things that we do or think that are getting in the way of reaching our goals. It can be much easier for someone on the outside to objectively see the patterns in our thoughts and behaviors. The more habitual our behaviors, the less likely it is that we notice ourselves doing them.

Additionally, maintenance of a habit requires that your reward circuits perceive on-going benefit from completing the habit behavior. If you can end the perceived benefit of the habit, thus removing the reward for the behavior, then the drive to do the habit will fade. Often, in thinking about ways to eliminate reinforcement of a habit, people focus on ways of changing their external environment. For example, one might stop associating with friends who encourage and praise a bad habit. But these sorts of external rewards are often hard to control. A recent study in songbirds, however, suggests that reward circuits also respond to internal assessments of one's own performance (Gadagkar et al., 2016). Specifically, when researchers distorted the sound of a bird's singing, the bird's dopamine neurons were inhibited, signaling to the bird's reward learning circuits that his singing behavior did not result in the beautiful song he was seeking. This shows that internal perception of one's own performance can also influence habit learning. If the habit behavior does not produce the expected results, habit circuits will decrease motivation to repeat it. This internal performance evaluation system creates other possibilities for eliminating rewards for a habit. If you can change your understanding of the goal of the habit or revise your evaluation of the typical outcome of the habit from positive to negative, then your internal performance monitoring system may stop reinforcing the habit and disfavor repeating it. Several approaches have been developed to encourage patients to reconsider their assessment of the outcome of their habit as a benefit. For example, Motivational Interviewing techniques help patients to consider ways in which the outcome of a habit conflicts with prioritized goals, and Normative Feedback techniques show patients that their habit is neither normal nor accepted, nor socially beneficial to do amongst their broader peer group. The clinical effectiveness of these formal psychotherapy techniques demonstrates the power of changing how we internally evaluate the results of our habitual behaviors, thoughts, and responses.

Cognitive behavioral therapy, another formal psychotherapy approach, teaches that with practice we are able to revise the mistaken assumptions we tend to habitually make in our thinking. Correcting these assumptions helps us make more objectively accurate health-related decisions. Cognitive behavioral therapy is designed to change thoughts and behaviors that are important to health. It has an enduring effect in the treatment of major depression and anxiety disorders and reduces the risk of relapse (Hollon et al., 2006). This enduring effect is particularly evident in comparison to treatment with drugs for anxiety and depression (anxiolytics and antidepressants). Cognitive behavioral therapy is also an effective treatment for chronic pain, insomnia, substance use disorders, eating disorders, and other health problems with a behavioral component. To get started, let's consider some of the most common methods used to change inaccurate expectations.

Reframing: Adopting a new perspective
Our psychological responses and emotions depend not so much as what happens to us as the way we think about things. Our thoughts about health behaviors and situations tend to become patterned and habitual over time. The habits we acquire that involve relatively automatic actions, tying one's shoes, brushing one's teeth, shaving, or preparing the morning coffee, are paralleled by mental habits we acquire. However, the prefrontal cortex can also redirect these physical and mental habits. In the language of contemporary psychology, in particular cognitive-behavioral therapy, the term "reframe" is used to describe a process of rethinking our assumptions, generally for the purpose of modifying all forms of habits. Reframing involves the practice of reconsidering your initial reaction to a situation or behavioral choice to broaden your perspective. By reframing your beliefs about an opportunity, you may discover new reasons or motivations for not doing unhealthful or doing healthful things. This concept and practice is at the core of highly effective cognitive therapies that have been developed and tested for a wide variety of health problems (Beck, 1976).

Rather than thinking about the effects of a behavior or situation as a whole, we often focus on only one aspect of the situation and ignore the other effects. When we habitually think of only the good aspects of an unhealthful behavior or only the bad aspects of a healthful behavior, these thought patterns can encourage us to act in ways that harm our health. Stepping back from our initial thoughts and reactions and considering other aspects of the situation can help us make a more objective and balanced assessment of the costs and benefits of doing a behavior. Simply taking another perspective can help fix the errors we make when we value a given opportunity.

For example, someone's first thoughts about going to the gym might be habitually negative. "I'm already busy and it is going to take time that I don't have to work out." "I'm going to get all sweaty and soggy and I hate that feeling." "All the really in shape people at the gym will make me feel bad about myself." "Exercising makes my muscles hurt and takes effort." If these thoughts are the only ones you have when you consider going to the gym, then chances are you won't go. Why would you go if it is going to be a miserable and negative experience? If you catch yourself having negative thoughts about a good behavior, pausing and trying to reframe can both encourage you to go to the gym and help break these unhelpful thought patterns. Reframing is in many ways simple. All you need to do is ask yourself "Why would I want to go to the gym?" "What good things are there about exercising?" Then brainstorm answers and see if they make sense to you. How might I reframe my thoughts about going to the gym? "Exercise will help energize me and help me think more clearly, so even though it takes time, I may be more efficient in getting things done." "Sweating will clean out my pores and make me feel really clean and fresh after I shower and change." "There are a lot of nice people at the gym and it can be fun to talk with them or make new friends as we exercise together." "Exercise makes me stronger and will keep me from getting tired and sore from my everyday activities." You may not only find that you can counter all your own arguments against going to the gym, but also come up with additional reasons to go. "If I work out for an hour, I can have that slice of cake I've been dying for without gaining weight." "I've always wanted to learn a headstand, and the yoga instructor says I'm only about a month of practice away from succeeding." "I've been having back pain lately, and my doctor says that building core strength and losing some weight is my best bet for preventing it from becoming chronic." Bringing positive thoughts about a healthful behavior to the forefront will encourage you to make a healthful decision. In this case, reframing may increase the chances you decide to go to the gym. It will also shape your experience at the gym. If you are thinking about the positive aspects of going to the gym, you will notice the positive aspects of going to the gym. Chances are you will have a much better experience when you are there.

While in principle the concept of reframing is simple, becoming good at it requires practice. For people who are really stuck in unhelpful thought patterns, it may be difficult to even come up with other ways of thinking about things. For this reason, it can be helpful get others involved in your early attempts to reframe. You could ask a friend, therapist, or members of a support group to point out when you are being overly negative or positive about a situation to help you learn to recognize when your biased thoughts are favoring bad choices. When you or your friend identifies such a situation, you can brainstorm together to come up with other ways of looking at the situation. This may generate a lot more ideas and thoughts than if you tried alone. If you take the time to think about your friends' ideas of other way of thinking about the choice, you may find that some of their thoughts ring true for you, even if you never would have thought of them yourself. I note that picking a friend that already does the behavior that you want to adopt can be particularly helpful. They obviously have some reason and motivation that keeps them doing that behavior. Someone who has the same behavior and thought patterns as you could wind up just reinforcing your current skewed perspectives. So, if you want to get fit but just can't think nice things about the gym, get a friend who does go to the gym to help you reframe. If you want to quit smoking, but all you can think about is how much better it will make you feel in this anxious moment, get a friend who has quit smoking to help you rethink that decision. Over time, as you practice reframing with a friend, you will find that you get better at both noticing when you are having unhelpful thoughts and coming up with alternate ways of thinking about things.

If you want to read more about how to reframe, we recommend the following online resources: http://www.mentalhelp.net/poc/view_doc.php?type=doc&id=9749&cn=353 and https://positivepsychology.com/cbt-cognitive-restructuring-cognitive-distortions/

To practice cognitive restructuring or reframing, see Exercise 1G (page 79).

Challenging expectations: Tackling irrational fears through graded exposure
Many of us have morbid fears; spiders, snakes, needles, and pain are common fears. Whether innate or resulting from experience, the amygdala and other centers of the brain make avoidance a natural consequence. Avoidance works in the short-term, but long-term avoidance of some fears, such as needles or dental drills, for example, can have long-term negative effects on obtaining medical and dental care. For phobic disorders in which one or more irrational fears interfere with a person's life, graded exposure can be a remarkably effective treatment.

Graded exposure is not to be confused with being called out in class for getting a poor grade. It is a clinical procedure in which a client is guided through the experience of the behavior and its consequences intentionally in a safe and reflective manner. Typically, the exposures will start with something totally unthreatening, for example, the word "spider," followed by something a little more threatening, for example, a picture of a spider. With each approximation toward the heart of the phobic disorder, the client is gradually able to extinguish this fear. Virtual reality systems that simulate contact with spiders have been developed, tested, and shown to effectively reduce fear and avoidance of spiders in people with arachnophobia or extreme fear of spiders (Cote & Bouchard, 2005). More generally, augmented or virtual reality systems have been developed for a variety of phobias and have been shown to be similarly effective to guided real-life exposures in clinical trials, providing a safe and effective option when real-life exposure is impractical (Hasan et al., 2023). Thus, guided exposure can be effectively applied to many different behavioral problems that stem from inaccurate beliefs or expectations about a situation or behavior.

Graded exposure is a particularly useful technique when a person has inaccurate or exaggerated fears or negative expectations about a healthful behavior. Having a friendly and more experienced person walk them through the healthful behavior (or do it with them) and encourage them to reflect on what they are actually experiencing on a moment by moment basis can be a powerful method for changing expectations.

This strategy can be used formally or informally. Something as simple as inviting your junk food-eating friend to try some of the more healthful, but unfamiliar food you brought for lunch (e.g., try a piece of my persimmon or my tofu bahn mi sandwich) could change their expectations through exposure and might increase the chance that they at least contemplate these options the next time they go to the grocery store. An office lunch workshop where a nutritionist brings in healthful lunch options that are available in the cafeteria or in nearby restaurants, explains their nutritional value in comparison to other choices, and then encourages people to sample each one and comment on their tastiness, would be a more formal version of the same strategy. Exposure interventions change expectations through experience and make people aware of choices that they could make or things that they could do that they may not have even considered before. In many cases, simply having a friendly and trustworthy face help us navigate the fear of the unknown is enough to change expectations and subsequently behavior through experience. Most people tend to think that anything they haven't done or tried already is bad, unpleasant, or at least at little scary. Improving their expectations about healthful behaviors makes them at least a bit more likely to do the behaviors in the future.

EXAMPLE: Applications for phobic or catastrophic responses to injury or pain

Notably, exposure is helpful for more than encouraging people to try something new. Exposure can also be extremely helpful in retraining or rehabilitating people who had a bad experience with something and now fear or avoid it unreasonably. For example, graded exposure has been used to great effect with chronic pain clients who have learned to fear movement. When someone is injured, he or she inevitably experiences pain and some loss of function around the injury. For example, if I sprain my ankle, it will hurt if I try to walk on it, and until my ankle completes the initial healing process, I will risk injuring it more if I try to walk. However, even after my ankle has healed enough for me to start moving it normally and walking again, my ankle will hurt when I move and walk on it, until I strengthen the surrounding muscles and ligaments and work out remaining inflammation and scar tissue that built up when I was immobile. But, I need to move my ankle despite the discomfort to get it back to its normal, functioning, pain-free state. Some people become so fearful about experiencing pain or reinjuring themselves that they never try to move during this later recovery period. This can lead to chronic disability and pain. Coaching people through the movements they fear and breaking expectations that movement will lead to excruciating pain or injury can be both highly effective and necessary to get chronic pain clients to recover.

This general strategy has been developed into a structured treatment plan for people with chronic pain and fear of movement (Vlaeyen et al., 2001). In short, chronic pain clients with fear of movement are helped to generate a list of movements that they are afraid to do or that they think might cause extreme pain or injury. The clients then rank these movements from lowest to highest in terms of fear and perceived danger. Treatment consists of the therapist working with the client to do the behaviors on the list. The therapist encourages the client to reflect on their pain and their ability to do the movements safely as they complete them. The treatment starts with the least scary movements and progresses as the client experiences success with completing less feared tasks. This treatment has been shown to be highly effective for reducing fear of movement and catastrophizing about pain in clients with chronic back pain in case-studies and trials (Woods & Asmundson, 2008; George et al., 2008; Leeuw et al., 2008). The treatment also tends to improve pain-related disability, although perhaps not any more so than other effective physical and behavioral therapies. The treatment changes clients' expectations about the danger and negative consequences of doing the movements and other activities required to recover. These changes in thoughts and beliefs tend to lead to healthful changes in behavior, even in people whose beliefs may be based on negative experiences in the past.

Comparing against others: Correcting perceptions through normative feedback
Correcting biased perceptions of what other people do can help encourage behavior change. Interventions may help people understand that (1) the unhealthful behavior that they do is not common in the broader population of their peers or (2) a healthful behavior is common among the broader population of their peers. These interventions are referred to as *normative comparisons*. They typically consist of:
1) Assessment: asking people about the details of their current behavior, and
2) Feedback: providing them factual information about how their behavior compares to that of other people like them in the general population.

For example, you might ask a person how much he or she drinks, and then provide him or her with information on the percentage of people of their age and gender that drink more or less than they do. Interventions using normative comparisons have been shown to be effective for preventing or reducing alcohol use and risky sexual behaviors in college-age populations, and dietary fat intake in adults (Moreira et al, 2009; Chernoff & Davison, 2005; Kroeze et al., 2008).

To use this strategy, you need factual information on how people behave in the general population. Epidemiologists have collected this information for some behaviors. Tools to help people use such information have been made to help change specific behaviors. For example, a web-based computer program is available that will provide feedback comparing individual student use of alcohol and marijuana to rates of use in the U.S. student population overall (i.e., http://echeckuptogo.com/). However, it can be hard to find epidemiological data for some behaviors. Lack of information to provide accurate feedback can be a barrier to using this type of intervention.

Notably, this strategy has the potential to change behavior in undesirable directions. Normative comparisons can also make unhealthful behaviors appear normal. Feedback about norms in the general population may increase unhealthful behaviors in people in particularly healthful social groups. For example, a teenager who does not drink alcohol and has no friends that do, might be more likely drink alcohol after finding out that she drinks less than many other people her age. Thus, it can be important to target these interventions to people with relatively uncommon, unhealthful behaviors. Americans on average do some pretty unhealthful behaviors, and generally our goal is not to get all people to this mediocre state. Interventions that teach people with extremely unhealthful behaviors that most people act differently from them can be very effective for encouraging them to drift towards the more healthful norm. If these same interventions teach people with extremely healthful behaviors that most people act differently from them or stigmatize their exceptional behaviors in some way, then we are doing them a disservice. It is hard enough to keep up healthful behaviors without professionals pointing out how rare it is to do. Thus, these interventions should be saved and used selectively for people identified as being on the extremely unhealthful end of the bell curve.

Revealing internal contradictions between our behavior and our values and goals

Thoughts about a given situation or behavior, for example, overeating, can be particularly powerful motivators when one can identify a contradiction between the behavior and personal values or goals. We all have images of how we ideally would like to be and how we would like to act. But our behaviors frequently do not match up with our ideals. In many cases, we are not aware of the disconnect between how we do behave and how we want to behave, or what we do and what we are trying to achieve. We may be doing things that prevent us from reaching our goals or from being the person we want to be. When we consider our individual behaviors in the context of our personal values and goals, we may find that we would like to make different choices. This may increase our motivation to alter our habits. When we recognize the connection between our behavioral choices and our values and goals, we may change our assessments of our opportunities and start acting in ways that are consistent with our long-term goals and personal ideals. By relating our current choices to our longer-term goals for ourselves, we may drastically change our estimation of the value of a short-term reward opportunity. We may not find feeling better in the moment as appealing if we are clearly aware and consider the fact that it will cause us problems and prevent us from reaching goals that are really important to us. Helping people to recognize when their behaviors are in conflict with their values and goals and using this to motivate behavior change is an explicit component of several highly effective therapies for promoting behavior change, specifically *Motivational Interviewing* (Miller & Rollnick, 2002) and *Acceptance and Commitment Therapy* (Hayes et al., 1999*).

Motivational interviewing, for example, highlights the disagreement between a client's actual behaviors and their stated goals to help motivate change. In this therapy, the provider is taught to provide simple, objective feedback to the client about how their choices or behaviors may be opposed to their stated goals. The provider encourages the client to explore these discrepancies so that association between the client's unhealthful behaviors and his goals become explicit and clear to the client. By asking the right questions, the provider can let the client give the reasons for doing the behavior then arguments against doing the behavior. The client's own reasons are likely to be the most persuasive—they are the ones the provider can effectively repeat to the client. The provider does not tell the client that the unhealthful behaviors are a problem that they must change, but instead gives the client enough objective information about the behavior and its typical consequences to allow the client to reevaluate whether the unhealthful behavior is worth doing. In essence, the provider simply provides missing or ignored information that may change the client's judgment of the value of an opportunity and allows the client to readjust their ideas about the value of the behavior themselves. Because our decision of whether to do a behavior depends strongly on our estimation of the value of making that effort, new information that greatly increases or decreases our estimates about the value of anticipated rewards can have a dramatic impact on our subsequent choices. Overall, motivational interviewing enhances drive to change behavior. *This increased drive may be particularly powerful and sustained because it stems from personal, internally generated reasons for change rather than the encouragement of a health professional.*

Motivational interviewing also avoids arguments between the client and provider by acknowledging that there is a choice involved in doing or withholding a behavior. This choice involves benefits and risks on either end; only the individual making the choice can decide which outcomes are more valuable to them. Doing a behavior may solve a short-term problem (e.g., help you deal with anxiety) but stop you from reaching your long-term goals (e.g., to stay healthy and active). For example, smoking might help you relax when you are immediately stressed but cause a myriad of health problems that will cause much greater stress in the coming years. Similarly, doing a behavior may cause a short-term problem (e.g., disappoint or start and argument with a friend) but help you reach your long-term goals. For example, I (J.T.) might have to turn down the homemade cookies my friend baked last night to keep my gestational diabetes under control and reach my longer-term goal of having a safe delivery of a healthy baby. Since the longer-term consequences are both probabilistic and potentially far into the future, choosing the behavior that helps in the short-term could wind up being the better choice. If I am hit by a bus on the way to work today, I might as well have had that cookie. By respecting the difficult decisions made by our dopamine system, Motivational Interviewing helps promote more trusting, less confrontational and more collaborative relationships between a provider and client.

EXAMPLE: Using Motivational Interviewing to encourage undervalued health behaviors

To illustrate, let's consider how Motivational Interviewing might be used by a health professional to encourage a client to make an effort to change a behavior. Let us imagine an overweight client with diabetes and back pain who has repeatedly failed to make dietary changes despite poor diabetes control and dire warnings from their doctor about their need to manage their diet and lose weight to prevent diabetes complications. The client has come to the clinic complaining of worsening back pain, despite the pain medications that were prescribed at the last visit.

Health Professional: *So Mr. X, what brings you here today?*

Client: *My back is killing me. I can't concentrate. I'm angry and tired all the time, and it is hard to work. Those pills that you gave me last time barely helped at all.*

Health Professional: *I'm happy to try to come up with a pain management plan that will work better for you. Could you tell me a bit more about your goals? Knowing that all pain treatments have their strengths and weaknesses, what are your priorities? What would you consider a success?*

Client: *I just want the pain to stop interfering with my life. I want to be happy and able to focus on my family and job instead of the pain in my back.*

Health Professional: *That seems like a very good goal. There are a few things that we could try that might help in that regard. Most simply, I could increase the dosage of your medication. But, that will also increase the side effects and may make you more tired and make it even harder to concentrate. It may also not be effective. Roughly one-third of people who try these medications don't find them effective at tolerable doses. Alternatively, one of the most common contributors to back pain is being overweight, and losing weight and exercising can substantially reduce back pain while also increasing energy, improving mood, and helping with your other health conditions, like your diabetes. A better, but more challenging solution, would be to try to start a diet and exercise plan to lose the weight that may be maintaining your back problems. Of course, this will take longer and require more effort, but this eventually should make it more likely that you will be able to keep up an active, social lifestyle. Alternatively, we could try a mix of the two. You could start a diet and exercise plan, and I could give you more powerful pain medication that you could use before you exercise, so that your back pain doesn't prevent you from doing the things that should eventually make it strong and pain free. It's your choice. I can play around with the medications and dosing and I can connect you with programs and people who can help you with the diet and exercise, but the choice is ultimately yours and you are the one who will have to do the work. Does any of this sound helpful?*

Client: *The medication really didn't help that much with the pain and in other ways made me feel worse. I'm not so sure I'll be able to lose weight, but I suppose it wouldn't hurt to try the program you mentioned. How about we try the both option? Could you give me some more powerful medication and sign me up for the diet and exercise program?*

Health Professional: *Of course. Let's do that now, and plan to check back in a couple of weeks to see how this new plan is working for you…*

The clinician focuses on getting the client to clarify his goals, and then presents factual information and choices that the client might consider as they relate to the client's own goals. The clinician highlights that the choice and responsibility to change behavior are the clients alone. The clinician can help but can't do it for them. Then the clinician lets the client make his decision. Because the clinician hasn't pushed any particular choice on the client, there is nothing for the client to argue or push back about. This prevents him from becoming defensive. While there is obviously lots of additional work to do to help the client change behavior in a lasting way, the health professional has now linked weight loss with something that the client cares about, specifically stopping back pain from interfering in his life, thus increasing the expected value of a diet and exercise program. By focusing on the client's goal, rather than the provider's priority, which might be to get his client's diabetes controlled, he has helped the client to prioritize weight loss.

Motivational Interviewing has been used to effectively manage diabetes, risky alcohol use, nutrition and obesity, physical activity, and smoking. For example, Motivational Interviewing improves weight loss in women with type 2 diabetes (West et al., 2007) as long as the therapy is an adjunct to regular medical care. It outperforms traditional advice-giving in the treatment of a broad range of behavioral problems and diseases (Rubak et al., 2005). Motivational interviewing need not involve an actual interviewer; online Motivational Interviewing, in the form of assessment and individualized feedback, is also effective (Webber et al., 2008).

To practice in identifying values and goals and using these to foster behavior change, see Exercise 1H (page 87).

Brain Challenge #1 Exercises

Exercise 1A: Practice Creating Positive Expectations

From a practical point of view, health professionals can reduce the degree to which their clients experience pain or increase the benefits of a treatment by creating positive expectations. There are different ways the same treatment can be framed by a health professional to a client that may produce very different reactions and health behaviors.

Part 1: Helping To Reducing Pain
A child is being given a potentially painful vaccination. What do you say to him or her?

_____
_____
_____

Example 1: "This is going to hurt, so hold still or I'll have to get someone to pin you down."

Example 2: "Remember how yucky it is to be sick and tired? The medicine I have here will prevent you from catching a type of bug that makes you really sick. You are really lucky to be able to get this medicine. Could I have your arm to give it to you?"

Example 1 is paraphrased from a truly terrible medical doctor I (J.T.) visited as a child, who did pin me down and give me the injection. Since that visit, it has taken substantial cognitive effort for me to overcome my emotional aversion to doctors and needles. My lack of control over this minor pain turned a simple injection into a traumatic experience that continues to influence my thoughts and behaviors 30 years later.

Example 2 is roughly what I told my 3-year old son before his last round of vaccinations. We practiced giving shots to a stuffed animal, and then he willingly and happily got his vaccinations and proudly told us all that evening that he had got the medicine that would make him healthy.

Review the statement you generated at the beginning of this section. Do you focus on the negative consequences or the positive outcomes? How can you re-word it so that the client feels informed and in control of what is going to happen to them?

_____
_____
_____

Part 2: Helping To Quit Smoking
Your client continues to smoke despite five previous quit attempts including liberal use of nicotine replacement therapy. They are discouraged and feel like there is no point in trying again. You decide to suggest a new medication for nicotine dependence. What do you say to the client?

_____
_____
_____

Example 1: "I know quitting smoking is hard work, so I'm really impressed with all the effort you have been devoting toward this important health behavior. The average person requires 7 quit attempts to learn all the skills they need to be able to stop smoking, so you are well on your way. I'd like to be able to help you. There is another medication that was approved to help people quit smoking. It is a pharmacologically sophisticated drug that specifically targets the brain circuits that drive you to smoke. In trials, people receiving this medication quit smoking at higher rates than those receiving other treatments for smoking cessation. Would you like to try it?"

Example 2: "Quitting smoking requires a lot of effort. Maybe you just aren't ready to quit yet. There is another medication I could prescribe to help you quit smoking, but it works similarly to nicotine replacement therapy and that didn't work well for you. Would you like to try it?"

While the content of both examples are true, Example 1 helps create an expectation that a quit attempt will eventually be successful and more likely if the client keeps trying and uses a fancy new drug. Example 2 echoes the client's belief that even with a new medication the outcome of another quit attempt will be another failure.

Review the statement you generated at the beginning of this section. Do you focus on the negative consequences or the positive outcomes? How can you re-word it so that the client feels informed and in control of their efforts toward behavior change?

_____
_____
_____

Part 3: Other Medical and Surgical Examples
Below are a few more examples of situations where you may be able to increase treatment success or decrease pain by fostering the client's expectation of benefit. Brainstorm different ways of discussing these treatments, focusing on creating positive expectations about treatment effects and making the client feel in control of their own behavior and mood.

You believe a combination of a selective serotonin reuptake inhibitor plus 12 weeks of cognitive behavior therapy would benefit your depressed client. What do you say to her?
Response 1: _____
_____
_____

Response 2: _____
_____
_____

Response 3: _____
_____
_____

A client presents with low back pain that began three days ago. They want an MRI and think they need surgery. You think that they are likely to get better with some anti-inflammatory medications and healing time. What do you say to them?

<u>Response 1:</u> _____

_____

_____

<u>Response 2:</u> _____

_____

_____

<u>Response 3:</u> _____

_____

_____

A client is about to go into surgery and is very scared about being in pain afterwards. What do you say to them?

<u>Response 1:</u> _____

_____

_____

<u>Response 2:</u> _____

_____

_____

<u>Response 3:</u> _____

_____

_____

Review the different responses for each of the examples above. Which ones focus on the negative consequences or the positive outcomes? Do you talk about wellness, model positive outcomes, and provide hope? How can you re-word it so that the client feels informed and in control of their efforts toward behavior change?

Exercise 1B: Identify Positive Associations for Behavior Change

Associations between rewards in your life and people, settings, things, thoughts, or situations can develop that encourage or discourage unhealthful behavior, thoughts, or moods. If you can identify these associations and become aware of them, you can take advantage of them to alter your exposure or response to these situations.

Part I: Identify Positive Associations

Try to keep a behavior or mood diary for at least a few days. Design your own method for recording this information easily and conveniently (e.g., in a small notebook or on an electronic device). Below is a list of what you should record, as well as a table you can modify to best record your own goals and associations:

1. Write down the mood, thought or behavior that you want to change.
2. Record the date and day of the week.
3. Regularly throughout the day, record the following:
   a. The intensity of the feeling or the drive to do the behavior you want to change.
   b. Things you notice in the environment/situation and people that are present.
   c. How you respond to the environment/situation and people that are present.
   d. Anything else you observe or think of at that time.

Target Feeling/Behavior:

Date:				
Time	**Intensity**	**Surroundings**	**Response**	**Other**
Date:				

Part 2: Minimize Negative Associations

Review the diary to look for patterns or situations in which the feeling or desire to do the behavior is more or less intense. This will provide clues to help you identify associations that encourage that feeling or behavior. You may find it helpful to have someone else look at the diary with you. They may be more open to noticing patterns that you do not see. Once you have found things that tend to make you feel or behave in ways that you are trying to change, you can work to alter your exposure to those cues.

Exercise 1C: Cues You Can Use

Consider one or two of your health-oriented goals. Think carefully about the cues that encourage your healthful activities. What reminds you to eat wisely, get regular physical activity or relax to manage your emotions during emotionally distressing events? Fill your everyday environments with cues that you associate with healthful actions and you will find you do them more often. Think like an advertising executive and expose yourself to sites, sounds, phrases, memories, and other reminders of your wellness goals to trigger healthful practices throughout the day.

To get you started, we provide some ideas that we have found helpful:
1. **Written Cues:** A notebook where weight, body fat, physical activity and other health data are recorded once a day, reminds me (W.G.) to stick to a diet and exercise plan.
2. **Visual Cues:** It is easier to take pills if they are in plain sight than if they are hidden in a medicine cabinet. My (W.G.) 90-year-old mother keeps her pills on the kitchen table so she unfailingly takes them at breakfast. In particular, photographs can be powerful visual cues. Pictures of places where you have hiked or pictures of yourself in optimal states can serve as daily reminders to emulate or recreate those states.
3. **Verbal Cues:** Asking a close friend or family member to remind you of your goals, particularly during times of weakness, can be helpful. Having my spouse remind me of the dessert I (J.T.) had at lunch when I am contemplating ice cream after dinner can help me moderate my diet.
4. **Musical Cues:** If you workout to music, you can create playlists that you associate with previous exercise highs to help keep you going. I (J.T.) successfully used my favorite dance music first to stay positive and productive at work during extreme pregnancy-induced nausea that otherwise had me vomiting 4+ times/day, and then later to keep me going through 42 hours of labor with my first child.
5. **Tactile Cues:** Put aside the clothes in which you would like to be able to fit, or the clothes you plan to use to take an exercise break, or wear the kind of shoes you would like to use for walking at a time when you are able to "get away from it all". You can also remove negative cues; for example, donate clothing that is now too large.
6. **Social Cues:** Find others who enjoy the activities you do and surround yourself with them as often as possible. Spend time with those with whom you can walk, cycle, play or cook healthfully, and you will be more likely to do these things regularly.
7. **Digital Cues:** Schedule your computer, cell phone or other digital devices to send you reminders of what you wish to accomplish on a daily or weekly basis. Numerous programs exist to remind and also to help you monitor what you eat, how much and in what kind of physical activity you engage, and how you feel after doing these.
8. **Scheduling Cues:** The paradox is that many of us take better care of cars than ourselves. Treat your daily health-related decisions like necessary maintenance rather than choices and put them in your appointment book or computer datebook to provide automatic reminders.

What works for you is likely to be different than what works for another person. Use the worksheet on the next page to help brainstorm cues you can use and come up with plans to incorporate them into your daily life.

WORKSHEET: Your Healthful Behavior Cues

Review the list on the previous page and then use the chart below to brainstorm cues you can use to promote your health goals and develop actionable plans to incorporate these cues into your life. How can you place these cues to create cravings for wellness activities? Bombard yourself with advertising for activities for a healthier you.

Type of cue	What are the desired cue(s)?	Where will the cue(s) be?	What will the cue(s) trigger?

Exercise 1D: Researching Your Own Personalized Normative Feedback

A common intervention technique used to target both individuals and populations is to provide normative feedback; in other words, to look up facts and statistics for what is actually "normal" for similar individuals or in your community. One of the ways in which this method has been used is to decrease alcohol consumption on university and college campuses by providing data on the drinking rates for the "typical college student". The goal is to correct over- or underestimated social norms by demonstrating that unhealthful behaviors are not as common or healthful behaviors are more common than may have been believed. Of course, this plan can backfire and reinforce unhealthful behaviors if it turns out unhealthful behaviors are more common or healthful behaviors are less common than expected.

For this exercise, we cannot provide you with normative feedback without knowing your target behavior or the social norms of the communities in which you live. However, with the Internet at your fingertips, it should be easy to find some hard facts from respectable websites such as the Centers for Disease Control and Prevention (e.g., https://www.cdc.gov/datastatistics/index.html) and the U.S. Department of Health and Human Services (e.g., https://catalog.data.gov/organization/hhs-gov). You may be able to look up more local data for you state, county, or city as well. You can either look up the unhealthful behavior you wish to decrease (e.g., smoking) to show it is less common than you or your client think or look up the healthful behavior you wish to increase (e.g., exercise) to show it is more common than you or your client think.

Here are some questions to consider when researching normative habits:
- What percentage of people engages in this behavior?
- How often do people typically engage in the behavior?
- How much do to people typically engage in the behavior (e.g., number of cigarettes)?
- What are the success rates of quitting (or starting) this behavior?
- What are the health consequences (or the health benefits) of this behavior?
- What is the average life expectancy of people who do (or do not) engage in this behavior?

Feel free to add to the list. What would change your mind about a health behavior? When considering the questions above and any others you may generate, we encourage you to jot down your own guesses about the correct answers before looking up the actual data. You may be surprised to see how much your social norms have biased your perceptions of certain behaviors.

Exercise 1E: Identifying Social Enablers versus Disablers

It is not uncommon for people in close relationships to discover that their spouse or partner is unwittingly sabotaging efforts to help achieve a health-related goal. That social influence may be even greater when it comes in social situations. For example, the social norm of finishing one's plate, of eating more when in groups, of eating more when in restaurants and of eating all of what is served, pits social norms against individual healthy choices. However, social pressure can also support healthy choices. Working out with others who support and enjoy similar healthful activities promotes greater physical activity, more opportunities to work out, longer participation and greater enjoyment.

Consider a health behavior you want to change, and then think about times that you feel pressured or tend to do the behavior in social situations. Are there specific social situations where you do or do not feel pressure to do the behavior? If so, what? Are there specific people that encourage or discourage you to do the behavior? If so, who? Brainstorm situations and people that encourage you to continue your bad habit.

Part 1: Situations That Encourage Bad Behaviors
To get you thinking, here are some social situations that tend to encourage bad behaviors in some people:
1) When I'm around someone I want to impress who does the bad habit.
2) When I'm around family or old friends who expect me to act like my old self.
3) When I'm celebrating.
4) When I'm around someone who is really nice to me when I make mistakes or feel bad.
5) When I'm around someone who benefits when I do bad behaviors.
6) When everyone else is doing the bad habit.

Now write some social situations in which you have trouble with a health behavior here:

_____

_____

_____

_____

Pick one of the social situations when you have trouble acting healthfully. Consider ways in which you can either avoid being in the situation or, more likely, act differently in the situation. Think of new things you could say or do when you feel pressured to do your bad habit. Find a supportive friend and role-play the situation. Practice these new responses so they seem easy and natural when you are in the real situation.

Part 2: People That Encourage Good Behaviors
Consider ways in which you might be able use social support to improve health-related activities. Are there people who encourage your healthful behaviors? What could loved ones, friends or colleagues do to support your healthful behavior? How might you encourage your social contacts to support you? To get you thinking, here are some ways you may increase support from existing social contacts:

1) Include friends in your attempt to change behavior (e.g., quitting smoking or going to the gym together).

2) Express your appreciation for their support, letting them know how important this change is for your health and well-being.

3) Encourage them to reward your good behavior.

4) Find new contacts that already do or encourage your new healthful behavior.

Now brainstorm some ways you can deploy social support to enhance your goals to change your health behavior:

_____

_____

_____

_____

Exercise 1F: Visualizing Social Networks that Enable and Disable Health-Related Habits

It is far easier to attain goals of fitness, weight, and managing difficult emotions when you have others who support you and who actively participate with you; for example, exercising together, eating the same healthful diet, or having emotionally intelligent discussions about feelings of anger, anxiety, or sadness.

As we have discussed, social interactions can contribute substantially to overvaluation of unhealthful behavior or undervaluation of healthful behavior. Identifying unhealthful behavior patterns in your family or social network can help you modify or reframe social interactions to make it easier for you to keep up more healthful behaviors.

For many people, it is easier to recognize patterns of social interaction and behavior when they are described visually. Drawing out connections between people that include their nature and quality can help describe a family or social network. You can then add symbols or codes to represent whether each person has a given behavior or health concern, and how they react to your behavior. The resulting pictures may give you a sense of the networks that do and do not support a given behavior pattern. This can help you identify existing social support for your healthful behavior. It can also warn you of groups or situations where it is likely that you will be encouraged to act unhealthfully.

Part 1: Informal Visualization

Draw an informal visualization using a simple set of symbols that you make up. For example, if I (J.T.) wanted to identify support for a vegetarian diet in my family, I could draw a family tree to 1) color code the symbols to indicate each person's behavior and 2) draw lines to indicate their support for my diet. In the box on the next page, I go through this exercise to create a visual representation of the familial support I do or do not receive for my vegetarian diet. Each square represents a male family member, each circle a female family member. The colors inside the symbols indicate what each family member eats. The black lines indicate family relationships as done in a standard family tree. The colored, dashed lines indicate the reactions I tend to get from family members regarding the lack of meat in my diet. I am the green circle at the bottom right.

As you can see, my husband, my son, one of my sisters, and one of my first cousins are vegetarian. Another first cousin is pescaterian, vegetarian plus fish. We are all very supportive of each other's diets and work together to ensure family dinners include vegetarian options. My other sister and first cousin both eat standard meat-heavy diets, but are supportive of other diets and consider others' food needs when we get together. My parents, grandparents, aunt, and uncle all eat meat-heavy diets but vary in their reactions. My father and grandparents seem somewhat incapable of even acknowledging that we do not eat meat. They regularly try to put meat on our plates, include meat in vegetable dishes, and make comments indicating distaste for our diets. My mother and uncle are verbally supportive as long as we do not try to make them eat what we are eating. My aunt is mostly supportive, but sometimes expresses concern that we might be damaging our health.

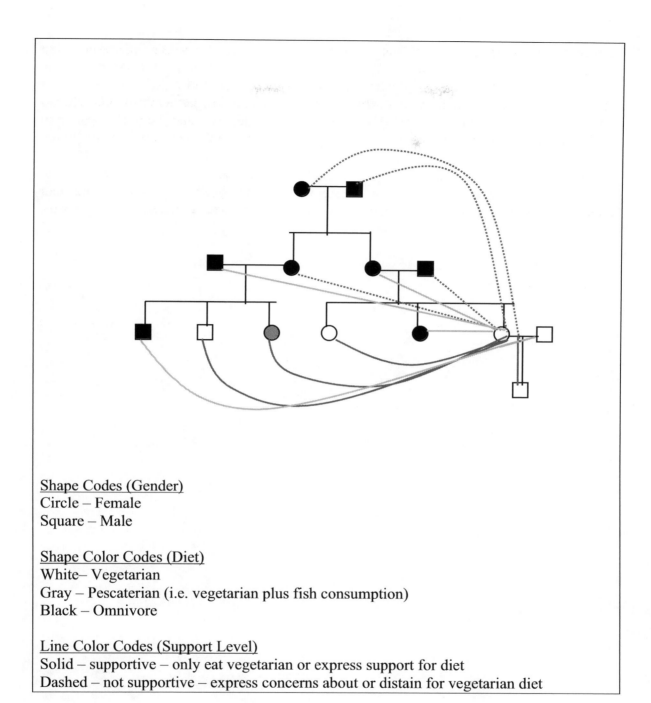

Shape Codes (Gender)
Circle – Female
Square – Male

Shape Color Codes (Diet)
White– Vegetarian
Gray – Pescaterian (i.e. vegetarian plus fish consumption)
Black – Omnivore

Line Color Codes (Support Level)
Solid – supportive – only eat vegetarian or express support for diet
Dashed – not supportive – express concerns about or distain for vegetarian diet

This diagram clearly indicates social support within my family that helps me eat vegetarian, and warns about potential pressure from older generations that may make it more difficult to follow my health choices.

In making such informal visualizations, you should feel free to describe connections between people in whatever way you think makes most sense. If you were interested in relationships at your work, you could start by using the floor plan of your office to describe how people in your building interact. Alternatively, you could draw out supervisory hierarchies to initially describe relationships (like the black lines on the family tree) and then indicate less formal relationships or behavioral interactions between individuals (like the colored lines on the family tree). Another possibility would be to simply draw connections between each person that talks to each other. These lines could be color coded to show the type of interaction (e.g., friendship, supervisor, job partnership). You should feel free to be creative in drawing up maps of social connections and their relationship to health behavior. Follow your instinct in choosing what you think is important to include.

Try drawing a picture of social interactions around a target behavior of your choice. On the next page, first brainstorm your coding system then sketch your visualization using that coding system. Which people do you want to include and on what dimensions do they vary (e.g., how they are connected, whether they do the behavior, level of support)?

Coding System:

_____
_____
_____
_____
_____

Visualization:

Look at your visualization. Are there parts of your network that appear more supportive of healthful behavior? Are their groups of people you may need to be very careful around? Do you need to reach out and seek additional support?

Part 2: Formal Visualization

There are several more formal techniques for assessing interconnections between people and their relationship to health or behavior. Scientists and health professionals use these techniques to depict and study interpersonal relationships and their impact. There are software programs to help draw and analyze these relationships, and they use relatively standard symbols and structures to indicate relationships and behavior. If you are interested in using these more formal techniques, below are some links that describe these techniques (specifically, genograms and social network), and examples of software programs available to help draw, build, and analyze these social interconnections.

Genograms

http://www.genopro.com/genogram/

GenoPro is a software program for drawing family trees and genograms. Genograms are family trees with additional information about relationships, behaviors or diseases included. This website does a good job of describing and showing examples of genograms and links directly to their software product if you are interested in using it.

Social Network Analysis

http://en.wikipedia.org/wiki/Social_network

Wikipedia provides a nice overview of social network analysis to get you oriented to its use, techniques and tools.

http://www.analytictech.com/networks

This website includes a description of various types of social network analysis, history of social network analysis, and detailed information on how to collect data, depict it, and analyze it. There are links to software programs to help if you are interested.

Exercise 1G: Modifying the Thoughts that Undermine Our Goals: The Power of Cognitive Restructuring or Reframing

How much we value healthful versus unhealthful behaviors is greatly influenced by our thoughts and expectations about the situation and our behavior. Psychologists have developed exercises to help people recognize when they are having thoughts that encourage or overvalue unhealthful behaviors or discourage or undervalue healthful behaviors. Once you recognize these thoughts, then you can evaluate them to determine whether they are accurate and helpful. When you identify unhelpful thought patterns, you can develop and practice alternative thoughts that lead to more balanced, healthful decisions.

Practices that help you identify unhelpful thought patterns and develop new helpful patterns are typically called cognitive restructuring or reframing. You can find many examples of these exercises in self-help or therapy manuals that use a cognitive-behavioral perspective. In this exercise, we will provide a general example of cognitive restructuring for changing health behavior. If you are having trouble relating this exercise to your own problem, you may find it helpful to look at exercises in a self-help or therapy manual written specifically for the health problem you are experiencing. These manuals will include specific examples of thoughts and expectations that are commonly held by people with that health problem (e.g., Burns, 1989; Antony & Swinson, 2008).

To begin, we will walk you through three steps of the restructuring or reframing process. During the exercise, we provide two different worksheets to assist you in the process. We use examples throughout so that you will have a sense of how to tackle your own health behavior goal.

Step 1: Identify Unhelpful Thoughts
To change thoughts that overvalue unhealthful or undervalue healthful behaviors, you first need to be aware of your own unhelpful thought patterns. It is essential to know precisely what thoughts you return to in given situations and how they influence your feelings and behavior. Often thoughts occur automatically and go by without notice. By monitoring your thoughts, feelings, and behavior in various circumstances, you can identify thoughts that encourage bad behaviors.

It can be difficult to accurately remember thoughts even immediately after you have them, let alone specific thoughts you had days or weeks ago. Thus, the first step is to develop an accurate and consistent method of monitoring your thoughts around your target health behavior. We provide you with a Thought Monitoring Form that you can use to record the thoughts you have about your target health problem, along with information about (1) when or in what situation you had the thoughts, (2) what your behavioral response was in that situation, (3) what happened when you did that behavior, and (4) the thoughts you had about the outcome of your behavior. Once you have a record of the thoughts you have habitually, the contexts in which you have them, and their impact on your health behaviors, then it will be possible to begin to evaluate their accuracy and change them if they are unhelpful.

Spend the next several days to weeks monitoring thoughts you have associated with your target health behavior in various situations. Record your observations in the Thought Monitoring Form, and take special care to record thoughts that you have repeatedly. We will come back to evaluate your records in Step 2.

Example: J.T.'s thought monitoring about sticking to her low-carbohydrate gestational diabetes diet.

Situation	Thoughts	Behavior	Consequences	Thoughts
I really want dessert and my husband and son are eating ice cream.	"I already had to skip the pasta and bread at dinner and now I can't have any ice cream either. It isn't fair. Pregnancy is miserable. I hate being a woman. Everyone around me is completely inconsiderate for eating carbohydrates all the time."	Feel bad for myself. Complain to my family about being pregnant. Notice all of the other unpleasant pregnancy sensations I am having.	Upset my husband and son by making them feel guilty about my being pregnant and anxious about my complaints. Make all my pregnancy symptoms seem more severe.	"I'm a terrible wife and mother. I wish I could go into hibernation until this pregnancy is over. I never want to be pregnant again."

WORKSHEET: Thought Monitoring Form

Directions: What were the automatic thoughts that occurred when you were considering your target health behavior? What did you do in response to your thoughts? What was the consequence of your action? And finally, what were your thoughts after the consequence of your action?

Date:

Situation	Thoughts	Behavior	Consequences	Thoughts

Date:

Situation	Thoughts	Behavior	Consequences	Thoughts

Date:

Situation	Thoughts	Behavior	Consequences	Thoughts

Date:

Situation	Thoughts	Behavior	Consequences	Thoughts

Notes & Observations:

Step 2: Identify Cognitive Errors

David Burns, MD (1989) devised a chart of common cognitive errors that he observed in his clients. W.G. adds a parallel set of cognitive errors that may be found in individuals who fail to take action to address a health risk. Below are two tables with these errors. People tend to make these thinking mistakes in general and sometimes being stressed and tired can make people more prone to them. I (J.T.) have included examples to go along with my low-carbohydrate gestational diabetes diet example from above. After reviewing the two tables of common cognitive errors, consider your Thought Monitoring Form. Are they biased by these thinking errors? Note thoughts and situations on your Thought Monitoring Form where you think you may be making these thinking errors.

Common Cognitive Errors (after Burns, 1989) and Examples During Attempts at Behavior Change (i.e., J.T.)

Thinking Error	Description	Example
Overgeneralization	Assuming that the outcome from a specific event or situation will occur in a large range of situations.	"Everyone else gets to eat whatever they want during pregnancy. I fail every medical screening test I'm given. I must be some sort of freak."
Catastrophizing	Focusing only on the worst, most extreme possibility regardless of how likely it is to occur.	"If my blood glucose levels are a little over target, I'll set my daughter up for a dangerous birth and a life of fighting obesity, diabetes and cardiovascular risk."
All-or-None Thinking	Focusing on only the extreme "best" or "worst" of a situation without regard to the full range of alternatives.	"If I can't eat exactly what I'm craving, I cannot enjoy anything I eat."
Jumping to Conclusions	Interpreting a situation with limited information and without a rational evaluation of its likelihood.	"Since he hasn't called back, my doctor must be avoiding me because he thinks I'm a hopeless case."
Selective Attention	Selectively attending to negative aspects of a situation while ignoring any positive aspects.	"Pregnancy messes up my normal diet, makes me tired, unable to do my normal exercise, gives me back aches, and generally ruins my body."
Negative Predictions	Assuming the worst will happen in a situation.	"If I don't perfectly follow health recommendations, my baby will die, be really sick, or hate me for the rest of my life."
Mind Reading	Assuming what people are thinking instead of finding out what they are really thinking.	"My husband wants to get away from me when I'm complaining about my pregnancy because he doesn't love me anymore and doesn't want the baby."

There are other categories of maladaptive thinking that occur in those reluctant to change behaviors that are also worth exploring. In this case, let us consider cognitive errors that might have stopped me from managing my gestational diabetes.

Additional Cognitive Errors (proposed by W.G.) and Examples That May Prevent Attempts to Modify Health Behavior (i.e., J.T.)

Thinking Error	Description	Example
Denial	Assuming that the outcome from a past set of events will not occur in the future.	"Just because my body couldn't process the glucose in the lab test doesn't mean I have a problem. The lab test is totally artificial. I'm healthy, I'm sure my body will handle sugar fine when I eat normal meals."
Positive Illusions	Assuming that things are fine in spite of significant evidence to the contrary.	"Although my doctors say I'm at high risk of pregnancy complications and I've screened positive for gestational diabetes on two lab tests, I don't need to change my eating patterns. I've never had health problems before."
Indecisiveness	Concluding that there are too many possible scenarios to make a decision or take action.	"There are so many different foods, I couldn't possibly keep track of how much sugar there is in each. Why even try to make low-carbohydrate meals when I'm sure to make mistakes?"
Rumination	Continuing to gather information or recycle one's thoughts without being able to determine when enough has been gathered to make a decision.	"Maybe I should get back on the internet and read more about this disorder. Each clinician told me slightly different ways of managing my diabetes. I clearly need more information to determine which is really the perfect strategy."
Helplessness	Assuming that you have no control over the problem and thus there is no point in trying to fix it.	"This is just one more example of my miserable genetic inheritance. You can't change what you were born with, so why bother to fight my biology?"

Step 3: Generating New and More Helpful Thoughts

After you have identified mistakes in your thought patterns, the next step is to come up with new more helpful thoughts to correct them and support more healthful behaviors. To generate these new thoughts, it can help to look at your specific thoughts more closely and challenge the logic behind each one. Is the thought based on facts or assumptions? It can be helpful to check the accuracy of the facts and assumptions included in your thoughts. Oftentimes a quick Internet search of good medical websites can help correct false beliefs that can lead to inaccurate thoughts and thinking errors. Below is a table with example questions to help you challenge your thought patterns. Challenge the thoughts in your Thought Monitoring Form with these questions and note places where they might be wrong and ideas for other ways of thinking about the situation.

Challenge	Specific Questions
What is the evidence?	What is the evidence to support these thoughts, assumptions, or conclusions?
What are the alternative views?	Are there other ways to think about the situation? How might someone else view this situation? If this were happening to someone else, how would you view it?
Is the thinking narrow?	Are there other aspects of the situation that you are ignoring? If you pay attention to other things going on at the same time would you think about it differently or see different ways of responding?
Is the thinking distorted?	Are you only attending to the dark side of things? Are you assuming that you can do absolutely nothing to change things?
What action can you take?	Where does thinking like this get you? If you thought something different or had a different response, how would that change the situation? What can you do to change the situation or how you feel?

Lastly, you can use the Cognitive Restructuring Form to systematically respond to your unhelpful thoughts by first identifying the specific situation, then tracking your immediate thoughts, identify the cognitive errors involved, imagining the outcome that will ensue if you engage in those thoughts, and then generating alternate coping thoughts that will help you avoid the undesirable outcome and engage in the healthful one. On the next page, we provide a sample of the worksheet that continues with J.T.'s low-carbohydrate gestational diabetes diet. On the page following that, we provide the blank worksheet for your use.

Example of the Cognitive Restructuring Form

Situation: I am pregnant, have been diagnosed with gestational diabetes, and have been put on a very low carbohydrate diet and strict blood glucose monitoring schedule to prevent birth complications and reduce health risks for my baby. I know the diet is important and that even little indulgences will throw my blood glucose off substantially. However, I really want dessert and my husband and son are eating ice cream in front of me.

Immediate Thoughts:

1) "If my husband and son really cared about me, they wouldn't eat anything that I'm supposed to avoid."
Type of Thinking Error: Mind Reading
Outcome: Frustrated at the fact that my husband and son are enjoying the ice cream I crave, I become angry watching them. I yell at them for having horrible health habits, being gluttonous and never taking my feelings into account. They get upset and try to avoid me for the rest of the evening.
Coping Thought: "My husband and son don't need to try to be me to care about me. They are different people. My husband and son have no metabolic problems, exercised a ton while I sat at work, and they love ice cream. Having a little is fine for them. There are lots of treats I can have that won't hurt my health and I should make choices that are good for me."

2) "Pregnancy is tiring and stressful and ice cream would make me feel better. I deserve to be spoiled. If I don't get ice cream, I'll feel punished."
Type of Thinking Error: All-or-None Thinking
Outcome: Frustrated at the perceived unfairness of the situation, I start to rationalize why I deserve ice cream and why sticking to the diet isn't that important. I give in to my craving and down a big bowl of ice cream in minutes. My blood glucose goes way above target for hours and I feel guilty and terrible for not taking care of my developing daughter.
Coping Thought: "Pregnancy is stressful and it is important that I feel cared for and have ways to deal with stress. But ice cream is a bad choice. I should do something else that is nice for me."

3) "This diet is a challenge, but it is important to keep my pregnancy and future daughter safe."
Type of Thinking Error: This is not an error in thinking; it's realistic.
Outcome: Recognizing the importance of the diet and my need to not feel deprived, I walk away from the table and make myself a pot of my favorite herbal tea. When I return with my warm, tasty cup of non-carbohydrate-containing tea, I'm content enough to enjoy the moment with my husband and son. They tell me fun stories from their day at the museum.
Coping Thought: "What can I do to take care of myself and my feelings and stick to my diet?"

WORKSHEET: Cognitive Restructuring Form

Directions: In the space provided, write out the situation where you found yourself having negative thoughts. List the negative thinking errors and replace them with coping thoughts. Write the likely outcome with both negative thinking errors as well as more realistic, coping thoughts.

Situation:_____

_____

_____

_____

Immediate Thoughts:

1) _____

Type of Thinking Error:

Outcome:

Coping Thought:

2) _____

Type of Thinking Error:

Outcome:

Coping Thought:

3) _____

Type of Thinking Error:

Outcome:

Coping Thought:

4) _____

Type of Thinking Error:

Outcome:

Coping Thought:

Notes & Observations:

Exercise 1H: Turning Values and Goals into a Plan of Action

How do we recognize thoughts and behaviors that are do not align with our values and goals? A first step is to be aware of our own values and goals. While we all have values and goals, we may not have thought about them and laid them out explicitly. If our values and goals are only hazy concepts, we may be less likely to factor them into our decisions. Taking time to identify and describe our values and goals can help us get started towards making choices that lead toward our dreams.

Recognizing the relationships between your specific thoughts and behaviors and your values and goals can help you reevaluate the benefits and costs of those thoughts and behaviors and potentially motivate change. Doing this, of course, requires that you are aware of your own values and goals. Only then can you start to consider whether your behaviors are helpful or contradictory to the things you are trying to achieve.

Step 1: Identifying Your Values
Psychologists and life coaches have come up with a variety of exercises to help you think about and identify your values. The main goal of these exercises is to help you consider what matters to you and what you value about yourself. It is fine to simply brainstorm on your own and write down what you think. Alternatively, you may find some of the thought exercises are helpful for identifying values that are important to you.

Allport-Vernon Classification
The Allport-Vernon classification of values (Allport et al., 1970) categorizes six major types of values and was designed to help people explore their own tendency toward different domains. Conspicuously missing from this classification is the value of Health, to which the attainment of all other objectives is secondary. Without our health, we are not fully functioning in our capacity to engage with and follow through on our personal values. However, the framework may still be useful to in identifying some of your own values and goals. The classifications are as follows:
1. Theoretical: Interest in the discovery of truth through reasoning and systematic thinking.
2. Economic: Interest in usefulness and practicality, including the accumulation of wealth.
3. Aesthetic: Interest in beauty, form, and artistic harmony.
4. Social: Interest in people and human relationships.
5. Political: Interest in gaining power and influencing other people.
6. Religious: Interest in unity and understanding the cosmos as a whole.

You can explore your values in these areas by taking the online test at:
http://webspace.ship.edu/cgboer/valuestest.html

Thought Experiments
Additionally, we have generated some thought experiments to help you make a list of values that you feel play some role in your life. You may find it helpful to phrase your values in terms of "I" statements.

1. Imagine someone is going to give a speech about you in the future (e.g., a eulogy, a retirement party, a 50th wedding anniversary party, an 85th birthday party). What would you like them to say about you? How do you hope they see you and your life accomplishments? What matters to you most?

2. List 5 people you highly admire. Why do you admire them? What do they have in common? What aspects of these people lives or behaviors do you wish to share? What about these people do you value?

3. Pretend you are writing a resume for a dream job of your own design. What will you do in your dream job? What will you accomplish? What will your day-to-day work look like? What makes you perfect for this job? What do you want a prospective employer to know about you?

4. Imagine you could achieve your "best self," whatever that means to you. How would you live your life? What would you seek to accomplish for yourself and for others?

Step 2: Prioritizing Your Values

Once you have generated an initial list, it is important to prioritize the values you identified. Often your values will be competing for time, energy, and resources. Understanding which values are more important to you will help you design goals and action plans that avoid compromising one value to achieve another one. In this step, we will attempt to order our values based on their personal importance.

To start, let's say I (J.T.) came up with this list of personal values after doing the exercises above:
I am healthy.
I am surrounded by happy people.
I am learning new things.
I am making the world a better place.
I can provide for my family and myself.
I am not wasting resources.

Now consider these values in pairs and think about what you would do if you had to choose between them. Go through each pair and mark the one that you would favor if you had to choose between them. For example, if forced to choose between being healthy and being surrounded by happy people, I would choose to be healthy around grumpy folks. So, I would give one point to "I am healthy". If forced to choose between being healthy and learning new things, I again would choose to be healthy and stuck with my current knowledge and abilities. So, I would give a second point to "I am healthy." After going through all the comparisons on the list, add up the points given to each pair of comparisons. This should clarify how you prioritize the values in your life. Although all of the values you list may be important to you, life requires choosing between them at various points. By understanding how you choose between your priorities, you can better predict places where your values may contradict and avoid creating goals and action plans that pit one value against another one.

For example, consider my (J.T.'s) choices in graduate school. While in graduate school, I had virtually endless opportunities to learn new things. There were always seminars on exciting new topics, and evening classes about new fields I never even considered. I could always keep working on my own research projects, carrying out experiments to give me answers to questions I identified. Graduate school was like a candy store for my inner nerd and I was a shameless binge eater. As encouraged by my program, I began graduate school focused on that one value (i.e., learning new things), but found myself getting more and more unhappy over time. I eventually got to the point that I did not really want to be in graduate school at all. Recognizing that I did not feel well and was not paying close attention to my health, I made some changes in my priorities, goals, and behaviors to reflect my high priority on being healthy. I made myself leave the school at 5:00 to go work out at the gymnastics gym down the street. I stopped going to evening classes with less than nutritious dinners and started cooking for myself every night. With these changes, I was much happier, healthier, and still learning new things, perhaps slightly more slowly, but now not at the expense of my other values. By recognizing the priorities among my values, I was able to fix my goals and behaviors so that they were in line with my values and their relative importance to me.

This example not only demonstrates the importance of prioritizing values, but also in developing goals and action plans that match these values. Just knowing that I care more about being healthy than learning new things does not help unless I come up with concrete goals and plans for becoming healthy that I can carry out in my life. Clarifying my values told me what I needed to focus on, but goal-setting, and action planning was required to turn that into specific changes in behavior (i.e., going to the gym at 5:00 and cooking my own dinners). Thus, after you have clarified your goals it is essential that you take what you find and turn to the process of goal-setting.

Step 3: Turning Your Values into Goals and Action Plans
While your values may be conceptual, hazy, and subjective in nature, it is important that your goals and action plans are concrete and measurable. Goals need to be specific and objective so that you can determine how to achieve them and when they have been met. As you develop a goal and an action plan to meet that goal, focus on making the goals and action plans specific, feasible, doable, and verifiable. What exactly do you want to achieve? Is that goal something you could realistically achieve? Is there a behavior you could do to bring you closer to achieving your goal? Is there a way for you to know (1) when you have done the helpful behavior and (2) when you have achieved your goal? If your goals and action plans meet these criteria, then they will be useful in helping you live according to your values.

We provide you with an Action Plan worksheet to help guide you in developing a goal and an action plan to meet it. It will also help you document your goals and plans so that you are more likely to stick to the plan and help you when you encounter problems. On the next page is a sample worksheet that describes a goal and action plan to help me (J.T.) meet my value of "being healthy". On the page following that is a blank worksheet. After you read through the example, pick one of your values and use the worksheet to develop a goal and action plan to help you live according to that value.

Sample Action Plan

The healthful change I want to make is: to eat more fruits and vegetables

My goal for next month is: to start every dinner with a salad or vegetable dish

The steps I will take to achieve my goal are (what, when, where, how much, how often):
1. I will go to the local farmer's market on Saturday and purchase fruits and vegetables for these salads/dishes for the upcoming week.
2. I will prepare a salad or vegetable dish for each dinner.
3. I will not eat anything else for dinner until I finish my serving of the salad or vegetable dish.

The things that could make it difficult to achieve my goal include: I do not have a lot of experience making tasty salads or vegetable dishes. It could be hard to think of things to make or decide what and how much to buy at the farmer's market.

My plan for overcoming these difficulties includes: I will purchase several cookbooks with seasonal recipes for salads and vegetable dishes. Before I go to the farmer's market, I will pick at least three recipes a week to try and will write down the ingredients.

Support/resources I will need to achieve my goal include: I will need time to go shopping on Saturday, so my family should not schedule other things that require my help during that time. Also, it would be helpful to have my family's support regarding eating more vegetables for dinner. It will be harder to stick to the goal if they complain about the food at every dinner. I will talk with them about my goal and see if they wish to help in choosing recipes, preparing food and shopping.

My confidence level (scale from 0-10, 10 being completely confident that you can achieve the entire plan): 7

What can you do to increase your confidence? If I find difficulty in following this plan then I will re-assess it after two weeks. I can change it to 2 recipes a week or invite a friend who is more experienced at preparing these dishes to help me learn how to make them. I know that if I keep revising the action plan I can make it work.

Plan for feedback and monitoring:
> How will you monitor actions? I will write down our dinner menu every night in a notebook.
> When will your actions be reviewed? My best friend (who is attempting the same action plan) and I will meet once a week to review our successes and failures, problem-solve difficulties and share solutions.

WORKSHEET: Action Plan

The healthful change I want to make is:

My goal for next month is:

The steps I will take to achieve my goal are (what, when, where, how much, how often):

The things that could make it difficult to achieve my goal include:

My plan for overcoming these difficulties includes:

Support/resources I will need to achieve my goal include:

My confidence level (scale from 0-10, 10 being completely confident that you can achieve the entire plan):

What can you do to increase your confidence?

Plan for feedback and monitoring:
        How will you monitor actions?

        When will your actions be reviewed?

Adapted from Jason M. Satterfield, Ph.D., University of California at San Francisco.

Brain Challenge #2
Enriching Your Life to Tame the Need for Immediate Gratification

Challenge Introduction

I can't get no satisfaction
I can't get no satisfaction
'Cause I try and I try
And I try and I try. . .

In the song, "(I Can't Get No) Satisfaction," Mick Jagger laments his ability to find contentment while noting that he attempts to do so repeatedly ("Cause I try, and I try, and I try and I try") despite the futility. As is often the case, artists first express what scientists later explain. When we are deprived of opportunities to make life better, we are programmed to start compulsively, and even obsessively searching for immediate relief. We try, and try, and try, and try to feel better right now, neglecting all the things we need to do to create a healthful, productive, enriched life in the Future. Like the singer, many who find satisfaction elusive will become focused on feeling better in the Now. They may develop a mentality that the only thing worth working for is something that benefits them immediately.

When you are down and out, the promise of instant gratification is likely to outweigh the hope of a better future in return for years of work towards an education, job, family, or network of impressed colleagues. When a person is not sure that he can take care of his short-term needs – when his brain perceives his life as impoverished – his brain will rewire to be impulsive and focused on immediate gratification.

Humans have adapted to survive in a wide variety of physical and social environments. We may hold high status in our community or have abundant food and resources available. Alternatively, we may have low social status or live in an environment where the things we need to survive are difficult to obtain. Our ability to shift our focus between immediate and longer-term needs contributes to our adaptability. But when we live in an environment where even those of low social status have high access to calorie-rich foods, rewarding drugs, emotionally arousing media, and sexually explicit images, the tendency to seek immediate gratification when we are relatively–deprived can lead to serious health and social problems.

Our ability to change our behavior depending on the prevalence of social and physical resources is key to our adaptability. A king and a serf would likely react differently to being offered a loaf of day-old bread. Similarly, an unemployed single parent would be more likely to agree to clean toilets for $50 than would a bank CEO. Sir Mick Jagger, who has secured over a billion dollars in royalties, versus Mick Jagger, the starving musician, no longer needs to compulsively seek immediate gratification. In Challenge #2, we will discuss ways to reprogram our brains to be less focused on immediate gratification, allowing us to put more effort into opportunities with longer-term benefit. In Chapter 2.1, we explain how medium spiny (MS) neurons in the nucleus accumbens hold back habits and play a key role in impulse control, what happens when these neurons are weak, and how they become strengthened. In Chapter 2.2, we present various ways in which you can enrich your life so your brain detects more opportunities and strengthens MS neurons. In

Chapter 2.3, we discuss how individuals differ biologically in their ability to strengthen MS neurons and how these differences can increase risk for addiction, mood disorders and obesity. We will also discuss how regular exposure to excessively large rewards, beyond those found in the natural environment (e.g., addictive drugs, processed food), can impair impulse control. Lastly in Chapter 2.4, we explore tested methods for increasing the experience of healthful pleasure in your daily life. Understanding the biological underpinnings of impulse control and need for immediate gratification will allow you to shape your environment to fit your biology.

Chapter 2.1: Reining in Maladaptive Habits: Strengthening Impulse Control

When you have lots of opportunities to make your life better, you can be picky. You can act on only those opportunities that offer a large pay-off for minimal work, and still obtain all you need. You can afford to bypass opportunities that provide short-term benefits but cause long-term problems. For example, you could turn down that fast-food burger and ask your personal chef to prepare a gourmet grilled vegetable sandwich and salad instead. When opportunities are sparse, however, you need to quickly and consistently act to take advantage of whatever opportunities are present. If it is likely that you will not have other options, then you had better accept the low-paying job and lunch on the burger and fries, despite your doctor's recommendations.

Our brains are wired to adapt our behavior based on relative availability of rewarding opportunities in our environments without our having to be conscious of this logic with each new opportunity. Our reward system keeps track of how many opportunities we encounter and adjusts our responses appropriately. When opportunities are rare, our reward system becomes very excitable and works very hard for immediate rewards. When opportunities are plentiful, our reward system becomes slow and sluggish, leaving decisions about whether to act on opportunities to other parts of the brain, such as the prefrontal cortex. With plentiful opportunities, only large rewards are sufficient to drive us to habitually work for immediate rewards. Thus, living in a world that seems to offer few opportunities will increase your drive for immediate gratification and encourage automatic quick reward-driven behaviors. Conversely, living in a resource-rich world will lead to choices that are made more deliberately by brain circuits that consider long-term benefits and consequences as well as short-term rewards and punishments.

By now, you may be wondering: what rewards will I obtain from reading this chapter—why bother? Our answer is that we will show you how to become less impulsive and improve your control over your habits by increasing the number of ways your brain can find "satisfaction", enriching your life, challenging your mind, and recognizing new opportunities. This will free you to focus on your long-term goals and avoid long-term negative consequences from short-sighted, reward-seeking decisions.

Learning to apply the brakes on reward-seeking behavior
In Challenge #1, we discussed the function of dopamine neurons that project to the nucleus accumbens, showing how they deliver information about the value of opportunities for immediate reward. We discussed the importance of training your dopamine neurons to accurately value health opportunities. Now we will consider the function of the nucleus accumbens neurons, a collection of neurons in the striatum, a brain region thought to play an important role in reward, pleasure, addiction, aggression, fear, and the placebo effect.

Your nucleus accumbens neurons make choices about whether to do a habit when you have an opportunity for quick reward or relief. Your nucleus accumbens neurons listen to your dopamine neuron's estimates of reward value and make decisions about whether to seek reward or ignore each identified opportunity. They control whether or not you habitually act when provided a chance for immediate gratification.

The nucleus accumbens neurons use a system of opposing controls, not unlike a car. The Direct Pathway acts like an accelerator. Direct Pathway nucleus accumbens neurons express the D1 dopamine receptor. Input from dopamine neurons excites these Direct Pathway neurons, pushing them toward sending a signal to initiate reward-seeking. The more input from dopamine neurons, the faster these direct pathway neurons start immediate reward-seeking behaviors.

Conversely, the InDirect Pathway acts like brakes on the Direct Pathway. InDirect Pathway nucleus accumbens neurons express the D2 dopamine receptor and inhibit or slow down the Direct Pathway. Input from the dopamine neurons turns on the InDirect pathway, applying the brakes on immediate reward-seeking so that your brain can consider other options. We are going to talk about this pathway extensively, and thus a quick abbreviation to refer to the D2 dopamine receptor-bearing, InDirect Pathway nucleus accumbens neurons will be helpful. So with deference to the psychologists of yore, I will refer to these inhibitory InDirect pathway neurons as ID brakes.

Under normal conditions, the Direct and InDirect pathways balance each other, providing an accelerator to drive habit behavior to improve immediate well-being and address needs, and brakes to keep decision-making to a safe, controlled, and adjustable speed. There are a variety of situations where the indirect pathway can become weak or unresponsive, effectively cutting the brakes on immediate reward-seeking. When the InDirect pathway (ID brakes) is weak, decisions to reward seek become too fast and easy to trigger. Without ID brakes, every little opportunity for an immediate reward will put your habit system into motion, carrying out behaviors to get a quick benefit. Moreover, decisions to reward- or relief-seek get going so quickly that other parts of the brain don't have time to weigh in on the choice. The reward-seeking has started before there is time to consider the possible consequences or alternative responses. When the ID brakes are weak, a person will behave impulsively, reacting blindly to opportunities for immediate benefit or relief. This reward/relief-seeking will become insensitive to punishment and consequences. Without strong ID brakes, the Direct Pathway makes choices before parts of the brain that attend to punishments and long-term goals and plans can provide input. Reward or relief-seeking is initiated before other options and outcomes are considered. Thus, having weak ID brakes sets up your brain to develop one of the cardinal symptoms of addictive disorders – the tendency to compulsively reward-seek despite negative consequences.

If you have a strong ID brakes, you will gain conscious control of your habits. You can think of your nucleus accumbens as a door to the striatum – the dopamine neurons come knocking with a reward opportunity and the nucleus accumbens decides whether or not to let the striatum release the habit to perform the behavior and receive the reward. While you may still act out of habit when a really valuable opportunity arises, your ID brake neurons will slow down your reward system's habitual responses and give the rest of your brain time to consider other options. But if these ID brake neurons are weak, your reward circuits will dominate your decision-making, habits will be given free rein, and you will seek immediate gratification at nearly every opportunity. The puff of the cigarette, the sip of alcohol, the extra cup of coffee, the extra bite out of that cookie, the one more episode on Netflix, the giving in to social pressure, the one last check of your e-mail, are held in check by these circuits located in the nucleus accumbens and striatum.

Since the neurobiology of this system is fairly complex, it is helpful to have a clear image of the process before getting into the details (see the Figure below for further details).

The striatum, originating in the limbic brain, is capable of storing and retrieving habits we perform without much thought, including everyday addictions, such as munching on that cookie. If the ID brake neurons in the nucleus accumbens are weak then we may still act without much conscious thought. Conversely, if they are strong then they give our conscious brain regions a chance to remind us why we may not want to perform those habits. In the case of a cookie, strong ID brakes let us contemplate before we bite.

FIGURE: Projections to and from the nucleus accumbens

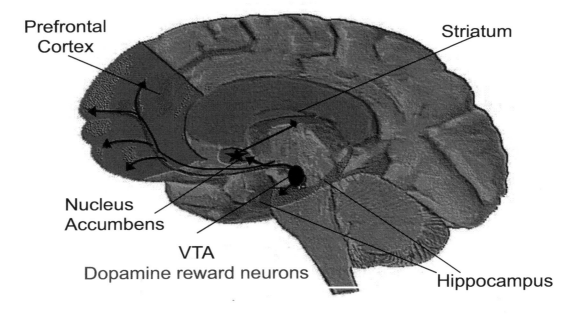

Legend: As we described in Challenge #1, the dopamine reward neurons in the VTA project to the limbic reward system and the prefrontal cortex (black arrows). These projections also go to the nucleus accumbens, located just anterior and superior to the amygdala, which determines how much work to put into seeking a potential reward. The neurons of the nucleus accumbens (depicted here as a black star with projections to the striatum) drive choices on whether to initiate the behaviors encoded by the striatum, the brain region that has learned and mastered our reward-seeking habits. The nucleus accumbens Direct Pathway acts as the accelerator on choices to initiate a reward-seeking habit, while the InDirect Pathway acts as the brakes.

What makes ID brake neurons fail?

As you can imagine, strengthening your ID brake neurons will be helpful for getting compulsive unhealthful habits under control. If we are going to be around temptation all the time, we want to have a strong set of ID brakes or we will impulsively over-consume quick rewards, such as food, addictive drugs, social approval, or relief from pain or anxiety. With weak ID brake neurons, you would eat everything on your plate or drink the whole bottle of wine. You would also seek relief from discomfort immediately. For example, you might be very sensitive to peer pressure and have trouble disappointing people even when it is not in everyone's best interest over the long-term. You might have trouble telling your boss that you must leave work on time today to make it to your class at the gym. You would have trouble persisting in uncomfortable social or physical situations, even when you know that the discomfort is a needed step towards an important goal. For example, with weak ID brake neurons you might find it hard to make it through the painful exercises in physical therapy, even when you understand the need to strengthen injured body parts to recover.

So, what makes ID brake neurons weak? As Mick Jagger described, when we "can't get no satisfaction," we will "try and try and try and try" to get what we can. In other words, when we are not exposed to enough opportunities for immediate gratification we become more willing to try for whatever we can get. ID brake neurons don't try to stall the reward-seeking, letting us automatically chase every opportunity for quick benefit that we recognize. Only when a lot of opportunities are presented to the striatum do our ID brake neurons develop the strength to hold back reward-seeking habits. Notably, this strengthening changes how we respond to the prospect of immediate rewards in general. It is not simply learning how to restrain oneself in specific instances. When we are presented with enough opportunities, the ID brake neurons in our nucleus accumbens will develop the ability to hold back other habits as well. For example, if you were to expand your access to immediate rewards by learning better social networking skills, this should strengthen your ID brake neurons. This strength should make it easier for you to skip getting a second helping at dinner or keep going on a jog when your legs start to hurt a bit. Exposure to frequent options for immediate gratification will make us less impulsive over time. When our lives are enriched with the ability to take care of our immediate needs and solve our immediate problems, our ID brake neurons become powerful enough to keep our drive toward immediate gratification-seeking in check.

To fully understand how the sum total of reward experiences modifies our ID brake neurons and our responsiveness to opportunities for immediate gratification, it is important to further explain the underlying neurobiology. As we discussed, dopamine neurons that project to the nucleus accumbens indicate the presence and value of opportunities for immediate reward through their firing rate. Because firing of dopamine neurons causes them to release dopamine, the amount of dopamine release in the nucleus accumbens over time provides information about the number and value of opportunities that you encountered recently. If you were to tally up how much dopamine was released in the nucleus accumbens, then the summary it provided would indicate the total value of all opportunities that you encountered in a given period. Our ID brake neurons do this tallying. As we mentioned, ID brake neurons have special D2 dopamine receptors that are activated when dopamine hits them. When dopamine activates D2 dopamine receptors, these receptors trigger changes in the responsiveness of the ID brake neurons. Specifically, they make these ID brake neurons fire more readily and make them harder to turn off (Dong et al., 2006). Thus, the total value of opportunities that you have recently encountered in your environment gets translated into the strength or excitability of these ID brake neurons (Trafton & Gifford, 2008). The more rewarding opportunities you encounter, the better your ID brakes get at stalling the Direct Pathway accelerator neurons from starting reward seeking. Repeated, small input in the form of opportunities to make life better, release dopamine onto dopamine receptors. This signal instructs the ID brake neurons to get stronger, such that they stall reward-seeking decisions more each time they are applied. Exposure to opportunities to improve yourself, strengthens the braking system that allows conscious, deliberate, slow, and reasoned choices about whether to reward or relief seek.

What do ID brake neurons do when they are on?
ID brake neurons are inhibitory, which means they prevent other neurons from firing. Specifically, these other neurons are the accelerator neurons that drive neurons in the striatum that encode well-trained or habitual motor programs. The striatum circuits have memorized all the behaviors that you can do without thinking, like riding a bicycle, chewing gum while you walk, or eating while you watch television. Health-related habits are also part of this repertoire, such as when you wake up in the morning and manage to brush your teeth without memory of having done so. In addition, there is evidence that the striatum is involved in processing rules for automatic speech. When someone says, "thank you" and you say, "you're welcome," your striatum circuits are involved (Dominey & Inui, 2009).

The key point is that for you to carry out a habitual behavior, you need to turn on the striatum to perform the habit using your Direct Pathway accelerator neurons. In an immediate sense, encountering an opportunity increases the chance that you will carry out a habitual behavior to try to get a quick reward (Taha & Fields, 2006). The ID brake neurons slow down the accelerator neurons, stalling or stopping decisions to trigger a habit. Firing of ID brake neurons prevents you from doing well-trained or habitual behaviors impulsively. Strengthening ID brake neurons so they fire more readily makes habitual behaviors harder to elicit.

What does this process look like at the neuronal level? You can visualize the way this system works by considering a simple circuit (Keeler et al., 2014). Here, VTA dopamine neurons provide input to both the Direct (accelerator) and the InDirect (brakes) pathway neurons, firing when reward opportunities are present. The Direct accelerator neurons sum up the input from the VTA neurons, and when the sum reaches a threshold, the neuron turns on the reward-seeking behavior. The ID brake neurons inhibit the Direct accelerator neurons, which functionally increases the sum needed to reach the threshold. When the ID brake neurons are active, it will take a longer time for input from the VTA to turn on Direct accelerator neuron activity to the point that the neurons initiate a habit behavior.

As an analogy, you can think of the habit behavior as a purchase with a price that the Direct accelerator neurons need to pay to trigger the behavior. Here, the VTA dopamine neurons provide income to the Direct accelerator neurons. The greater the expected value of opportunities, the more the VTA neurons pay the Direct accelerator neurons. In this analogy, the ID brakes are the tax collectors. For every dollar of income that the VTA provides to the Direct accelerator neurons, the ID brakes take a proportion. While the ID brakes are collecting taxes, it will take the Direct accelerator neurons longer to save up enough money to pay for the habit. Stronger ID brakes, the equivalent of higher tax rates, will slow down the Direct accelerator neurons and make it less likely that the habit behavior is initiated.

How do opportunities change the accelerator and brakes?
In addition to immediately affecting whether a habit is triggered in response to an opportunity, dopaminergic input from the VTA encourages the strengthening of both the Direct accelerator neurons and the ID brake neurons. Exposure to frequent opportunities will make the Direct accelerator neurons more efficient at reaching the threshold to initiating a habit, speeding up their decisions. But it will also strengthen the ID brakes, making them better at stalling the Direct accelerator neurons. Exposure to reward opportunities enhances the function of both the Direct and Indirect pathway neurons, but the net effect is to enhance the ability to stall habit decisions (Keeler et al., 2014).

To use our money analogy, with few opportunities for reward, Direct accelerator neurons are paid relatively little (e.g., $10/hour), but ID brakes apply a low tax rate (e.g., 5%, or $0.50/hour). With more frequent opportunities for reward, Direct accelerator neurons get paid more (e.g., $15/hour), but the ID brakes apply a higher tax rate (e.g., 50%, or $7.50/hour). So long as the ID brakes are healthy and functional, it will take the Direct accelerator neurons longer to collect up enough money to initiate a habit in the frequent opportunity case, accumulating money at $7.50/hour instead of $9.50/hour. By strengthening the two pathways as they respond to opportunities, the system improves its ability to regulate habit behavior. Habits can be initiated even faster when needed, but the ID brakes have greater control and ability to slow decisions when taking time for careful consideration of consequences and priorities is appropriate.

Neuroscientists have a pretty good understanding of the detailed cellular mechanisms that underlie these immediate and learning effects, but explaining them in detail is beyond the scope of this book (For an overview, see Trafton & Gifford, 2008 or Keeler et al., 2014). The main point is that opportunities for reward immediately alter the rate at which Direct and Indirect pathway neurons fire and change the way they respond in the future.

On a very short time scale (milliseconds), opportunities change the immediate behavior of these nucleus accumbens neurons, altering the information that they send to the neurons in their network. Additionally, opportunities release neuromodulators, brain chemicals that alter the properties of the neuron by either modifying the existing proteins in the neuron or changing the type or amount of proteins the neuron produces. Because proteins function as the machinery of the neuron and determine how it responds, this changes how the neuron behaves and what it responds to later.

In short, repeated exposure to opportunities to make your life better will change the structure and function of neurons in your reward circuits, making them less reactive to the prospect of immediate gratification. Enriching your life with skills and social networks that allow you to solve problems will strengthen the ID brakes that prevent you from impulsively seeking immediate gratification. When your reward system is toned down in this way, your brain will have more time and flexibility to think about non-habitual options and long-term goals. Your brain will be rewired to be more rational and less impulsive.

Exposure to opportunities for reward will alter the responsiveness of your nucleus accumbens neurons. Enriching your life by increasing your options for bettering yourself should strengthen your ID brakes and help you focus on long-term plans and goals.

Chapter 2.2: How Can I Enrich My Life: What Does the Nucleus Accumbens Recognize as an Opportunity?

How do you strengthen your ID brake neurons? Anything that adds immediate opportunities to your life will strengthen your ID brake neurons. If we want to increase our exposure to opportunities in our lives, the first thing we need to do is define "an opportunity" as our dopamine neurons recognize them. In its most basic description, dopamine neurons see anything that provides a chance to improve our immediate well-being, our "satisfaction", as an opportunity. But how can we achieve this?

The easiest opportunities for most people to conceptualize are basic rewards like food and water. Such primary reinforcers include air, water, food, sleep, and sex. Similarly, social approval, money and increased social status also provide immediate reward, making your life better by improving how other people treat you. These are known as secondary reinforcers. The situations that you perceive as providing these secondary reinforcer rewards are learned through experience and observation rather than hardwired. Your reward system is as likely to be excited by abstract or culturally created rewards, such as money, gold, or diamonds, or by the rewarding value of transformative ideas and continuing education, as by satisfying your appetite with cheeseburgers and Twinkies.

Opportunities for improvement also include situations where you can remove yourself from an uncomfortable or dangerous state to a more comfortable or safe state. This could include anything that provides relief from stress, pain, boredom, or anxiety. It could also include solving a problem that was presented to you. Thus, challenging situations and solvable problems operate just like opportunities to get something nice and earn positive benefits. These problems provide the opportunity to find and apply a solution to make life better.

In sum, anything that increases your awareness of how to have nice things happen to you, anything that increases the amount of social approval you expect to receive, or anything that increases your exposure to problems that you are capable of resolving quickly will strengthen your ID brake neurons and reduce your drive for immediate reward. There are obviously many ways to increase opportunities in your life, and we will discuss interventions designed to do this and provide exercises to achieve this.

Social skills training and communication skills
The most readily available rewards in our environment are social rewards from others, for example being shown respect or approval during a social interaction. Social approval, a smile, kind words, helpful advice, assistance with a problem, respect, sympathy, appreciation, and so forth from others can be highly and immediately rewarding. Depending on our social and communication skills, we may find ourselves the recipient of these social rewards all the time or rarely at all. One of the best ways of expanding opportunities and enriching our lives is to improve our social and communications skills. When we know how to interact with other people in positive ways, we not only create possibilities for pleasant, rewarding interactions with them, but also possibilities to gain access to resources and other more tangible opportunities that these people control.

Social skills training is a behavioral therapy designed to help people improve their social and communication skills. The goal is to elicit more positive responses from others. While it was designed and is primarily used to teach people with mental health disorders or clinically significant behavioral problems how to interact in ways that promote better emotional and behavioral health, the strategies and practices included in the therapy can be helpful for anyone, regardless of their starting level of social and emotional ability.

The first step in social skills training is to assess and determine the individual's actual difficulties in relating to other people. Once general problems with a social behavior are identified, the therapist can help break down the overall behavior into its smaller components. These can be worked on individually and in order of difficulty. Once specific components of behaviors are identified then they can be worked on using a variety of techniques including instruction, modeling, role-playing, and feedback. As with all behavior change techniques, successes should be reinforced.

Described more simply, a therapist, group member, or friend could tell you ideas for improving your social interactions (instruction). They could demonstrate how you might react in a situation that you find difficult (modeling). You could then pretend to be in that situation and act out how you would behave (role-playing). Others could join the role-play as needed. A therapist or others could then give you an analysis of how you behaved, telling you things you did well, things that you could have done better, and suggestions for improving your behavior on the next try (feedback). This process can then be repeated as needed.

For example, perhaps you recognize that you feel uncomfortable around groups of people you do not know when you are trying something new. This leads you to sit around watching television in the evenings instead of trying that Tai Chi or ethnic cooking class you thought sounded interesting. Last time you tried to go to a class you snuck in the back at the last minute, did not talk to anyone, could not really see what was going on, got really confused and left within ten minutes. You could break down your needed skills into: 1) expressing your interest in learning to an expert, in this case most likely the instructor; 2) sharing your nervousness and asking for support, 3) introducing yourself to others in the class, 4) observing the full range of expertise in the class (i.e., that there are other beginners like you) rather than comparing yourself only to the best person in the room, 5) reflecting on what you learned and how you improved during your time in the class. You could then make a plan and practice each of these skills, ideally with a supportive therapist or friend, until you are comfortable with your behavior. With a clear plan and confidence in your ability to turn going to new class or group meeting into a positive experience, you can then go to that Tai Chi or ethnic cooking class with a much better chance of having fun, meeting new friends, learning something new, and going back the next week, than you had before.

Psychologists have found that being passive or aggressive, as opposed to assertive, in one's communication with others is a common and harmful enough problem for people that they have designed programs that directly address this social skill. Such programs are typically called "assertiveness training". They focus on helping people learn how to express themselves and ask for what they need without being accusing or demanding, how to stand up for themselves in social interactions, and how to respect both themselves and others in their communications. The approach and techniques are basically the same as those used for other social skills training. These programs can be generally helpful for teaching communications skills that open opportunities in one's life, particularly for people who tend to feel unsure of themselves or not respected in their day-to-day life.

To practice improving social or communication skills, see Exercise 2A (page 119) and Exercise 2B (page 123).

Progressive behavioral shaping: Breaking down a problem into smaller, solvable steps

While many of us are good at identifying final goals, rewards, or things that we would like to acquire or achieve, we may have trouble figuring out the steps involved in reaching our goals. The ultimate behavior that meets the goal or gets the reward may seem impossible when considered from your current perspective. Most goals require learning and mastering numerous smaller behaviors first, or meeting many intermediate goals before the ultimate goal can be achieved. Creating opportunities in your life requires that you begin to notice, work toward, practice and master these intermediate steps so that you can make progress toward your larger goals.

Psychologists have described a process for training complex and difficult behaviors by breaking the behaviors down into smaller, simpler parts and encouraging practice and rewarding success on these intermediate behavioral pieces. They refer to this process as progressive behavioral shaping. The basic idea is to break down a behavior into its component pieces. Then you provide rewards for completing the simplest components of the behavior correctly and repeat these rewards until the behavior is mastered and automatic. At this point, you can add another component to the behavior to make the performance more difficult again. You then reward completion of the new behavior or combination of behaviors until that has been mastered. This is repeated until the whole complex behavior has been learned. The process involves only simple reward-learning processes, but used correctly, it can be extremely powerful for shaping behavior or learning complex skills.

EXAMPLE: Progressive behavioral shaping to achieve a complex behavior

To illustrate how progressive behavioral shaping can be used to teach complex, impossible-seeming behaviors, let us consider an example from my (J.T.'s) gymnastics coaching days. Most people are fairly intimidated when I suggest to them that they could learn a back handspring (i.e., back flip). In fact, if they just attempted it, even with my help, the most likely outcome would be their landing painfully on the floor in some unpleasant position, potentially with me underneath. Thus, I always break up back handsprings into at least three component parts. These do not need to be completed in sequential order. It can be easiest to start with the end of the trick. First you need to learn to support yourself in handstand and pull your legs down to return to standing. This could be broken into many sub-steps, but most of my gymnastics students have already learned all of those parts before we ever contemplate a back handspring. So first, we will practice kicking to handstand,

---

arching slightly, and then snapping our feet back toward the ground to return to standing. This is a relatively safe but not easy exercise and can take a while to learn correctly. I will work with my students, encouraging and praising them as they make progressively better attempts toward doing this piece of the trick. While this piece itself is not a recognized gymnastics trick and would get no credit or points in a gymnastics competition, it is nevertheless crucial to learning a back handspring and other tumbling skills. Thus, as a coach, I must find ways of providing artificial rewards for practicing and mastering this piece of the trick since it may not be independently rewarding. Once this part has been mastered, I will then switch to teaching the students the very beginning of a back handspring. They must learn to bend their knees to push off as they start falling backwards. If they lean forward instead, as is most people's tendencies, they will jump in the wrong direction and not make it safely to their hands. So second, we practice this initial falling backwards action against the wall or onto a mat. I again praise improvements until this piece is mastered. Only then do I let students start to put the behaviors together as they learn the middle piece (i.e., jumping backwards from their feet to their hands). At this point, I can ensure that they safely complete this transition, knowing that they will be jumping in the right direction and are capable of finishing the trick once their hands make it to the ground. This allows us to practice the whole behavior safely until it is mastered. By breaking the trick down into pieces, a behavior that is difficult and dangerous to even try can be learned safely and consistently by the vast majority of dedicated people.

The two crucial components of using progressive behavioral shaping are: 1) breaking down your goal behavior into learnable pieces, and 2) creating rewards or reinforcers to encourage these intermediate pieces.

To practice progressive behavioral shaping, see Exercise 2C (page 124).

Enrichment activities
Getting involved in new activities will provide new opportunities for reward. New activities inherently provide new challenges and new social networks, which creates new opportunities to succeed and gain social approval. Enriching your life with new activities can seem challenging. First you must identify activities that sound interesting to you. Next you have to find ways to learn and get involved with those activities. A trip to the library or some Internet exploration can help you find new ideas and connections. To get you started, we have provided a couple of helpful websites that provide ideas about new activities and ways to get started. Take a look, and give something new a try!

https://hobby-finder.com
This website provides information on how to get started on over 300 different hobbies, from crochet to motorcycles. It includes descriptions of the hobby, suggestions for beginner books and videos, and other helpful resources for getting going on your new hobby. Explore, pick something interesting, and get started!

http://www.hipsfinder.com/
While this page is set up with links to programs in the United Kingdom rather than the United States, this collection of information on Hobbies, Interests, Pastimes and Sports

(HIPS) provides lots of new ideas for things to do. You pick an energy level, age range, environment (e.g. on the water, urban area), type of activity (i.e. individual, group, couple, family), and competition category (non-competitive, zany, competitive) and they suggest ideas, complete with links to additional information, clubs, organizations, and classes. It is a fun site because it provides suggestions far beyond the standard mix. For example, we would not have thought of belt sander racing, laser clay pigeon shooting, and greasy pole competitions on our own. This is a great place to head to for both new activities or to be reminded of activities you already know, such as gardening, hiking, or hula hooping.

To increase perception of opportunities in your life, see Exercise 2D (page 125).

Chapter 2.3: Reward Deficiency Syndrome: Why Having Fewer D2 Dopamine Receptors Increases the Risk of Addiction, Mood Disorders, Obesity, and Suicide

There are substantial individual differences in how fast ID brake neurons strengthen in response to rewarding opportunities. In other words, it takes different people varying exposure to opportunities to strengthen their ID brake neurons to comparable levels. This variation is caused by differences in the number of D2 receptors on the surface of the ID brake neurons. As we have described, reward opportunities trigger dopamine neuron firing, which in turn dumps dopamine onto the dopamine receptors on the ID brake neurons. The dopamine sticks to and turns on these dopamine receptors, which then send a signal to the ID brake neuron telling it to change its responsiveness so it will be more likely to fire in the future. The more frequently D2 dopamine receptors are turned on, the bigger the change in responsiveness. If ID brake neurons only have a few dopamine receptors on their surface, each opportunity is less likely to transmit a signal (or will send a small rather than a larger signal) telling them to change their responsiveness, when dopamine is released. Without a lot of dopamine receptors, the ID brake neurons cannot detect that a lot of opportunities have been presented and will only change their responsiveness slowly. Thus, when ID brake neurons only have a few D2 dopamine receptors they strengthen very slowly and have trouble gaining control over our habitual behaviors. When D2 dopamine receptor levels or activation are low, it is difficult to halt, shift, or devalue behaviors that provide immediate reward or relief, even when that behavior is followed by punishment or loss (Zalocusky et al., 2016; Barlow et al, 2018; Johnson and Kenny, 2010). Low D2 dopamine receptor levels are thought to underly the behavioral pattern of repeated use despite consequences that comprises part of the diagnostic criteria for substance use. More generally, low D2 dopamine receptor or dopamine deficiency may underlie a variety of reward or relief seeking behaviors that people repeat despite their causing significant harm, consequences, or failure to meet long-term goals (Kenny et al., 2013; Gondré-Lewis et al., 2020).

Some people do not make as many D2 dopamine receptors because of a difference in their genetic code for the receptor. One of the versions of the D2 dopamine receptor gene is called the A1 allele. People born with the A1 allele of the D2 dopamine receptor produce relatively few D2 dopamine receptors on their neurons. Genetic studies have shown that people with the A1 allele of the D2 dopamine receptor are more likely to develop a drug or alcohol problem and have more trouble quitting once they have developed a substance habit (Comings & Blum, 2000). Among those with an alcohol use disorder, persons with the A1 allele of the D2 dopamine receptor are more likely to die earlier (Balldin et al., 2018). People with the A1 allele are also more likely to become obese or develop a gambling, gaming, or excessive internet use problem, demonstrating that in general they have more trouble controlling urges for immediate gratification. As we mentioned before, the limbic reward circuits cannot tell the difference between things that make life better and things that relieve immediate discomfort. People with the A1 allele also have more trouble dealing with stressful situations. They may favor quick fixes to obtain relief or avoid stressful situations. For example, a study in college students found that interpersonal stress increased risk of problematic gaming only in the subpopulation that had D2 dopamine receptor alleles that reduced expression of the receptor (Kim et al., 2022). Moreover, the effect was mediated by a tendency to use avoidant coping strategies when stressed. These associations suggest that having fewer D2 dopamine receptors makes people more prone to do automatic reward-driven behaviors. Over time this may lead to health conditions from chronic over-consumption of things that provide immediate reinforcement (e.g., cookies, alcohol, or drugs) or chronic avoidance or relief-seeking from stressors. Suggesting that these genetic tendencies can also increase risk of harm from relatively rare impulsive relief-seeking, several genetic studies found that D2 dopamine receptor genetic variants were associated with risk of making suicide attempts (Kimbrel et al., 2022; Genis-Mendoza et al, 2017; Suda et al., 2009). These findings also suggest that genetics can modify your risk of developing health problems due to compulsive reward-seeking.

Raised to be mild
It is important to remember that our genes alone do not determine our behavior. Although genetics clearly contribute to risk of impulsivity, the version of the D2 dopamine receptor gene that a person carries does not determine his or her tendency to seek reward on its own. For example, the A1 allele was shown to increase novelty-seeking, a personality trait associated with high-risk or impulsive behaviors such as substance use, in adults ages 24-39 only when they were raised in a punitive child-rearing environment. Interestingly, this same population of adults with the A1 allele was not at greater risk of novelty-seeking if they were raised in a more positive environment (Keltikangas-Järvinen et al., 2008). In other words, when children with this same genetic vulnerability were raised by parents who provided lots of attention, chances to succeed at things, and praise for their efforts, they did not develop a novelty-seeking personality. Likewise, adolescent girls who experienced more negative parenting by their mother were more likely to develop depressive symptoms if they had the A1 allele versus not; but those with the A1 allele did better when exposed to little negative parenting (Zhang et al., 2015). These studies highlight that genetics alone rarely control behavior, but rather modify people's reactions to their environment. People with the A1 allele may need a more enriched environment, with more frequent opportunities and dopamine release, than most to avoid being impulsive. But within such an environment, they may not develop a tendency to reward- or relief-seek.

Social hierarchy and need for immediate gratification
In addition to genetics, environment has also been shown to affect how many D2 dopamine receptors are made by your ID brake neurons. Some very clever experiments in monkeys suggest that your experiences, particularly in your social environment, may change the number of D2 dopamine receptors in your nucleus accumbens (Morgan et al., 2002). In this study, researchers started by keeping a group of macaque monkeys housed alone in cages – basically in solitary confinement – for several months. They then used positron emission tomography (PET) imaging to examine how many D2 dopamine receptors the monkeys had in their brains. They found that all the monkeys had low levels of D2 dopamine receptors in their striatum (the region of the brain in which the nucleus accumbens resides). They then moved the monkeys to a shared living environment where they could interact for a few months. Like humans, macaques are both very social and very competitive. A group kept together will create a dominance hierarchy very quickly. The

monkeys at the top of the dominance hierarchy get all the spoils of being top banana. They get first choice of food, and lots of positive attention and grooming from the other monkeys. The monkeys at the bottom do not have as pleasant a life. They get other monkey's leftovers, rarely get help picking off the parasites and, worst of all, bear the wrath of everyone else's bad days. The researchers observed the monkeys' behavior and determined each monkey's rank in the social hierarchy. They then put the monkeys back in the PET scanner and looked at their D2 dopamine receptors again. They found that the monkeys at the top of the dominance hierarchy had greatly increased the number of D2 dopamine receptors in their brains. The monkeys at the bottom had just as few D2 dopamine receptors as they did when they were housed alone. Being dominant and having lots of resources at their disposal increased the monkeys' D2 dopamine receptor levels! The researchers then looked at whether this change had any impact on the monkeys' desire for cocaine, a potent drug reward. They found that while the monkeys on the bottom of the hierarchy would make very liberal use of the cocaine they were offered, the dominant monkeys used much less and decreased their use over time. Apparently, the extra D2 dopamine receptors helped them adapt to become less and less interested in opportunities for immediate gratification. More recent studies have shown that measures of socioeconomic status are similarly associated with D2 dopamine receptor levels in healthy humans (Wiers et al., 2016), suggesting that social status in humans is also sensitive to, and perhaps driven by, differences in, D2 dopamine receptor expression in striatum.

Supranatural rewards
Natural everyday rewards of the kind humans were exposed to during most of their evolution, release only moderate amounts of dopamine from VTA dopamine neurons. Modern society has engineered supranatural rewards that release much larger amounts of dopamine from the VTA when encountered. As we discussed in chapter 1, these large dopamine signals will lead to over-prioritization of these supranatural rewards. But additionally, this outsized dopamine release leads to loss of ID brakes, essentially through overuse and resulting loss of D2 dopamine receptors. Addictive drugs have this effect, from heroin, cocaine, and methamphetamine, to alcohol, tobacco and cannabis (Volkow & Baler, 2014). Prescription medications from the opioid, benzodiazepine, barbiturate, and amphetamine classes also release large amounts of dopamine when they are absorbed quickly.

It was observed years ago that repeated use of addictive drugs results in a loss of D2 dopamine receptors in the nucleus accumbens. Stopping use of addictive drugs leads to recovery of normal D2 dopamine receptor levels over the course of weeks to months (Rominger et al., 2012). More recently, chronic exposure to other more extreme opportunities for reward or relief have also been shown to lead to loss D2 dopamine receptors and associated impulsive behavior. Specifically, chronic exposure to high-fat junk food has been shown to lead to loss of D2 dopamine receptors and impulsive behavior, even if total calorie consumption and weight is maintained within normal levels (Adams et al., 2015). Chronic consumption of processed foods in which rewarding components (e.g., fat, sugar, salt) have been highly concentrated results in similar effects on ID brakes as does use of addictive drugs. Additionally, injury and/or pain also actives VTA dopamine neurons intensely, training the habit system to learn strategies to gain quick relief, like guarding the injury, resting, seeking help from others, or taking medication. Injury-related dopamine release can contribute to loss of D2 dopamine receptors; Loss of D2 dopamine receptors will promote a tendency to compulsively relief-seek, even when these strategies prevent recovery. Recent studies have shown that patients with chronic non-neuropathic back pain also show reductions in D2 dopamine receptors in these circuits, consistent with loss of ID brakes (Martikainen et al., 2015). Use of prescription opioid analgesics or alcohol for pain relief from an injury may amplify the loss of D2 dopamine receptors, making loss of ID brakes more likely. Together, these studies suggest that when reward or relief opportunities get too big, ID brakes can lose their D2 dopamine receptors, along with their ability to slow down reward or relief seeking.

Why do large rewards lead to loss of D2 dopamine receptors and the ID brakes? This is likely due to the way that D2 dopamine receptors work. When they bind dopamine, the dopamine receptors send a signal. But in the process, they change shape and cannot send another signal until they go through a recycling process. Here, the D2 dopamine receptor is taken inside the neuron and chemically treated to return it to a functional state. This recycling process takes some time (e.g., roughly an hour), and isn't perfectly efficient; some receptors are destroyed in the recycling process. The neuron can make more D2 dopamine receptors from scratch, but that is also a slow process. With normal-sized natural rewards, the moderate amount of dopamine that is released activates a small proportion of D2 dopamine receptors. The large remaining population of D2 dopamine receptors is available to signal while the others recycle. Under these normal conditions, activity is moderate enough that the recycling and synthesis of new D2 dopamine receptors is fast enough to maintain a steady supply, with stable levels of D2 dopamine receptors on the ID brakes. Large, supranatural rewards, on the other hand, activate too many receptors at once, first temporarily desensitizing most receptors, and over time overwhelming the recycling process, such that overall D2 dopamine receptor levels decrease.

When supranatural reward or relief opportunities overwhelm and deplete the D2 dopamine receptor system, the ID brakes will not function effectively and habitual reward- or relief-seeking behaviors will become compulsive and punishment resistant. Eliminating exposure to the supranatural rewards will allow your neurons to catch up on recycling and synthesize new D2 dopamine receptors to return the system to a normally functioning state, though this process may take months to fully recover. Minimizing use of potentially addictive drugs and medications as well as consumption of junk food can help keep your ID brakes strong and functional, giving you time to consider and make conscious choices about whether to do a habit behavior.

Notably, if you have been chronically exposed to supranatural rewards like addictive drugs or junk food, recent studies suggest that you can increase levels of D2 dopamine receptor more quickly by engaging in normal everyday rewarding experience. For example, among methamphetamine users in behavioral treatment for their substance use disorder, supervised exercise (1 hour/day, three days/week for 8 weeks) significantly increased D2 dopamine receptor levels in the striatum (Robertson et al., 2016). So, avoiding supranatural rewards and adding in natural reward opportunities may head you more quickly down the path towards habit control and achieving long-term goals.

Dopamine deficiency and consuming passions

The US economy is driven in large part by consumption, based on the notion that having more goods and services will make us happier. This is fueled by over-valuation of a wide variety products that our reward centers have been conned into purchasing. Interestingly, compulsive buying, a condition known as oniomania, is related to dopamine activity. In clients with Parkinson's disease, a disorder of rigidity and tremor related to loss of dopamine neurons related to movement, drugs that increase total dopamine activity are also associated with compulsive buying, gambling, and sexual activity (Weintraub, 2008; Lee et al., 2009). Drugs such as these that modify overall dopamine levels have revealed greater insights about the relationship between dopamine and risky behaviors.

Dr. Larry Koran, a Stanford psychiatrist, had the opportunity to test clients who had been identified as compulsive shoppers by setting them loose at the Stanford Shopping Center, a vast mall near Stanford University. Citalopram, an antidepressant that inhibits the uptake of serotonin (i.e., a selective serotonin reuptake inhibitor or SSRI), also increases expression of the D2 dopamine receptor. Clients receiving this drug significantly reduced compulsive buying (Koran et al., 2002). This suggests that compulsive buyers have low dopamine activity and, like others with dopamine deficiency, compulsively reward-seek, in this case buying objects in hopes of instant gratification. A similar effect was observed by using haloperidol, a drug that mimics dopamine deficiency by blocking the D2 receptors. In pathological gamblers, haloperidol increased the self-reported rewarding effects of gambling and the desire to gamble (Zack & Poulus, 2007). These studies suggest that dopamine deficiency may contribute to our financial decisions, potentially encouraging risky financial choices as well as risky health behaviors.

Why would you want to be more driven by need for immediate gratification?

If impulsivity is risky and self-destructive, why aren't our brains simply wired to be risk averse? There are times when it makes sense for your brain to focus on the short-term. Think about the circumstances in which your MS neurons become weak. You become driven by immediate needs when you have few rewarding opportunities in your life or are at the bottom of the social hierarchy. When you are in a situation where you may not have many chances to make your life better, or chances that you have right now may not be available next week, your brain readjusts itself to make sure that you take advantage of all the opportunities that appear. When you may not get another opportunity to get food for dinner, impress your higher ups, or make yourself feel better, you do not stop to think about whether taking that opportunity is really the best in terms of meeting your long-term goals. You take the opportunity while it is there. Only when you have plenty of opportunities to make your life better does your brain bother to stop and ponder which of the options is best for your future. Our brains are wired to let our reward circuits take over when we are in a resource poor environment, or at the mercy of our dominant peers.

But what about those people who are born with a genetic predisposition for reward-driven behavior (i.e., have the A1 allele of the D2 dopamine receptor)? We cannot know for sure, but possibly their ancestors lived in an unstable environment, where plentiful opportunities could quickly disappear. For example, food and water might be plentiful in summer but sparse in winter. In this case, you would not want to start worrying too much about how you look in your swimsuit in the summer. You would eat while you can and store up fat and supplies for the winter. You would not leave those nuts on the trees just because you already had plenty to eat today. You would pick them and store them, either as fat or preserved for later. If the number of opportunities in your environment could rapidly decrease, you would not want to reduce your drive for immediate rewards too much while they are present. Thus, when times are bad your brain will want to more slowly strengthen your MS neurons and reduce your tendency to work for immediate reward only slightly when times were consistently good.

In other words, in environments where resource availability is unstable, it is beneficial to seek out and consume or store as many resources as possible during times of plenty, as you will need these resources later when resources are scarce. Consider a temperate northern environment with a productive summer growing period with lots of food and resources followed by harsh winter with little to eat. Those who ate or collected lots of food during the summer will be more likely to survive the winter than those who sought out only what they needed in the summer. In such an environment, people with the A1 allele will do better. In environments where resources are consistently plentiful, however, those who only seek out and consume what they need will do better, as they avoid the health problems caused by chronic over work or over consumption. Consider a tropical rain forest where food is plentiful and available all year round. People who felt compelled to eat or even collect and store all the food they could possibly find would eventually suffer from obesity or at least exhaustion from never-ending hard labor. Here, those without the A1 allele will do better. As modern society turns most environments into ones where resources are consistently plentiful, those with the A1 allele are having increasing tendencies towards health problems.

The problems arise when your brain is wired for impending scarcity, but you live in an environment where reward opportunities are everywhere all the time. This mismatch is obviously problematic when you think about positive reinforcers like food. Habitually eating most of what you come across is a good idea if you live in an extreme environment and food is scarce. But, this strategy will leave you morbidly obese if you live in a place where food is always available and you are bombarded with advertising to remind you of that fact. The same problems occur when you have a genetic tendency towards reward-driven behavior and relief opportunities are everywhere. Let's say you live in a high-pressure environment where potential threats are everywhere. You run into people you do not know and thus do not really trust all the time. You have deadlines for being everywhere (e.g., your work, your kid's soccer game, closing time at the grocery store). News media lets you know about every upsetting problem that is occurring anywhere in the globe. If your brain habitually spends its time trying to escape from or solve every one of these problems that it encounters, you will wind up spending all your time hiding from, fleeing from, or obsessing about threats that you could realistically ignore. You may wind up with an anxiety disorder. The point here is that having a genetic predisposition for reward-driven behavior is not really a problem of having a mis-wired brain, it is a problem of mismatch between your environment and your brain's expectations of the environment. Society in the United States is not well-designed for people with the A1 allele of the D2 dopamine receptor. Consistent exposure to too many opportunities is problematic for people genetically designed to survive in unstable and potentially dangerous environments.

Aesop's fable "The Ant and the Grasshopper" can be a helpful allegory for remembering these biological tendencies. On a warm sunny day, a grasshopper sits in the sun, playing music and enjoying himself while a troop of ants toil away storing up food in their nests. The grasshopper encourages the ants to play and the ants retort that they can't because they need to store up food for the winter. They suggest that the grasshopper does the same, but he replies that he can't be bothered as winter is a long time off and there is lots of food. When winter comes, the grasshopper is starving and begs the ants for food. The disgusted ants reply that he played all summer and he can continue to play now and do not share their food with him. The point of the story is to teach the virtue of hard work and preparation.

FIGURE: Match between D2 dopamine receptor genetics and local environment

	Unstable Resources (e.g., summer versus harsh winter)	**Stable High Resources** (e.g., tropical rain forest with year round harvest)
A1 allele (slow adaptation to plenty)	Compulsively consume when resources are plentiful. Use reserves during scarce times. **Excellent Chance of Survival**	Compulsively consume all the time. Develop problems related to over-consumption. **Poor Chance of Survival**
No A1 allele (rapid adaptation to plenty)	Consume only what is needed when resources are plentiful. Starve during scarce times. **Poor Chance of Survival**	Consume only what is needed all the time. Stay balanced and healthful. **Excellent Chance of Survival**

Legend: Different versions of the D2 dopamine receptor are well-suited to different environments. The A1 allele of the D2 dopamine receptor is a common genetic variant. People with this genetic variant produce fewer than average D2 dopamine receptors, and thus their neurons adapt less when they receive dopamine signals. Because D2 dopamine receptors are involved in readjusting reward-seeking tendencies based on the availability of resources in the environment, persons with the A1 allele adapt more slowly when resources are plentiful. They will continue to seek and consume rewards, such as food, even when there are lots of opportunities to get more later. People without this genetic variant will rapidly reduce their search for and consumption of rewards when opportunities to get more are plentiful. These different patterns of behavior are either useful or problematic depending on the characteristics of the environment in which a person lives.

As we just discussed, those with the A1 allele are wired to tend to behave like the ants. Regardless of the plenty around them in summer, they will continue to work compulsively to collect up all the rewards around them, assuming that those rewards will not be available at a later time. Those without the A1 allele tend to be more like the grasshopper. In times of plenty, they lose the drive to work for quick rewards, and may spend their time attending to less necessary things. But our world is no longer set up like the harsh insect kingdom where resources are sometimes plentiful and sometimes scarce.

Ironically, it is those of us with the biological tendency to act like ants that are more likely to have health problems in our current society. Surrounded by opportunities for immediate reward, the ants among us will have trouble not over-consuming or over-avoiding. They may over-eat, over-shop, or over-work, or develop social anxiety or depression as they over-avoid perceived threats. While we value the virtue of effort and preparedness, we have set up a society where the tendency to behave like this can lead to health problems. All the advertising and pervasive opportunities for reward in our capitalist society are endangering our ant-like peers, putting them at risk of obesity, stress-related disease, addiction, and anxiety disorders.

A scientific consensus is emerging that the origins of many chronic adult diseases are found in the developmental and biological disruptions occurring during the early years of life (Shonkoff et al., 2009). Living in environments where there is an abundance of stress and emotional abuse and few resources to advance or cope, has a strong relation to the risk of developing alcoholism, substance abuse, depression, hypertension, diabetes, and coronary artery disease. Arguably, the perception of scarcity in a society where images of prosperity are everywhere in commercials, also plays a fundamental role in encouraging desire for immediate gratification. Therefore, both the poverty of emotional and psychological support and the absence of culturally-defined resources, particularly in the presence of highly available non-nutritious food, addictive substances and stressors, are key in increasing long-term risk of chronic disorders.

Shaping your environment to fit your biology
What should you do if you or your client has ant-like tendencies? The key here is recognizing your biological tendencies and working to shape your environment into one that works with you rather than against you. If you are an ant, it is unreasonable to expect yourself to be able to learn moderation in an environment where you are exposed to possibilities for quick rewards all the time. Instead of trying to change your behavior within your existing environment, you will need to make efforts to reduce your exposure to unhealthful opportunities and cues that trigger unhealthful habits. If you are an ant and you want to lose weight, do not expect yourself to be able to eat less without changing your day-to-day environment. Get rid of the TV or only watch pre-recorded shows so you can skip the commercials and reduce advertising exposure that drives eating. Food commercials are prevalent on TV and they work. For example, in 2004, the average child watched 40,000 advertisements on TV, at least 70% of which were for food. Moreover, a community survey of adults found that each hour of watching television was associated with additional consumption of 136 calories per day (Jason and O'Donnell, 2008; French et al., 2001). Do not allow these commercials into your home if you have trouble with over-eating. Stock your kitchen with only healthful food options. If the grocery store is overwhelming, order food online or shop with a more grasshopper-like friend so that you do not have to resist the temptation of the bakery aisle or the ice-cream case. If you are an ant, do not stock a liquor cabinet or hang out at bars and expect yourself to drink in moderation. Leave your credit cards at home and do not carry cash when you are not shopping for pre-planned needs. When you do shop, make a list of what you will buy before you go. Do not experiment with drugs, because your biology will lead you toward addiction. People with the A1 allele, people with family histories of addiction, obesity, anxiety disorders, gambling problems, people with lots of room to climb on the social ladder, or people who have simply noticed that they tend to act like Aesop's ants, should not trust their behavior to willpower, or expect to be able to moderate their habits like they

may see others do. It is to your advantage to identify these characteristics within yourself so you can create or seek out the environments that work best for you.

If you or your client has this background, it is important to recognize your biology and shape your environment to be more like one for which you are adapted. Just because you have a friend that can have a wine cellar and only have 3 drinks per week, or who can buy a 5-lb. bag of mini-candy bars and keep them on her desk for co-workers without eating more than one, doesn't mean that you should be able to do the same. People are biologically different and suited for different environments. Don't waste your time trying to fight your biology and certainly do not feel bad or guilty for the behavioral tendencies you inherited. Recognize your biology and its strengths and weaknesses and shape your world to fit your genetics. Embrace who you are and do not let envy for other's biology drive you to expect the impossible from yourself.

To identify factors in your environment that encourage unhealthful behaviors and to shape your environment to encourage unhealthful behaviors, see Exercise 2E (page 128) and Exercise 2F (page 130).

It's worth noting that the 12-step program, which has been shown to be highly effective for treating addictions and maintaining healthful behaviors over the long-term (Humphreys, 2004), starts by encouraging people to accept a disease model of addiction. The disease model of addiction suggests that the compulsive use and avoidance patterns that characterize addictive behaviors stem from a biological origin and are exacerbated by environmental contingencies. The first of the 12-steps to recovery is admitting that you are powerless over your addiction. This program starts by encouraging people with addictive tendencies to stop believing that they can control their behavior in a setting that encourages their compulsive habits, and focus on surrounding themselves with people, places, and interactions that discourage unhealthful behaviors and encourage more healthful habits. Before we understood the biology underlying the disease model, creative people came up with effective ways of helping themselves and others reshape their environment to limit dangerous compulsive habits.

<u>WARNING: How guilt and self-stigma can drive self-perpetuating compulsive habits</u>

On the surface, perfectionism may seem like a good trait. Logically, if you are not satisfied with yourself or your behavior, then you should be really motivated to change, and that should protect you from destructive habits. But in reality, strong motivation to change isn't the key component to long-term behavior change; it takes environmental and social changes, and learning new behaviors and thought patterns, to make meaningful changes stick. And perfectionism, particularly feeling bad about yourself when you act unhealthfully, turns out to actually encourage bad habits by increasing the negative affect and stress that triggers compulsive habits in us all.

The dangers of feeling guilty about our unhealthful habits are delightfully depicted by Antoine de Saint-Exupery in his children's book *The Little Prince* (Saint-Exupery, 1943). In this book, a young boy visits a variety of planets, each inhabited by a single quirky adult.

On one planet, he encounters a man with an alcohol problem, and in his child-like way he asks him what he is doing. The man eventually explains that he is drinking to forget that he is ashamed of his drinking problem. While this circular logic is humorous in a story, it can be seriously problematic in real-life. For example, in one of our own research studies, we found that the tendency to eat things to feel better (e.g., have a piece of chocolate to cheer yourself up) was associated with being overweight only insofar as people reported feeling bad about themselves for the way they ate.

This suggests that eating to manage mood only leads to being overweight if you feel bad about the fact that you ate a treat. If you eat to feel better and then actually feel better, then it is not a big deal. But if you eat to feel better and then feel ashamed of eating, then you are going to have to eat more to treat your shame, creating a compulsive cycle of overeating. Supporting the dangers of guilt and self-stigma, a study of participants who had already completed a 6-month weight loss program showed that those randomized to then receive a day of counseling focusing on reducing self-stigma about weight showed greater improvements in body mass index three months later (Lillis et al., 2009). Being less critical about your own behavior and tendencies and accepting yourself for who you are is not a sign that you are giving up on your goals. Abandoning judgmental perfectionism is a key step to being able to develop and maintain healthful habits.

Delay discounting: How can we stop devaluing our future?

Having low numbers of D2 dopamine receptors in the nucleus accumbens has also been linked to increased delay discounting in both animal models and in persons with substance use disorders (Barlow et al., 2018; Ballard et al., 2015). Delay discounting refers to the tendency to value things less the longer you must wait for them. With delay discounting, people favor smaller immediate rewards over larger delayed ones. The extent to which one will choose a smaller value reward to get it more quickly is not only associated with D2 dopamine receptor availability and but is also exaggerated among those with substance use disorders. These findings suggest that delay discounting may be a behavioral consequence of having weak ID brakes. When one's InDirect Pathway neurons are weak, a person will take immediate rewards over later ones, even if the later reward is of substantially greater value than the one available in the moment. New research suggests practices that may influence delay discounting decisions. What can these teach us about how to effectively manage and limit impulsive behaviors?

Episodic Future Thinking (EFT) is an intervention where one plays through future events in one's mind, allowing one to pre-experience a situation. In EFT, one envisions personal future scenarios, describing plausible, personally relevant, future events in detail, ideally including vivid descriptions about both the internal experience (e.g., thoughts, feelings) and external occurrence of the event (e.g., what happens). Interventions eliciting EFT have been shown to reduce delay discounting in standard monetary choice tasks (e.g., asking "do you want $X now or $Y later?") and in health behavior related decisions and actions (e.g., about alcohol, smoking, snacking) in children, adolescents and adults (e.g., Stein et al., 2016; Bulley & Gullo, 2017; Dassen et al., 2016; Daniel et al., 2015). Several of these studies have found that EFT *related* to the behavior or goal of interest enhances the impact of EFT on delay discounting and is necessary to influence subsequent health behaviors

(Dassen et al. 2016; O'Donnell et al., 2017). As an example of these findings, smokers with intention to quit who engaged in an exercise of Episodic Future Thinking, imagining positive life experiences after they had stopped smoking, both showed less delay discounting in a standard monetary choice task and smoked fewer cigarettes in the subsequent week (Chiou & Wu, 2017). These experimental studies suggest that EFT could be used to reduce impulsive choices and encourage health behaviors where long-term benefits come from foregoing opportunities for immediate gratification.

While most of the studies of Episodic Future Thinking and its effects have focused on single brief decisions in experimental settings, observational studies have suggested that the tendency to think in terms of future experience and events may have broader effects, even reducing risk of addictive disorders over time in whole populations. For example, it has been observed repeatedly that adolescents who are more religiously affiliated and engaged are less prone to substance use. A recent longitudinal study of 131 adolescents over approximately 6 years, explored the association between higher religiousness in early adolescence and lower tobacco, alcohol and marijuana use in late adolescence (Holmes and Kim-Spoon, 2017). They found that young teens with higher religiousness were more likely to endorse afterlife beliefs in middle adolescence, and having afterlife beliefs was associated with a greater future orientation in one's thinking. This greater future orientation in middle adolescence was associated with less substance use in late adolescence. This suggests that the beneficial effects of religiousness on reducing risk of addiction may stem from the focus of many mainstream religions on the future impact of one's current behavioral choices; these religions present a clear vision of the positive long-term effects of healthful choices and the negative long-term effects of unhealthful choices through vivid depictions of consequences in an afterlife. This may help simplify and make salient the future scenarios associated with a given choice and help generalize future scenarios across health behaviors. This emphasis and simplification may facilitate regular episodic future thinking. Simply put, picturing burning in a tortuous hell because of drinking may provide a more moving and quick future-focused vision than an attempt to think through what it would be like to slowly die of alcohol-related cirrhosis. Likewise, floating in peaceful bliss with people you love might be easier to imagine than the experiential and situational benefits of sobriety and abstinence. Moreover, being involved in a social group that focuses on the afterlife may encourage one to consider future effects more often. This points to ways for making lasting improvements in health decisions regardless of one's spiritual beliefs. Creating powerful personal imagery for positive future states you desire and negative future states you wish to avoid in relationship to your health decisions may help you delay gratification and avoid poor choices.

To practice Episodic Future Thinking related to your health behavior goals, see Exercise 2G (page 133).

Reward or Choice Bundling is another strategy which may help to reduce delay discounting. In choice bundling a series of decisions regarding whether to do a behavior are aggregated into a single choice (Ashe and Wilson, 2020; Rung et al., 2019). For example, rather than making individual decisions about whether to drink alcohol with each meal, one could decide whether they will drink alcohol this month.

Choice bunding may help prevent preference reversals, where a choice between a smaller more immediate reward and a larger delayed reward flips as the immediacy of the smaller reward is greater. For example, say I offered someone a choice between a donut tomorrow or $15 in a week. Probably, they would choose the $15, as they could purchase numerous donuts with that money and both rewards are perceived as distant and thus discounted. But, come tomorrow, if I offered the same choice, "would you like a donut now or $15 in 6 days", a subset of those same people would change their preference, and take the immediate donut over the later $15. Now that the smaller donut reward is more immediate, it becomes discounted substantially less, such that it may now be valued greater than the larger, but still substantially delayed and thus discounted reward. Such preference reversals can significantly frustrate attempts at health behavior change and have been particularly associated with risk and relapse in addictive disorders (e.g., Satyal et al., 2023; Turner et al., 2021).

Conceptually, choice bunding may help link together choices between a smaller more immediate reward and a larger more delayed reward, such that the decision is considered from the less immediate framework. Thinking of a choice as a subscription of sorts may help keep the comparison between rewards in a more distant frame, where differences in delay discounting between the smaller and larger rewards are not so dramatic (Monterosso and Ainslie, 2006). Considered in a subscription model, while delay discounting may make the smaller but immediate reward to be perceived as higher value on day one, in subsequent days, both rewards would be relatively discounted, and the larger-later reward would again be estimated as higher value. Bundling these choices causes the decision maker to sum across each of these decisions. Over those bundled choices, the exaggerated value of the smaller immediate reward of day one is outcompeted by the preferred larger-later rewards on future days. Taking the prior example, choice bunding would make the decision between receiving a donut each day for a month starting today, or $15 a day for a month starting in 6 days. Summarizing makes this a choice between 30 donuts received over the next 30 days or $450 received over the next 36 days. This bundled frame can help to make the larger later rewards win out despite the delay in reward receipt.

Monterosso and Ainslie (2006) argue that the first step of 12-step programs for substance use disorders (e.g., Alcoholics Anonymous) is a foundational argument that establishes choice bundling into decisions about substance use. Step one declares "We admitted we were powerless over our addiction - that our lives had become unmanageable". It implies that decisions to use substances are inherently linked and cannot be separated. One needs to give up the hope that one can make a choice once and not have that choice repeat indefinitely. By starting the process of recovery by bundling today's choice regarding whether to use substances with every future choice, one can flip choice preference away from the smaller immediate reward (i.e., substance use) back to the larger later reward (i.e., recovery), thereby maintaining abstinence even in the presence of opportunities for immediate substance use.

While the ability of choice bundling to shift decisions towards larger-later rewards can be demonstrated in rodent, pigeon, and human experiments (Hofmeyr et al., 2010; Ainslie and

Monterosso, 2003; Stein et al., 2013; Ainslie, 1974), research into how to best use this quirk of decision-making clinically to reshape reward and relief-seeking habits is scarce. But understanding the concept can help make it easier to create effective plans to change habit behaviors. If you want to eat less meat, you'll likely be more successful if you decide to eat vegetarian for a month, rather than try to favor vegetarian options at every meal. If you want to exercise more, you may be more likely to succeed if you decide to schedule a walk every day at 4:00 for the next month, rather than try to choose a walk over rest every afternoon. Understanding the challenges caused by preference reversal (i.e., the tendency to choose smaller-sooner rewards over larger-later rewards when the small reward is available immediately), can help you recognize these tendencies in yourself and clients and design choice bundles or behavior subscriptions to prevent this threat to our long-term goals.

Chapter 2.4: Increasing Pleasurable Activities in Everyday Life.

As we discussed, experiencing a dearth of small everyday rewards can lead to a reward or dopamine deficient state in which habits that provide immediate relief or gratification are overly favored. While there are many ways of increasing recognition of and engagement with opportunities for immediate improvement in well-being, simply learning and incorporating habits that bring instant joy and pleasure is intuitively appealing. A variety of techniques for increasing experience of pleasure in life have been developed and studied and provide exercises towards the effective pursuit of happiness.

Savoring

Recognizing that reduced salience of natural rewards was a core problem in patients with addiction and chronic pain, Garland and colleagues developed a therapy entitled "Mindfulness Oriented Recovery Enhancement (MORE)" that includes exercises to explicitly increase attention to, engagement with, and valuation of natural rewards through savoring skills (Garland, 2016). Savoring skills involve purposefully orienting and attending to sensations associated with one's environment, along with any positive emotions, thoughts or meaning associated with the experience. For example, sitting here writing in my living room, I might simply attend to the light from the window bouncing off my blue walls, and reflect firstly on the way the light plays across everything else in the room and then how much I love the color. I then might reflect on how it reminds me of the blue sky on warm sunny days, and the feelings of contentment and pleasure that I've experienced on days outside in perfect weather. From there, I might remember the effort I put into picking the color and repainting my walls, glorying in my ability and success in beautifying and bettering my environment in ways that matter to me. Intentionally directing attention to the sensory experience, positive associations, and personal meaning associated with something as simple and everyday as light reflecting off a wall enables me to find immediate pleasure and a sense of achievement and self-efficacy in something I could have easily not noticed at all. In MORE, patients explicitly practice this integration of mindfulness meditation techniques with intentional savoring and reappraisal skills to learn and habituate this strategy to extract moments of joy within everyday life. In MORE, savoring practice may start with guided practice around experiences that are commonly found pleasurable, such as viewing and smelling flowers, with the goal of learning to attend to and experience deep appreciation in fleeting moments of life.

Consistent with intent, when studied in a clinical trial of smoking cessation, MORE led to changes in response of anterior cingulate cortex and ventral striatum to both cigarette cues and positive images, with those trained in MORE showing reduced activation in these brain regions per fMRI imaging in response to cigarette images and more activation in these same regions in response to positive images (Froeligner et al., 2017). Additionally, the increased response to the positive images predicted improvements in positive affect and reductions in smoking among study participants. Likewise, participants on long-term opioid analgesics for chronic pain randomized to receive MORE rather than supportive group therapy showed increased autonomic responses to natural reward cues; this increased response to natural reward cues was responsible for the positive effect of MORE on reducing anhedonia among participants (Garland et al., 2023). Together, these suggest that practice in savoring everyday experience enhances valuation of natural rewards, increasing pleasurable experience and positive emotions and improving ability to shift behavior away from habits that cause harm or pain.

Self-Soothing

Self-soothing refers to the ability to comfort oneself in the face of distress, though soothing techniques can be used to provide reward or comfort even in the absence of need for relief. Oxytocin is a neuropeptide that has been shown to mediate numerous forms of self-soothing, providing reward or relief in reward circuits, reducing anxiety and physiological responses to stress, and facilitating social affiliation. Oxytocin is released when sensory neurons are activated by gentle touch or warmth, such as during mother infant interactions, sexual contact, and warm interactions between people or people and pets (Uvnas-Moberg et al., 2015). Oxytocin can induce dopamine release in nucleus accumbens reward circuits and reduce stress response in the hypothalamic pituitary adrenal axis (Insel et al., 2003). It thus can have beneficial effects on reducing reward/dopamine deficiency and minimizing stress effects on habit behaviors. It may increase social reward opportunities by increasing trust and encouraging positive social interactions (Uvnas-Moberg et al., 2015). Learning and using strategies to induce oxytocin release can increase experience of natural rewards. Understanding what causes oxytocin release can help one develop a set of go-to strategies and habits to provide relief or pleasure during everyday life.

Gentle touch and skin to skin contact is the most studied method of inducing oxytocin release. Warm touch, hugs, massage, sexual contact, and other consensual physical contact between people can all elevate oxytocin levels and provide reward (e.g., Tomosugi and Koshino, 2023). But what if there aren't loved ones available to cuddle? Self-soothing touch may provide similar benefits. In an experimental setting, simple self-soothing touch, consisting of 20 seconds of self-chosen touch, such as putting a hand on your heart or belly or stroking your upper arms, was found to prevent increases in cortisol level and heart rate caused by a social stress test, just as a hug did (Dreisoerner et al., 2021). Likewise, physical contact does not have to be between two people. Stroking or snuggling with pets produces similar effects. Music has also been shown to increase oxytocin levels. When patients on bed rest after heart surgery were provided music, their oxytocin levels increased and they experienced a sense of relaxation (Nilsson, 2009). Finding self-soothing practices that are readily available and create a sense of warmth, safety, and connectedness (e.g., taking a moment to breathe with your hands on your belly, holding a warm drink, stroking your arms, head, or a pet) may help increase natural rewards in your environment and reduce the negative impacts of stress.

Some therapies include exercises that explicitly foster self-soothing skills. Dialectical Behavior Therapy (DBT) (Linehan, 1993) explicitly encourages development and practice of self-soothing skills. For example, DBT encourages taking time to engage each of your 5 major senses and focus on something pleasurable or comforting. One might take time to view something they find beautiful, listen to music or sounds of nature, such as ocean noise or bird-song, smell something enjoyable such as cooking spices or flowers, taste a favorite or comfort food, or experience gentle touch by taking a bath, putting on moisturizer, or sitting in the warm sun. PositivePsychology,com provides a practical review of techniques and practices that can be helpful for encouraging effective self-soothing practices (Nash, 2022). A second example, Compassion Focused Therapy (Gilbert, 2014; Gilbert, 2009) includes an intentional focus on development of cognitive skills to enhance motivation to collaborate with and support oneself and others and experience a sense of contentment and safety. Here, in addition to exercises designed to reduce self-shame and criticism, the therapist uses mindfulness, imagery, and exposure techniques to help patients develop and practice the ability to feel compassion towards others and themselves. Meta-analysis of small clinical trials and observational studies of Compassion Focused Therapy found that the therapy moderately increased the ability to self-soothe, providing early evidence that this approach can increase the ability to self-soothe across clinically (e.g., patients with eating disorders) or non-clinically targeted populations (e.g., teachers) (Vidal and Soldevilla, 2023).

Smiling

Experimental studies suggest that the motion of making a facial expression provides feedback to brain circuits that interpret emotional experience, increasing the likelihood or intensity of experiencing an emotion congruent with the facial expression (Coles et al., 2019). The act of smiling itself can increase the experience of pleasure and reduce the experience of stress in everyday life! For example, holding a pair of chopsticks sideways between your teeth forces your mouth into a high-level smile position, referred to as a Duchenne smile. Kraft and Pressman (2012) used this manipulation of facial position to examine the effect of facial posture on affect and stress response. Compared to holding chopsticks vertically in their teeth in a neutral facial expression, persons watching humorous or pleasant videos in the chopstick-forced Duchenne smile position experienced greater positive autonomic arousal. Likewise, when asked to hold a hand in ice-cold water (i.e., a pain tolerance task) or trace lines in a mirror with a non-dominant hand (i.e., a frustrating task), those forced to hold their face in the Duchenne smile had lower heart rate after the stressor and less of a reduction in positive experience from the stressful task. Likewise, people mimicking a smile or a grimace using the same chopstick techniques experienced about 40% less pain and a lower heart rate upon a vaccination-like injection with a needle, as compared to those holding a neutral facial expression (Pressman et al., 2021). This literature suggests that practicing smiling throughout the day may help increase positive emotion and enhance the experience of reward in everyday life.

Obviously, carrying chopsticks between your teeth all day isn't a particularly practical approach to adding smiles to your day. Chen et al (2016) created a simple mobile phone application to encourage smiling, and randomized college students to practice one of several strategies, including prompting the students to (1) take a smiling selfie each day, or (2) take a picture of something that made them smile or feel happy to reflect on. Taking the pictures increased positive mood and arousal in both conditions, and qualitative interviews with participants suggested that the application was not only generally well accepted, but made participants feel better about themselves and the people and things in their lives. Adding intention to simply smile or engage with things that make you smile, with or without the help of the camera in your pocket, may augment natural rewards in your life, and add one more tool to combat dopamine deficiency and increase flexibility to change habit behaviors.

Brain Challenge #2 Exercises

Exercise 2A: Assertiveness Skills
(Adapted from Sorrell et al., 2005)

Social skills training is a well-tested and effective intervention for mental health disorders (e.g., Dilk & Bond, 1996), and the skills taught are likely to be helpful for most people. Because a majority of the available rewards in human culture are social or involve working with others, good communication skills are essential for creating opportunities to make your life better. Passive or aggressive communication styles can prevent people from creating opportunities. Here we will practice an assertive communication style.

A useful technique for practicing assertive communication is the SAS technique. SAS stands for:

> <u>State</u> the problem and its consequences.
> <u>Ask</u> for what you need.
> <u>Spell</u> out the advantages of cooperation.

The first step of assertive communication is to state the problem and its consequences. By clearly defining the problem, you eliminate confusion or assumptions about what the people involved are thinking or feeling. Thus, you should start your assertive communication by stating what the problem is from your perspective and how this problem affects you. Be objective and do not blame or judge the other person. Because you are explaining your side of the problem and not making assumptions about the other person's motivations or their side of the problem, you should find yourself using the word "I" rather than "you".

Once you have clearly presented the problem from your perspective, the second step is to ask for what you need in the situation. You should focus on being direct and clear so that there is no misunderstanding about what you want from the interaction. Be sure to be specific, but respectful of the other person.

The last step is to spell out the advantages of cooperation. Again, it is important to remain objective and accurately and clearly describe what will likely happen if the person cooperates with you. By focusing on the good things that will come out of cooperation rather than the bad things that might result if they do not, you reduce the chance that the other person feels manipulated, resentful or bullied into doing what benefits you.

Let us consider an example situation to illustrate this technique. Pretend you are at a business meeting with a session over lunch. You have special dietary restrictions and indicated these in the space provided on the registration forms for the meeting. The registration forms promised that special meals would be provided for those with dietary restrictions. However, at the start of the lunch session, the server delivers you the standard meal that you cannot eat and scurries off to the next table.

For comparison, let us consider what a passive or aggressive response might look like and the likely consequences of these types of communication:

A passive response would be to let the server go and sit there looking unhappy, not touching your lunch, and hoping someone will notice and intervene. The most likely consequence of this approach is that no one would notice your expression of misery, and you will end lunch feeling hungry, neglected, frustrated, and unfairly treated.

An aggressive response would be to call the server over immediately, tell him he messed up, state that you clearly outlined your dietary needs on the registration forms, and that you will complain to management if you do not get your special meal right away. This approach might successfully get you a suitable lunch, but it may upset the server, create a commotion, or make others around you think that you are not a very nice person for bullying the conference staff.

Let's walk through the SAS process and consider an assertive approach instead.

Step 1 of the SAS technique for assertive communication suggests that you should clearly state the problem and its consequences. You could get the server's attention and explain the problem from your perspective. For example: "Excuse me sir, but I have special dietary restrictions and cannot eat this meal without harming my health. "

Step 2 suggests that you should ask for what you need. You could clearly explain what you want. For example: "I had requested a low-salt, vegetarian meal on my registration because I can only eat food that meets these criteria. Could you check whether there is a special meal reserved under my name or ask the chef if there are lunch options that would meet these criteria?"

Step 3 suggests that you should spell out the benefits of cooperation. You clearly explain how this extra effort could benefit the server. For example: "If you help me get a meal that I can eat, I will enjoy this meeting much more and will recommend that we use this conference center for all our future meetings."

This approach is likely to get you your special lunch without conflicts that might upset you or others. The server is likely to leave the interaction feeling like he was able to do something special to help his company. Your colleagues are apt to see you as a nice person who stands up for yourself.

The SAS technique is relatively simple to use, but can require practice if you are not accustomed to an assertive communication style. In the beginning, it may feel uncomfortable or take effort to plan or carry out. Thus, practicing this style in relatively safe environments is key to becoming good at it and able to use it in more stressful situations. Your body language during the communication should match your words. Pay attention to your body language during the interactions. You should focus on listening to others, maintaining eye contact and positioning your body squarely toward the other person. You should maintain a confident but respectful posture, and speak firmly, clearly, positively and loud enough to be heard. You want to make sure that the other person acknowledges and respects you and feels like they are being acknowledged and respected as well. Directing your attention clearly on the other person and giving them time to interact and respond will help ensure that this happens and that the interaction goes well.

Find a friend or partner and role-play assertive communication styles with them. It may be useful to brainstorm situations in which you have previously been unable to articulate your needs. Try responding assertively to a request for you to do something you do not want to. Practice asking for something others did not notice you needed. Share feedback with your partner about the choice of words and body language during the interaction.

The form on the next page may be helpful for you as you begin to practice using the SAS technique by yourself or with a friend or partner.

WORKSHEET: SAS Assertive Communication Practice

In the space provided, write the situation, the **stated problem** and its consequences, **ask for** what you want, and **spell out** the benefits of cooperation.

"SAS" Communication Technique
State the problem and its consequences.
Ask for what you want.
Spell out the benefits of cooperation.

Date:

Situation	Stated Problem	Asked Wants	Spelled Benefits

Date:

Situation	Stated Problem	Asked Wants	Spelled Benefits

Date:

Situation	Stated Problem	Asked Wants	Spelled Benefits

Date:

Situation	Stated Problem	Asked Wants	Spelled Benefits

Exercise 2B: Tips For Resolving Disagreements

There are numerous books and resources on healthy communication styles. Although they differ in various ways, a consensus of experts in clinical psychology agree on the following "rules" of engagement that can facilitate communicating what matters in a way that leads to meaningful change (Reis & Rusbult, 2004).

1. Agree to discuss one particular issue at a time. When multiple issues are raised while trying to deal with the problem at hand, the discussions can become counterproductive.

2. Agree on a time and place to have the discussion.

3. Agree to take a break if the discussion gets heated.

4. Use the word "I" instead of the word "you".

5. Avoid attacking the other person; instead, discuss how you feel.

6. Avoid defending your own position, even or especially when you feel attacked.

7. Agree on rules of disengagement; for example, if after 30 minutes we cannot come to a resolution, let's resume at a later time to be agreed upon.

8. If you cannot agree on rules of engagement or if they fail, secure the assistance of a trained third party in whom you can both trust to help mediate and resolve difficult issues.

Consider the list and a recent disagreement you had with someone. How many of these rules of engagement did you follow? Are there things you would do differently the next time you have a disagreement with a close relationship or friend?

Exercise 2C: Progressive Behavioral Shaping

Important components of using progressive behavioral shaping are: 1) breaking down your goal behavior into learnable pieces, and 2) creating rewards or reinforcers to encourage these intermediate pieces. In the following exercise, we will practice these components for one of your goals.

Step 1: Identify the final goal.

_____

_____

_____

Step 2: Identify the behavior you need to do to achieve your final goal. This is your ultimate target behavior.

_____

_____

_____

Step 3: List all of the pieces of your ultimate target behavior.

_____

_____

_____

_____

_____

_____

_____

_____

Step 4: Reorder these pieces according to difficulty. If there are pieces that require that you have already mastered other parts of the behavior, list them as sub-parts of that piece of the behavior. You can do this by numbering the pieces you listed above.

Step 5: Choose a piece of the behavior to work on, ideally starting from the easiest, most independent piece that you have yet to learn. Will doing this piece alone benefit you? If not, set up an artificial system to reward you for doing this piece. This may mean getting a coach or friend to encourage you or setting up rules for rewarding your own success.

Step 6: Repeat step 5 until all pieces have been learned. Keep in mind that different pieces may take differing amounts of time.

Exercise 2D: How Can We Increase Perceived Opportunities In Our Life?

There are many ways to increase our exposure to and awareness of opportunities in our lives. Despite popular beliefs, winning the lottery, having your company go public or inheriting millions from your great aunt are not the best or most likely ways of enriching your life. A large bank account may or may not translate into day-to-day opportunities to improve your well-being. Adding healthful activities to your life is one simple way to expand your opportunities. Happily, these are accessible to all and do not require extreme luck, a favorable market or a blue bloodline.

Step 1: Identifying Health Opportunities in Your Life
What rewarding events can you count on in the next few days?
1.
2.
3.
4.
5.
(additional ideas after reading Step 2)

What rewarding events can you count on in the next few weeks?
1.
2.
3.
4.
5.
(additional ideas after reading Step 2)

What rewarding events can you count on in next few years?
1.
2.
3.
4.
5.
6.
(additional ideas after reading Step 2)

<u>Step 2: Additional Ideas for Health Opportunities</u>
Below is a list of some healthy pleasures. If these are things you do, or would like to do, make a check mark next to them. If you want, you can write a brief description next to the item as to when and where and with whom you might like to take advantage of it.

Physical/Recreational
Walking
Stretching
Working out
Gardening
Jogging
Cycling
Swimming
Hiking
Boating
Yoga
Tai Chi
Other meditation
Massage
Leisure bath/shower
Household tasks
Sit in the sun
Rest

Creative
Arts
Crafts
Listening to music
Singing
Playing an instrument
Going to the theatre
Watching a film
Writing music
Photography
Writing in your journal
Writing essays, books, or poetry
View a video about art/music/theatre

Charitable
Attend a volunteer group
Attend a religious meeting
Donate your time
Donate clothing, goods, etc.
Support non-profit organizations
Help others in need

Prosocial

Reaching out to a dear friend or someone you think might be lonely
Expressing gratitude
Inviting guests over
Sharing books, arts, crafts, healthy recipes
Playing golf, tennis, baseball, pickle ball, etc.
Playing board games or cards
Join a club, band, choir, or orchestra
Workout with a friend
Express love
Start a group
Start a non-profit
Make someone laugh
Comfort someone who is sad
Plan and take a shared vacation

Educational/Cognitive

Help someone solve a problem
Teach knowledge and wisdom
Acquire new computer skills
Acquire a new language
Take a class in something you want to learn or that will provide you valuable skills
Watch a how-to video on something you want to learn and try to do it yourself
Use an app to learn and practice a new skill or learn something about yourself (e.g., track eating or sleeping patterns, learn a new coping skill, practice a new type of puzzle)
Read this book

Step 3: Additional Health Opportunities in Your Life

Now revisit Step 1 and add to the lists for the next few days, weeks and years based on the additional ideas for health opportunities that you selected in Step 2.

Step 4: Incorporating and Remembering Your Health Opportunities

Looking at your compiled list in Step 1, which now includes both health opportunities you can count on in the next few days, months, and years as well as additional ideas for things you do or would like to do, you now need to come up with ways to remind yourself of these opportunities. This is not about convincing yourself to do something new, just reminding yourself of the things you already do or plan on doing.

Come up with a system to increase your perception of the goals you may take for granted. For instance, you could write your daily goals into your paper or electronic planner so that you have the satisfaction of crossing it off your list each day. You could keep a checklist on the wall of your kitchen or living room that you run through each day, month, and year. You could place sticky notes around your home or workplace. You could keep a diary to track your health goals regularly. Each of these serves as a tangible reminder of the ways in which you are actively involved in your own health – even if it does not feel as active as these behaviors become habitual.

Exercise 2E: Avoiding Non-Ideal Environments for an Ant

The main question to consider here is whether a strategy of moderation versus abstinence is right for you. Is moderation is realistic for you? Consider your past behavior and your family's habits. Do you or your relatives have trouble with alcohol, tobacco, substance use, compulsive spending, gambling, obesity, or mood disorders? Do you find yourself or relatives buying things you did not intend to when you go shopping, or overspending on your credit card? When you start eating or drinking, do you have trouble stopping? Do you compulsively work long hours, even though your family wants you home and you do not realistically need the money? If your honest answer to some of these questions is yes, then there is a good chance that you are biologically wired to act like Aesop's ant.

You may find that you must change or even give up some of your current lifestyle or friends, but with some effort you will find alternatives that are just as, if not more, enjoyable. Do not try to learn to eat less at the all-you-can-eat buffet, just do not go to all-you-can-eat buffets. Try a different restaurant that provides smaller portions or use small plates at home. Do not try to buy less when you go to the mall. Don't go to the mall and go for a hike in a park instead. Do not try to drink less when you go to the bar, just do not go to the bar. Try taking a class or going to a community event to be social. Yes, there are people who can go to buffets, watch the shopping channel and go to bars and not overeat, over-buy, or over-drink. But if you are not one of them, do not beat yourself up trying to be someone you are not. Just avoid those situations. Get out of there. Not all environments in this world are good for all of us. Is it possible for everyone to maintain a healthy weight? Yes. But is it possible for everyone to do so while eating at all-you-can-eat buffets every meal? No.

It can be daunting to think about avoiding or giving up all these familiar environments at the same time. If you know you tend to overindulgence or excess, you can work one by one to remove tempting situations from your life. Below we give you an opportunity to brainstorm some situations, and then start by picking one to change.

If you think you have this biology, think about situations where you tend to overdo it. List some of these situations here:

_____
_____
_____
_____
_____

Pick one of these situations and consider ways that you can reduce your exposure to these temptations. List ways you could avoid this situation here:

_____
_____
_____
_____
_____

Lastly, for the situation you should probably avoid, think up an alternative enjoyable thing to do. List this new, and hopefully safer, alternative and then give it a try. When you are ready for more change, return to your initial list and repeat for another situation.

_____

_____

_____

_____

_____

Exercise 2F: Creating an Ideal Environment for an Ant

Shaping your environment can be a powerful way to improve your habits. Here we will walk you through methods for changing your environment to discourage unhealthful habits and encourage healthful alternatives. Even subtle changes can shift your behaviors in healthful directions.

List the habit you want to limit: _____
Example: I want to stop eating a lot of sweets in the evening before bed.

1) Make it harder to do your bad habit.
If you increase the amount of effort required to do your bad habit and insert steps that slow down your ability to carry out the bad habit, you will disfavor your habit in two ways. First, your nucleus accumbens will be less likely to determine that the effort is worth the pay-off. Second, your prefrontal cortex will have more time to notice and actively inhibit you from doing your bad habit.

Consider ways in which you can add in purposeful inconveniences to doing your habit.

Describe ways that you could make the habit harder to do:
_____
_____
_____
_____

Example:
I could not keep sweets in the house and force myself to go out to get sweets for dessert. I could also find places to go out where I can get a reasonably sized single serving of dessert, so that my trips out are not that problematic. I could only let myself buy basic ingredients to make desserts, such as flour, sugar, baking soda, cocoa power, nuts, and fruit, so that I would have to cook or bake in order to have sweets to eat.

3) Make it easier to do the right thing.
If you reduce barriers to doing an alternate healthful behavior instead of your habit, you will increase the likelihood that you do the healthful behavior instead.

Consider ways in which you can simplify doing something healthful instead of doing your bad habit.

List the healthful behavior you want to do instead: _____
Example: I want to have a cup of herbal tea and some fruit for dessert.

Describe ways that you could make the healthful behavior easier to do:
_____
_____
_____
_____

Example:
I can buy a variety of appealing herbal teas and display them prominently in the kitchen. I can keep a teapot on the stove and fill it regularly so that I just have to turn on the burner to start the tea. I can purchase fresh fruit for the week, and keep it on the counter along with a cutting board and paring knife to encourage me to prepare and eat the fruit.

3) Remove cues that trigger your bad habit.

When you are reminded about the possibility of doing your bad habit, you must actively stop yourself from doing the habit. It is much easier to stop doing a habit if you never consider the habit in the first place. Removing reminders can reduce the frequency at which you consider doing your bad habit.

Consider ways in which you can remove reminders that encourage your bad habit.

List things that encourage or make you think about doing your bad habit:

_____

_____

Example:
Cookie sheets on the counter make me think about baking cookies. TV commercials make me think about eating something fun. Seeing my husband looking for dessert makes me start searching too. Feeling tired and hungry makes me start looking for food.

Describe ways that you could remove or hide these things in your environment:

_____

_____

_____

Example:
I could store the cookie sheets in the back of the cabinet. I could record my favorite TV shows and skip through the commercials, or not watch TV late at night. I could make my husband tea and fruit before he starts searching for food. I could eat more vegetables or drink more water at dinner so that I feel full longer after I eat. I could go to bed when I start feeling tired and just get up earlier to finish things, instead of trying to stay up late.

4) Add cues that trigger your good behaviors.

Adding reminders to do alternate healthful behaviors can help you to automatically initiate these good behaviors. And if you are already doing the alternative behaviors, you might not even consider doing the unhealthful habit.

Consider ways in which you could add reminders that encourage your healthful alternative behaviors.

List things that encourage or make you think about doing your healthful behaviors:

_____

_____

Example:
Seeing my teacup makes me think of tea. Feeling a bit chilly in the evening makes me want tea. Soft lighting and a soft chair make me want a cup of tea. Bright colors and tropical scenes make me want to eat fruit. Seeing trees makes me want to eat fruit.

Describe ways that you could add or showcase these things in your environment:

_____
_____
_____
_____

Example:
I can always leave my teacup on the counter, or in the living room. I can turn down the thermostat so the house is a bit colder. I can get lower wattage light bulbs with a warm color balance and put pillows and a blanket on the chair that I tend to sit in after dinner. I can decorate my kitchen or buy dishware with bright colors and images of fruit and tropical settings on them. I can put a small tree or maybe a picture of an orchard in the living room or kitchen.

5) Avoid situations where consuming or doing too much is encouraged or even possible.
There are many places that have been specifically designed to encourage gluttonous indulgence in our bad habits. Don't go to these places, or at least don't go often. Go somewhere else instead.

Consider places that encourage you to indulge your bad habit.

List these places here:

_____
_____

Example: All you can eat ice cream bar. The restaurant with the giant dessert portions. My grandmother's house. My friend's potluck dessert parties. The donut store.

Consider whether there is an enjoyable alternative place you could go.

Describe such places here.

_____
_____
_____
_____

Example:
The organic frozen yogurt place that has all sorts of fruit toppings. The restaurant with the better dinner food and smaller dessert portions. I could bring my grandmother to my house. I could encourage my friend to change up her party format, and help with suggestions and organizing. Maybe we could all go to a yoga class, do a group hike, or have an exotic fruit tasting. I could go to the bagel store instead.

Exercise 2G: Episodic Future Thinking: Imagining future experiences as they relate to your health goals

Vividly imagining ourselves in the future can help us value future rewards more and reduce impulsive behavioral choices in the present. The practice of imagining ourselves in future situations – thinking through what we would experience, what we would do, how we would feel, how others would react to us, etc. – is called Episodic Future Thinking (EFT). EFT reduces the amount that we devalue rewards that come at a delay (i.e., long-term benefits). Moreover, future thinking related to a specific health behavior goal can help change actual health behaviors away from immediate gratification and toward long-term health (e.g., less snacking or cigarettes smoked in the short-term).

Imagining your future self in terms of your health goals is a concrete way that you can encourage better long-term decision-making and reduce the temptation of immediate gratification. Setting and recalling these future visions in your everyday life can help to increase your orientation towards the future and reshape your behaviors to match those of your desired future self. We will walk through a couple of exercises to guide episodic future thinking about your own health goals, using examples to illustrate the points.

First consider what you want to change about your current state. Are there behaviors or situations that you need to change or overcome to achieve your ideal future? Describe your current state challenges here:

_____

_____

_____

Example 1 Current State: *I sprained my ankle badly playing soccer last month and since then have rested and mostly immobilized it. The swelling has gone down, and I can put weight on it, but now my ankle and my legs are weak from disuse. Moreover, I got hurt when a particularly aggressive and much larger player fouled me to stop me from shooting on goal. I'm scared of being reinjured, or even having to go up against larger defenders when I go back.*

Now, consider your goal. What do you need to do to reach your ideal future? Describe that here:

_____

_____

_____

Example 1 Goal: *To return to playing in my soccer league. This will require physical therapy, strength training, extra soccer practice, and confidence in my abilities in competition, so that I do not hesitate or play tentatively when I return to league games.*

Next, consider your ideal future, and describe scenarios where you behave in a manner consistent with your goals. The point in episodic future thinking is to imagine these future situations in graphic detail, attending to your emotions, thoughts,

141

feelings, reactions, and outcomes. Immerse yourself in the future experience, imaging how your ideal future self would feel, think, and respond, and what it would be like to live through that experience. Describe some scenarios that you could imagine to practice episodic future thinking:

For Example 1, below are 3 different scenarios that one could use to guide an episode of future thinking focused on achieving the example goal.

Example Scenario 1. *Imagine yourself successfully persisting in your physical therapy exercises and getting stronger. How does your ankle feel during the exercises? If there is pain, does it last long? How do you feel after you make it through a set? What do you think as you do the exercise? What do you think when you finish? What do you (or your trainer) say to yourself when you complete an exercise?*

Example Scenario 2. *Imagine yourself back in practice doing drills with both feet with power, strength, agility, and balance. How do you feel as you complete the drills? What do you think as you are moving through the movements? How does it feel to be strong and trust your legs and ankles as you practice? How do your teammates react to you?*

Example Scenario 3. *Imagine yourself back in a game, playing fearlessly, strong, and intelligently against skilled and aggressive opponents. What do you do when a defender runs at you? What do you think and feel? How do your legs respond when you try to execute a difficult move? What do you do and what is the outcome? How do your teammates react?*

To help further illustrate, below is a second example to help encourage goal-directed episodic future thinking.

Example 2 Current State: *I am painfully shy and timid with people I don't know. In new social situations I drift away from people and conversations, and wind up feeling lonely, unloved, misunderstood, and uncomfortable in the back of the room. I feel disconnected and start thinking about all the ways I am different and how I don't like my peers.*

Example 2 Goal: *To participate comfortably in social settings and stop avoiding interactions with new people.*

Example 2 Scenario 1. *Imagine yourself at a conference for your job amongst others in your profession. Some are presenting information about their recent projects. Imagine yourself starting up an interesting discussion with a presenter. What did you say? How did you present yourself? Did you make eye contact? How did they respond? Did they give you their full attention? Did you learn interesting things in the conversation? Did you offer up information about what you do? Were they interested? How did you feel during and after the interaction? How did others around you respond to the conversation? Did they join in or talk with you after? What did you think about yourself and the people you talked with after the conversation?*

Example 2 Scenario 2. *Imagine yourself feeling confident and having fun meeting new people at a potluck at your local community center or religious organization. Imagine introducing yourself to someone you don't know. What do you say? How do you feel? How do they respond? How do you keep the conversation going? Do you ask questions? Answer them? How do you show interest in the other person? Do you enjoy yourself and feel connected to the people you met?*

To summarize, think of situations where you are not happy with your own behavior or feel like you are not successful. Consider your goals. How would you behave in your ideal future? Imagine yourself living through situations you currently find challenging as your ideal future self. Dream yourself as you want to be in vibrant detail. Remember these visions, and they may help you to make choices that forgo your immediate impulses and benefit you long-term, bringing you closer to the ideal self you imagine.

Brain Challenge #3
Enhancing Resiliency to New Threats and Chronic Stressors

Challenge Introduction

Let's consider the last time I (J.T.) tried to stick to a diet. I started Saturday morning and got myself off to a great start. I made it through the whole weekend eating nothing but small portions of healthful food every few hours. I was committed to my goal of losing five pounds, was excited about all the fresh local produce I was going to be eating and felt great after two days of success. I went to work Monday morning with my food for the workday all packed, sure that it would be easy to stick to my diet locked in my office with nothing but good things to eat in appropriate amounts. I got to work, made myself a cup of tea, and started to go through my e-mail. First e-mail is a message from my boss in the national office. It is an absolute emergency. They need complicated data for a Congressional briefing by noon Eastern Standard Time, two hours from now, and my Californian programmers who know how to do the analysis won't be in for another hour and a half. I start to plan but stop to read another e-mail from a journal that has been reviewing a paper I submitted four months ago. The e-mail contains ten pages of frankly mean and not very constructive criticism about my last two years of work. I feel my anxiety rising. Maybe I would feel better if I have a snack. Next thing I know I've eaten all my food for the workday and it's not even 8 am. What was I thinking? What happened to my well-planned diet? How is staying fat going to help me when I'm at risk of failing at work and being rejected by the scientific community? Why did I turn traitor on all my long-term goals the second I was stressed?

Feeling stressed and helpless increases the value of all immediate reinforcement opportunities. Stress makes feeling better urgent, and more important than competing long-term plans. Developing resilience to stress can increase your ability to make good long-term choices and stick to your health goals. In Challenge #3, we will explain how stress can ruin even the most well intended plan and encourage you to act impulsively. In Chapter 3.1, we first describe stress and what triggers the stress response then discuss how stress increases your need for immediate gratification. In Chapter 3.2, we investigate why some people are more vulnerable to stress-driven impulsive relief-seeking. In Chapter 3.3, we discuss ways that you can become more resilient to stress. Patterning and pacing your activities can help. Moreover, learning that you have control, or the ability to keep yourself safe in the presence of stressors in your life, can buffer the effects of stress exposure.

Chapter 3.1: How Does Stress Increase Your Need for Immediate Gratification?

Why do we have a stress response?
Stress is a physiological response to being threatened. Situations that endanger your well-being alert your brain about the potential need to respond. When things in your environment or your physiological state indicate that your well-being may be at risk, your brain activates a series of protective mechanisms. We refer to these mechanisms as a stress response. This stress response alters your physiology and behavior to focus on addressing this immediate danger at the expense of other goals, thus ensuring that you prioritize getting yourself to safety.

This stress response changes hormone levels to redistribute energy to body systems needed to respond or escape. Body systems that focus on longer-term goals, like growing bigger and stronger, repairing damaged tissues, and having children, are slowed down to divert energy to these "fight or flight" systems until the threat is addressed. This part of the stress response is supposed to be a temporary and short-term change in response to an acute stressor and can have wide-reaching and negative effects on your health when stress becomes chronic (see Robert Sapolsky's *Why Zebras Don't Get Ulcers,* 2004 for a very enjoyable and accessible description of this stress response and its health consequences). When long-term maintenance and growth systems are neglected by chronic focus on emergencies, physical and mental health problems may develop.

In parallel with these hormonal changes, your brain activates circuits that make you seek immediate relief from the threat. Among other things, these circuits talk to your limbic reward circuit, including the nucleus accumbens, as described previously, and the amygdala, a structure involved in the rapid detection of threat even before one is conscious that a threat exists. When you are threatened, the brain decides that any opportunity to improve your well-being in the immediate moment is one you should take. Immediate rewards are prioritized over long-term goals. In the case of my diet, my lunch made me feel momentarily better when important people challenged me. This temporary relief was prioritized over my long-term goal of weight loss. The logic behind this brain response is simple. Why worry about the future when you are threatened now? If that threat is not addressed, there might not be a future. This logic is highly adaptive if the relief solves the problem. If I were stressed because I was starving, then eating my lunch would be a great response. If I was being attacked and I dropped what I was doing to run to safety that would also be helpful. *The problem is that stress prioritizes anything that will make you feel better right away, whether or not it actually eliminates the stressor.* Stress can make you drop your long-term goals, not to save your life, but for nothing greater than the fleeting feeling of calm offered by a quick treat or escape.

What triggers a stress response?
Truly threatening situations, like being attacked with a knife, nearing starvation, or being caught in the wilderness unprotected in a blizzard, will trigger this stress response. In these cases, it is obvious that this stress response is appropriate, helpful, and even crucial for your survival. However, many much more subtle and potentially threatening situations can

146

also trigger a stress response. Thus, having your boss give you a dirty look, getting stuck in traffic when you have an important meeting, speaking in public, or talking to someone you find attractive, can all also trigger a stress response. Moreover, very subtle changes in your bodily state will trigger a stress response. When you miss a scheduled meal, do not get enough sleep, let your blood glucose get too high or too low, or have your muscles work without enough oxygen, your brain will trigger a stress response. In these situations, you may not really be in any immediate danger, but your brain will start that same stress response just in case. Since such situations may occur every day or even multiple times a day, this can lead to chronic stress and thus consistent focus on short-term fixes rather than long-term plans. As we will describe later, most people learn to shut off the stress response when they feel they have control over these daily stressors. However, this chronic focus on the now can sabotage our attempts to improve our futures.

To assess whether your typical stress symptoms and their triggers, see Exercise 3A (page 159).

How chronic stress can alter your reward system to favor immediate gratification: The serotonin connection

Many of the behavioral effects of stress, such as depressive behaviors and altered response to reward, have been associated with the brain chemical serotonin. Notably, selective serotonin reuptake inhibitors (SSRIs), a class of medications that effectively treat depression and PTSD, modify the brain's serotonin system to produce their therapeutic effect.

Where in the brain are these serotonin neurons located? Neurons in the dorsal raphe nucleus (DRN) provide the majority of serotonin released in brain regions that regulate stress-related behaviors. The DRN is a cluster of neurons in the brainstem that connects with many other parts of the brain, including the limbic reward system and the prefrontal cortex (see Figure on next page for further details).

The DRN is activated by a variety of stressors. For example, the DRN is activated during social defeat where an animal's territory is invaded and an aggressive intruder defeats it, during inescapable pain, and when an animal is forced to swim without an escape route (Abumaria et al., 2006; Kirby et al., 2007). Note that in all the models, the animal is forced to endure social or physical threats, no matter how the animal responds to the situation. They have absolutely no control over their stressors. After experiencing these stressors and DRN activation, animals exhibit more submissive, helpless, and defensive behaviors, and increased anxiety (e.g., Cooper et al., 2008, Christianson et al., 2008). For example, DRN activity following these stressors has been shown to reduce social exploration in young rodents, indicating that they are more anxious in social situations (Christianson et al., 2008), and enhance anxiety-related startle responses (Meloni et al., 2008).

The same principle applies to humans. When stress activates the DRN, we become anxious, defensive, and less likely to stand up for ourselves. We become very sensitive to pain and will do things to make it go away quickly. This might include taking potentially addictive drugs, disengaging from our lives and interests, or doing directly self-destructive behaviors to activate our bodies' inner pain control systems.

FIGURE: Projections of the serotonin neurons in the DRN

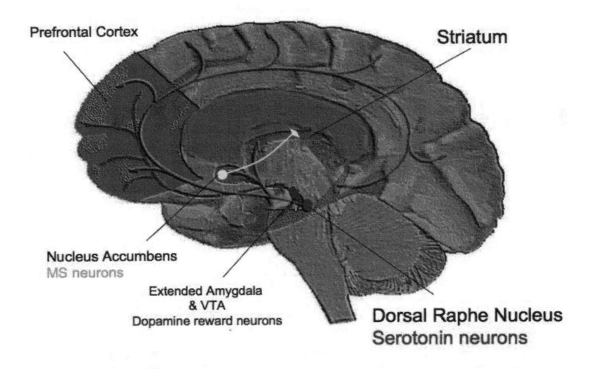

Legend: The dorsal raphe nucleus (DRN) is located in the brain stem, an area involved in basic functions such as attention, arousal, and control of autonomic functions such as breathing and blood pressure. The serotonin neurons in the DRN (in black) project to a variety of brain regions involved in reward learning, habit formation and habit inhibition including the nucleus accumbens and the prefrontal cortex.

We can now alter activity in the DRN and reduce these effects using SSRI medications. The way these medications modify the serotonin system may seem confusing at first. These drugs increase the level of serotonin by blocking the reuptake of released serotonin by the serotonin neurons. This, in turn, decreases the activity of the serotonin neurons because of their built-in feedback system: when they detect that serotonin levels are high then they decrease their activity. Thus, giving drugs that increase serotonin levels reduces the stress effects in DRN serotonin neurons. In other words, SSRIs reduce symptoms of anxiety and depression, at least in part, by blocking activity in the DRN.

How a sense of control over stressors prevents the effects of chronic stress
To help prevent everyday situations that are not really a threat from causing chronic stress, our brains have a circuit that can stop these potential stressors from making our reward circuits more focused on immediate gratification. This circuit is driven by the ventromedial prefrontal cortex, a part of the brain that may give us a "sense of control" over events in our lives. Some very important experiments in rats have demonstrated how this circuit is

activated and what it does, and recent imaging studies confirm that these lessons from stressed out rats can be applied to the human rat race.

Steve Maier and Linda Watkins have studied the psychological factors that determine the impact of stressors on behavior and physiology as well as the underlying brain mechanisms involved in influencing those states. They discovered that the degree of "control" which animals can exert over a stressor determines whether the stress will alter the brain and behavior. Exposure to uncontrollable stressors (e.g., a predator) sensitizes the serotonin neurons in the DRN, resulting in exaggerated release of serotonin in the areas of the brain to which the DRN neurons project.

Exposure to stressors can increase the expected value of immediate rewards (as in Challenge #1) and encourage reward-seeking behaviors. For example, stress is known to alter addictive reactions to drugs of abuse. This research team has shown that uncontrollable stressors, but not controllable ones, exaggerate the rewarding properties of opioid drugs such as morphine (Rozeske et al., 2009). In addition, they found that this effect is influenced by serotonin neurons in the DRN.

Maier and Watkins found that having control over a potential threat activates a medial prefrontal circuit that can turn off the DRN response. The researchers studied the effect of variable control on stress by setting up a system where rats would receive a shock to their tail to stress them (Maier et al., 2006). To study the difference between experiencing controllable and uncontrollable stressors, they connected rats in pairs so that they would both receive the exact same strength, pattern, and number of shocks. They gave both rats a wheel that they could spin. For one rat, spinning the wheel would turn off the shock. For the other rat, spinning the wheel would do nothing. Thus, both rats would get the same shocks, but only one rat would have control over the shocks.

The rats showed very different effects on their stress response and behavior. The rat whose wheel did not stop the shocks displayed classic signs of stress, such as anxiety, submissive behavior, and weight changes. In contrast, the rat that received the same shocks, but had control over when the shocks stopped, exhibited none of these signs of stress. Having control over the stressor prevented the shocks from causing these stress-related changes in behavior and physiology. This occurred even though the two rats experienced the exact same shocks. When the rat recognized that he had the power to turn off the shock, he realized that it did not actually pose a threat. Thus, the prefrontal cortex turned off the stress response.

Maier and colleagues then combined this shock stressor paradigm with a technique that turns on or off small brain regions to investigate exactly how having control over stress alters the response to stress. They found that activation in the ventromedial prefrontal appears to be both necessary and sufficient for control over the shocks to prevent the effects of chronic stress. Turning off the medial prefrontal cortex eliminated the control effects even when the rat actually had control over the shocks. Likewise, turning on the medial prefrontal cortex mimicked the control effects even when the rat did not actually have control over the shocks. Moreover, this part of the brain appears to be activated when a rat is given control over a stressor.

Interestingly, once a rat had been trained that it had control over the shock stress, the rat started to generalize its sense of control to other stressors. The rat acted as though it had control (i.e., does not show a stress response) even when the animal did not actually have control over the new stressor. Once a rat experienced a sense of control over certain stressful situations, it started to activate ventromedial prefrontal cortex in response to a variety of stressors, thus preventing the negative effects of stress exposure. In other words, when the rat experienced control over potentially dangerous elements of its world, it stopped viewing difficult situations it encountered as immediate threats. Supporting the hypothesis that humans respond similarly to stress and control, Kerr and colleagues (2012) studied the response of the ventromedial prefrontal cortex of people who feared snakes to anticipation of viewing videos of snakes, when the viewer did versus did not have control over whether the video played. Just as in the rats, ventromedial prefrontal cortex activity was associated with perceived control over viewing of the snake video, and this activity was linked to decreased activity in amygdala and other brain regions involved in stress and fear response. Together, this suggests that developing a sense of control over our own stressors may help protect us from responding to everyday stressors, even those that objectively are not within our control (e.g., traffic or bad weather). The experience of control over a stressor, through activity initiated by ventromedial prefrontal cortex activity, can make you subsequently resilient to future stressors and unpleasant events (Maier, 2015).

FIGURE: The effects of controllable versus uncontrollable stress

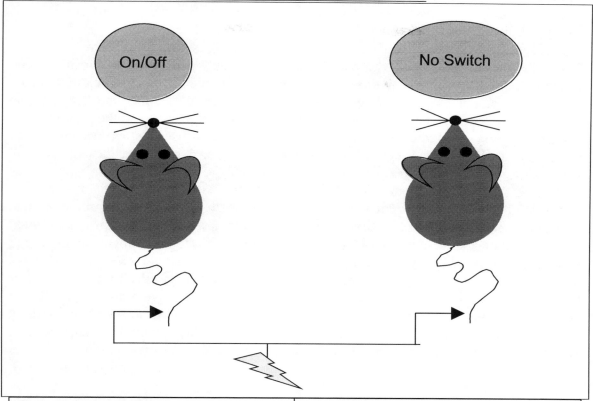

Control over stressor	No control over stressor
Little to no effect of stress exposure	Fear conditioning – *develop fear and avoidance of similar situations* Learned helplessness – *stop making efforts to solve the problem causing the stress* Exaggerated drive for immediate reward – *overvalue things that provide short-term relief or reward* Neglect of physiological responses that maintain long-term health and growth – *increase risk of chronic diseases and health problems, such as diabetes, heart disease, depression, cancer, and infertility*

Legend: Maier and colleagues (2006) experimental paradigm for determining the effects of controllable versus uncontrollable stress. The effects of this exposure are summarized in the table above. Pairs of rats were connected such that both would receive the exact same intensity and duration of tail shock. In addition, they were both provided with a wheel. For one rat, the wheel acted as a switch to turn off the tail shock. This rat was shocked, but was able to turn off the shock at will. For the second rat, the wheel was inactive and had no effect on the tail shock. This second rat was thus shocked exactly the same amount as the first rat but did not have control over when the shocks were turned off.

Posttraumatic stress: Horror frozen in memory

The effects of control over stress observed in rats are also observed in studies of people with posttraumatic stress disorder (PTSD).

PTSD may occur in people who experience or observe a terrifying or horrible event. Greater chronicity and severity of stress may increase the likelihood of developing PTSD after a trauma. For example, an estimated 31% of Vietnam veterans and 20% of Iraq veterans developed symptoms of PTSD (National Institute of Health and the friends of the National Library of Medicine, 2009). Rape, torture, natural disasters, car accidents, and other traumatizing events produce PTSD in a proportion of the people exposed, resulting in an estimated 7.7 million people with PTSD in the US.

PTSD is characterized by symptoms including: 1) feeling jumpy or on guard against impending threats or danger (hypervigilance), 2) avoiding situations or things that remind you of the traumatizing event (avoidance), 3) being unable to stop thinking about the event, oftentimes having nightmares about it (re-experiencing), and 4) feeling disconnected from people and your environment (numbing). People with a history of childhood abuse or neglect seem particularly vulnerable to developing persistent symptoms of PTSD. In addition to these symptoms, people with PTSD have been shown to have substantially greater than normal risk of developing other co-existing disorders, including substance and alcohol use problems, obesity, cardiovascular and metabolic disorders, and chronic pain (Ryder et al., 2018; Vieweg et al., 2007; Perkonigg et al., 2009; Defrin et al., 2008; Shipherd et al., 2007; Brady et al., 2000).

Notably, behavioral risk factors for all these co-existing disorders center around compulsive behaviors to feel better immediately. People with these co-existing disorders may tend to use substances and alcohol to feel better in the next few minutes, even though it makes them feel worse a few hours later and causes additional problems. They may eat a whole bag of cookies because they taste good for a couple of minutes, even though doing so may make them feel sick 20 minutes later and gain weight for life. They may eat processed food filled with sugar and fat rather than fresh fruits, vegetables, and grains. They may rest or take pain killers the minute they feel pain, even though they need to exercise and get involved in life to help recover from their injury. In all these disorders, the afflicted individuals choose short-term relief with long-term consequences over longer-term benefits. These behavior patterns may result from over-active reward circuits, stemming from under-activation of the circuits in the prefrontal cortex that cancel the impact of stress-related activation of the DRN.

Interestingly, a series of brain imaging studies have shown that potentially threatening stimuli evoke a pattern of brain responses in people with PTSD similar to that observed in the rats given uncontrollable tail shocks. As noted, the amygdala, a "watch dog" of the brain, is critically involved in sensing threat or danger, such as that signaled by a fearful voice or face. Researchers examined the response to fearful versus happy faces in trauma-exposed men with and without PTSD (Shin et al., 2005). Using fMRI, they found that the men with PTSD showed greater activity in the amygdala and lesser activity in the medial prefrontal cortex when shown fearful faces. Moreover, a greater severity of reported PTSD symptoms was related to a greater decrease in activity in the medial prefrontal cortex when viewing fearful faces. A similar pattern of brain activity was found using PET to compare responses to personal trauma stories in combat-exposed veterans with and without PTSD (Liberzon et al., 2003).

Recall that the amygdala also works as part of the limbic reward circuit to identify the importance or value of an opportunity to respond habitually, and greater activity in the amygdala indicates that you highly value and have an exaggerated drive to escape from terrifying situations. Meanwhile, the medial prefrontal cortex is activated when you feel you have control over stressors, and a lack of activity likely indicates that you feel like you do not have the ability to keep yourself safe in scary situations. Thus, when you have a lack of control over stressors, you will have a robust stress response that increases your drive for short-term reward when exposed to potential threats. The finding that the severity of PTSD symptoms is related to a lack of activity in the medial prefrontal cortex when a person is in distressing situations suggests that lack of activity here may be partially responsible for the disorder (Maier et al., 2006). A meta-analysis of findings from imaging studies of patients before and after they were treated with effective psychotherapies for PTSD found that PTSD symptom improvement following treatment was associated with reduced amygdala and increased prefrontal cortex activity (Malejko et al., 2017). Interestingly, some early studies also suggest that transcranial magnetic stimulation (TMS), which uses magnets to induce brain activity, shows promise as a treatment for PTSD when focused on the medial prefrontal cortex (Clark et al., 2015). This emerging research suggests that both current psychological treatments for PTSD and novel TMS treatments may effectively reduce symptoms of PTSD by increasing activity in prefrontal cortex to reduce stress and threat-related responses mediated through the amygdala – mimicking the effect of providing a sense of control over the stressor observed in rat experiments.

Just like the rats that had no control over when and how long they were shocked, people with PTSD have full-blown responses to threatening situations, even when they are not realistically in danger. This may lead to the exaggerated fearful and escape responses that are part of the disorder and may explain the co-occurrence of other disorders that include compulsive searching for immediate gratification. Extrapolating from the rat studies, these findings also suggest that people who do not learn that they have control over threats or stressors in their environment may be at greater risk of developing PTSD.

How great is your sense of control over the stressors in your life?
A useful way to consider a person's sense of control over what happens to them is their "locus of control", or their belief about what causes good or bad things to happen to them. People who tend to believe that they have control over what happens to them have an internal locus of control. Presumably, like the rat with the wheel that turned off the shocks, people with an internal locus of control have learned that decisions and actions they make can change what happens to them. In contrast, people who tend to believe that an outside power, such as a god, the environment, or fate, controls what happens to them have an external locus of control; they have learned that good or bad things happen to them regardless of what they do.

Many studies have examined the impact of having an internal versus external locus of control on changing health behaviors. In general, having an internal locus of control has been shown to be beneficial for changing health behavior when other factors for health behavior change are in place. For example, having an internal locus of control seems to be helpful if you: 1) understand and believe in the connection between the behavior and health outcomes, and 2) believe you are able to achieve the behavior (i.e., have self-efficacy for that behavior).

Locus of control influences health-related behavior in clients with chronic disorders. Cancer clients with an internal locus of control were more likely to take healthful steps that prevented recurrence of the cancer (Park & Gaffey, 2007), and having an internal locus of control predicted better attendance at dietitian visits for clients with diabetes (Spikmans et al., 2003). Having an external locus of control explained one-third of the association between experiencing socioeconomic adversity early in life and developing depression by age 18 (Culpin et al., 2015). Although locus of control is not the only factor influencing behavior, these studies suggest that people who believe that they can influence what happens to them are more motivated to try to change their behavior and more successful in their attempts to change. To some extent, this finding may seem obvious. Of course, people who think that their decisions change what happens to them are more likely to change their decisions to try to change their health. However, the rat research on controllability of stressors both gives us insight into how someone might develop an internal versus external locus of control and also helps explain how an internal locus of control might make behavior change easier. A sense of control over what happens to you, by increasing your resilience to stress, can reduce drive for immediate relief and thus allow you to make decisions that are more aligned with your long-term goals rather than your short-term desires. To assess your own locus of control for health in general (Forms A/B) or for a specific health condition (Form C), check out the Multidimensional Health Locus of Control (MHLC) Scales created by health researchers at Vanderbilt University: https://nursing.vanderbilt.edu/projects/wallstonk/

In review, the serotonin-driven dorsal raphe nucleus (DRN) plays an important role in overvaluing quick fixes during times when we feel threatened. Chronic activation of the DRN can lead to learned helplessness and stress-related disease. Further, the effectiveness of SSRIs for treating mood disorders may relate to their effect on serotonin activity in the DRN. The ventromedial prefrontal cortex can prevent activation of the DRN during stress, thereby preventing the negative effects of stress on health-related choices and chronic disease. The ventromedial prefrontal cortex is activated when one feels that they are in control of the stressors in one's life, and PTSD is a disorder that includes an impairment of ventromedial prefrontal cortex activity and a sense of not having control over the stressors in one's life. It is therefore not surprising that SSRIs are effective as a treatment for PTSD (Ipser, et al., 2006). Lastly, an individual's locus of control – whether he believes what he does can change what happens to him or that it depends on external factors beyond his control – also plays a role in how he responds to stress.

Chapter 3.2: The Effects of Early Childhood Experience on Stress Systems

The environment that you experience early in life can substantially affect how you respond to stress later in life. Early experiences and exposure to stress have lifelong consequences. Stress in early childhood contributes to childhood obesity and the subsequent risk of type 2 diabetes mellitus, hypertension, and coronary artery disease. Even high-quality health care is unable to eliminate the stress-mediated and significant disparities in health outcomes that stem from socioeconomic and racial inequalities (Marmot et al., 1984).

The brain is the primary organ that perceives stress, and chronic stress can leave an enduring effect on the hippocampus and prefrontal cortex. The effects of stress on these brain regions have enduring consequences for susceptibility to chronic anxiety, aggression, mental inflexibility and poor short-term memory.

Prolonged stress is associated with a reduction in the volume of the human hippocampus (Shonkoff et al., 2009). Further, chronic conditions such as diabetes, major depression, Cushing's disease and posttraumatic stress disorder can all impair the human hippocampus' ability to regulate short-term memory. The prefrontal cortex has been found to be smaller in individuals who self-report a lower socioeconomic status and in individuals with major depression. Changes in activation of the prefrontal cortex are also related to stress. Functioning in the prefrontal cortex can be impaired, at least temporarily, by increases in stress, such as that observed in medical students studying for their board examinations. Activation of the prefrontal cortex can lead to a sense of impending danger and increase blood pressure.

What prepares us for stress: The stress hormone cortisol

Adult conditions such as heart disease, stroke, diabetes, and cancer were once regarded as the result of adult behavior and lifestyles; however, advances in the understanding of the effect of cumulative exposure to stressful experiences, including prenatal events and traumatic childhood events, have made it abundantly clear that these disorders have childhood roots. Contributing to all these chronic conditions is the hormone associated with stress: cortisol. This hormone, while crucial for adaptively preparing us for fight-or-flight survival responses in the wake of tangible stressors, can also drive body systems into unsustainable states that wear out these systems and lead to damage over time. Cortisol endangers the hippocampus, making these neurons vulnerable to damage during otherwise survivable moments such as brief oxygen deprivation or seizures. Cortisol also suppresses the immune system, which can be beneficial for preventing acute inflammation following injury; however, chronic immune suppression leads to chronic immune-related disorders. Chronic elevation of cortisol is associated with narrowing the arteries supplying the heart and brain, and with hypertension, leading to both an increased risk of myocardial infarction and stroke (Sapolsky, 2004).

This basic stress-response mechanism developed to aid survival in an age of famine and scarcity, but now, in a time of plenty, causes disease by encouraging people to overeat to add to their fat storage and protect against the potential risk of insufficient food. Chronic stress and excessive cortisol activity leads to the accumulation of fat, especially at the midline (belly), which in turns greatly increases the risk of developing insulin insensitivity and type 2 diabetes. Onset of obesity and type 2 diabetes is occurring at earlier and earlier ages in our stressful society.

The enduring effects of maternal anxiety and separation

Research with animal models shows how the stressfulness of one's early environment influences how one's stress system develops and responds later in life. A key component of this environmental effect is the level of anxiety and type of care behaviors that one's mother shows early in one's life. If your mother acts highly stressed when you are young, you will develop exaggerated stress responses. Your response to stress adapts to match your mother's assessment of the stability and safety of your early environment. Because of this process, you tend to inherit your mother's reactions to stress. This inheritance is not genetic, but mediated through your early experiences with your mother.

Research on the effects of mothering style on children's stress resilience, or the ability to be healthful even in challenging conditions, has been beautifully reviewed by Champagne and Meaney (2001). Most studies of the effect of early environment have used a rodent model where newborn pups are removed from their mother for a short (15 minute) or long (usually hours) period each day. When the pups are only removed briefly, it is referred to as "neonatal handling", and when they are removed for a longer period of time, it is referred to as "maternal separation".

Interestingly, neonatal handling and maternal separation tend to have opposite effects on stress responsiveness and adult response to immediate rewards such as drugs of abuse. Neonatal handling reduces stress responsiveness, anxiety behavior and drug and alcohol use later in life. In short, rats removed from their mother for about 15 minutes a day become resilient to stress and less driven to obtain immediate rewards such as drugs or an escape from scary situations. Maternal separation increases these same behaviors. Rats removed from their mother for longer periods of time each day become more reactive to stress, showing larger, more prolonged stress responses and greater drive for immediate rewards or relief.

Maternal separation alters the development of the medial prefrontal cortex, a key brain region that we have described as critically involved in reducing stress effects when we feel in control. Specifically, maternal separation leads to changes in development of inhibitory neurons and changes in connections from serotonin and dopamine neurons in the medial prefrontal cortex (Helmeke et al., 2008; Braun et al., 2000), increases reward-seeking with preference for places where the rat was previously given opioid drugs such as morphine (Michaels & Holtzman, 2008), increases self-administration of alcohol and cocaine when the rats are adults (Moffett et al., 2007; Roman & Nylander, 2005; Francis & Kuhar, 2008), and increases response to a painful tail pinch, showing that these rats are more driven to escape from stressful situations (Brake et al., 2004). Maternally separated rats cope with social defeat by showing more passive or submissive behaviors and fewer proactive coping strategies (Gardner et al., 2005).

Differences between brief versus long maternal separation

So, what is the difference between repeated brief separations versus long separations from one's mother? Why would a little time away from your mother make you more resilient but a longer time away make you more vulnerable to stress? It turns out that when pups are briefly removed and then returned to the cage, most mother rats greet their returned pups by fawning over them, licking and grooming them and giving them protected time to breast feed. Thus, the brief separation gains the rat pups extra attention from their mothers and makes them more resilient to stress. In contrast, when the pups are removed for longer periods it means more time away from mom and less attention. With longer separations, the pups receive so much less attention during the separation that a bit of extra grooming upon return cannot make up for the time away. This suggests that the level of care and attention the pups receive from their mothers might alter how they respond to stress later in life.

To test this possibility, researchers used natural differences in the attentiveness of mothers to examine the relationship between amount of licking and grooming and later stress response without actually removing any of the pups from the cage. Pups raised by mothers who were highly attentive and naturally licked and groomed their pups a lot were more stress resilient, just like those who had been exposed to neonatal handling. Pups raised by mothers who were not very attentive and ignored or avoided the pups a lot, were less stress resilient and extra responsive to stress as adults, just like the pups who had been exposed to maternal separation. Notably, when the pups grew up and had pups of their own, they tended to mother just like they had been mothered. If they had received a lot of attention, they did a lot of licking and grooming. If they had received less attention, they in turn paid less attention to their pups. Mothering style appears to be passed down from generation to generation.

Does this mean that mothering style is genetic? It turns out that it is not. If you cross-foster the pups so those born to less attentive mothers are raised by more attentive mothers and vice versa, then the pups mimic their foster mother and not their birth mother. In other words, if pups born to less attentive mothers were raised by very attentive mothers, they grew up to be resilient to stress and very attentive to their own pups (Huot et al., 2004; Champange & Meaney, 2001). Moreover, a study in monkeys showed that changing environmental conditions can affect mothering styles. If changes in the environment make it harder for mothers to care for their young ones, then the mothers pay less attention to their children and these children then grew up to be more anxious and show signs of stress (Rosenblum et al., 1994). Just by varying how hard the mothers had to search to find food, the researchers changed both the mothers' ability to dote on their babies and their babies' later responses to stress. Growing up with a mother who is stressed all the time, either because the environment is difficult or because the mother was trained to be anxious and highly reactive to stress when she was young, will encourage your brain to respond more to stress and be more focused on short-term choices.

How do you escape your past?

Is there anything you can do as an adult to make your stress system less responsive if you did grow up in a stressful environment or with an anxious mother? We do not know if you can reverse the changes in the brain that encourage larger responses to stress. But you can certainly pay extra attention to developing the other redundant systems that dampen the effects of stress. For example, you can learn to attend to and recognize your control over stressors to better activate your medial prefrontal cortex. This perception of control will decrease the impact of the stress. You can also learn to recognize, make use of, or increase opportunities in your environment to strengthen the MS neurons in your nucleus accumbens (see Challenge #2). As we previously described, this increased exposure to opportunities for immediate reward will reduce your drive to respond to short-term rewards, and make it easier to consider longer-term goals.

Increasing opportunities for reward can reduce the effects of early life neglect on stress response and behavior. With the rodent models, enriching the cage environment of pre-teen rats that had been "maternally separated" as pups normalized their stress response and reduced their anxiety behaviors when they were adults (Francis et al., 2002). Notably, these changes in stress response and behavior occur without changing the effects of "maternal separation" in the brain. In other words, the brain changes that occurred as a result of the "maternal separation" were still apparent in the adult rats after environmental enrichment. While adult enrichment did not erase the developmental changes produced by less attentive mothering, it did correct the body's response to stress and reduce anxiety behaviors. The neurobiological "memory" and stress vulnerability from early stress were still there, but the brain compensated for them and they no longer caused unhealthful effects on the body or behavior.

From a public health perspective, we can help future children grow up to be resilient to stress by supporting programs that reduce stress on mothers and give them more time to attend to their babies. Observations suggest that mothering style in humans is similarly related to stressful environments. For example, a study of mothers in the WIC program found that those that reported greater levels of stress, depression or anxiety fed their children in a less attentive, supportive manner (Hurley et al., 2008). While it has not been directly tested, we would expect that better maternity leave policies and programs to ensure that new mothers have food, shelter and support would reduce their stress, increase their attention to their children, and decrease later stress in their children.

Chapter 3.3: How We Can Develop Greater Stress Resilience

Since stress can sabotage our ability to focus on long-term goals, finding ways to avoid stress can make it easier to stick to healthful behavior plans. While obviously you cannot stop all your daily activities to avoid many stressors, there are several relatively easy things you can do to greatly reduce stress in your life. We describe three stress control techniques that have been successfully used in psychological interventions to facilitate behavior change.

Scales to assess the magnitude of life events that produce stress emphasize that life changes can create many challenges. At the top of the list of stressful events are the death of a spouse or child, followed by divorce and marital separation. Positive events can also be stressful, including an impending marriage, marital reconciliation, and retirement. Increasing the predictability of stressors or our control over them can improve our ability to manage stress. The techniques explained below can increase your ability to experience a greater sense of control over important events in your daily schedule and overall life.

Pacing, scheduling, and self-care: The sleep connection

Our bodies and brains do their best to predict when we will eat, sleep, be active or rest. This allows our bodies to prepare for these events so that they produce less change in our physiology and thus less stress. For example, if our brains expect a meal to come soon, they can plan and release insulin to ensure that our cells are ready to absorb the sugar we eat as soon as the meal is eaten. This prevents this sugar from floating around in our blood where it might react with proteins and trigger inflammation. The easiest way for our bodies to know what is coming is for us to follow a regular schedule, especially for sleep.

Not following a regular schedule has been associated with health risks, including premature death, mood disorders, learning problems, cancer, and reproductive dysfunction (Evans & Davidson, 2015). This has been studied in shift workers, whose inconsistent schedules lead to greater rates of sleep disturbances and altered eating patterns. Studies have found that shift workers, especially those with night work, have higher rates of gastrointestinal problems such as irregular bowel movements, dyspepsia, heartburn, abdominal pain, flatulence, chronic gastritis, gastroduodenitis, and peptic ulcer (Costa, 1996). In addition, some studies have suggested that shift workers also have higher rates of cardiovascular problems, such as hypertension, angina, myocardial infarction, and other heart disease, but these are less conclusive.

Additionally, not following a regular sleep schedule may lead to poor decision-making. For example, sleep deprivation changes the way the brain, including the ventromedial prefrontal cortex, makes decisions in a gambling task (Venkatraman et al., 2007). Specifically, sleep deprivation increased activation in the nucleus accumbens and made it more sensitive to risky decisions. This suggests that lack of sleep exaggerated the value of immediate rewards. At the same time, sleep deprivation made the prefrontal cortex less sensitive to losses, thus reducing avoidance of losses and increasing the likelihood for risky behavior. Both changes would encourage higher-risk, short-term decisions at the potential expense of longer-term benefit. Similar effects are observed during food deprivation, when people are more likely to choose an unhealthful (junk food) versus a healthful snack (fruit) when they were hungry (hours after lunch) versus not (immediately after lunch) (Read & Van Leeuwen, 1998). A simulated night shift caused people to favor high-fat foods at breakfast (Cain et al., 2015). Again, this is consistent with people making more short-term decisions when their bodies are stressed.

Habitual lack of sleep has been associated in some epidemiological studies with becoming overweight or obese (Marshall et al., 2008; Patel & Hu, 2008). These findings are particularly strong in children (Magee & Hale, 2012). Presumably, this is because being over-tired is a stressor, and people tend to over-eat while stressed. Partial loss of sleep (i.e., sleeping 5-6 hours instead of 7-8) can disrupt a variety of hormone levels, disturbing maintenance of safe levels of glucose in the bloodstream and altering levels of the appetite hormones leptin and gherlin to favor increased hunger (Knutson & Van Cauter, 2008). These hormonal disruptions might not only increase the risk of weight gain, but also the risk of developing Type II diabetes. Notably, associations between sleeping for less than 5 hours a night and developing diabetes have been observed (Gangwisch et al., 2007). Young adults who frequently interrupted sleep with smartphone use, slept 48 minutes less on average and had higher body mass index than those with fewer nighttime interruptions (Rod et al., 2018). Among overweight or obese dieters on a targeted 600 calorie per day reduction in consumption, longer sleep duration and higher sleep quality predicted greater fat loss over the 15 to 24 week program (Chaput & Tremblay, 2012). A shift towards risky, short-term decision-making when sleep-deprived may have long-term consequences for health, potentially contributing to obesity and metabolic disorders, and making weight loss more difficult. While good long-term studies still need to be done to prove this hypothesis, we would expect that fixing one's schedule to allow for sufficient rest and sleep should reduce risk for a wide variety of problems related to making short-term decisions focused on immediate gratification.

<u>WARNING: Do not let consistency turn into monotony</u>

One common pitfall in trying to develop a consistent schedule of healthful practices is confusing regularity with repetition. Doing the exact same thing every day is boring. Very few people can do the same thing over and over without craving something new. Monotony will lead you back to unhealthful patterns simply for the thrill of novelty. The key here is that it is important to have a consistent pattern to your health behaviors, not repeat the same behaviors over and over. While it is good for you to eat at the same times everyday, it is important to add variety into what you eat. The consistent pattern will allow your body to be prepared for the work of digestion, and the novelty in your actual food choices will keep your life full of the variety and flavor that we all require to stay interested and challenged. Similarly, it is important to exercise consistently every day, so developing a stable schedule where you do some sort of physical activity at a set time each day will do wonders for your health. But if you try to walk on a treadmill in your living room everyday at 6 for an hour, there is a good chance that you will be bored to tears with exercise within a few weeks at best. Take that same idea of walking for an hour every evening and vary aspects like the setting, companionship, and pace, and you will find that the pattern brings new exciting challenges, relationships, and places to your life. Monday, hike through a park you have never explored. Tuesday, briskly walk through the mall with a friend you have not seen in a while. Wednesday, chase your kids (or your neighbors' kids) around the playground. Thursday, take a social dance class. You will still be exercising every day at 6 for an hour, but you won't suffer the déjà vu and misery from tedium that brings an end to so many well-intentioned attempts to develop patterns that promote wellness.

Because maintaining a consistent schedule is important for reducing stress, many successful behavioral interventions have included a focus on improving consistency in one's schedule. Cognitive Behavioral Therapy for Insomnia (CBT-I) has been developed to help reduce sleep disturbances and insomnia that can lead to sleep deprivation. CBT-I uses simple behavioral techniques to effectively reduce insomnia and normalize sleep patterns. These techniques include ensuring your bed is only associated with sleep, restricting sleep time and napping to ensure that you are tired at bedtime, relaxation training, reducing use of substances (e.g., caffeine, alcohol, sleep aids) and exercise shortly before bedtime, and using cognitive strategies to reduce anxiety about sleep and insomnia. These strategies help people make the most of the time they leave for sleep. CBT-I has been shown to be effective in randomized controlled trials and is strongly recommended for use as the initial treatment for chronic insomnia disorder in clinical practice guidelines (Qaseem et al., 2016, Schutte-Rodin et al., 2008; Morgenthaler et al., 2006). Even better, CBT-I techniques avoid the use of medications to induce sleep. Use of sleep medications can lead to greater sleep problems over the long-term. Digital versions of CBT-I have been developed and shown to reduce insomnia and related depression symptoms as well as traditional face-to-face CBT-I therapy (Lin et al., 2023) Digital CBT-I applications can make these effective treatments more accessible.

To assess your need for better sleep habits, see Exercise 3B (page 160).

The detrimental effects of overwork and sleep deprivation
Of course, treating insomnia and improving sleep efficiency will only solve sleep-deprivation-related stress problems if you give yourself enough time to sleep. In our fast-paced society, it is very common for people to convince themselves that they do not have time to sleep and must keep working when they should be resting. The unspoken assumption underlying these decisions to forgo rest and overwork is that one will be able to keep working effectively and get more done if they keep going. In many cases this assumption is wrong, and the extremes of this problem are obvious. Overworking can lead people to make bad decisions that at a minimum can be difficult and time-consuming to correct. Overworking can lead to injury that can take months to rehabilitate. Overworking can lead to mood disorders (e.g., depression) that can reduce productivity for weeks to months. Pushing yourself when you need rest can be dangerous and can lead to difficult-to-correct problems. Even when overwork problems are not as extreme and obvious they can lead to similar problems. Working too hard one day will tend to make you require more rest or be less efficient the next. Moreover, the consequences of overworking can be exaggerated if you have a chronic health condition.

Concerns about overwork have been formally recognized and incorporated into effective cognitive behavioral therapy programs for a variety of chronic health problems. These programs focus on teaching clients how to pace themselves and help them learn to recognize how much work they can do without worsening their disorder or becoming tired and inefficient. The therapist then helps the client design a work-rest plan that optimizes their ability to get things done and minimizes exhaustion and worsening of health as a result of work.

The concept that being unrested can worsen efficiency and safety is leading several industries to experiment with on-the-job naps to improve work quality and efficiency. A number of hospitals are encouraging nurses and physicians with long hours or inconsistent shifts to take sleep breaks in special designated rooms in an attempt to reduce medical errors and increase client safety. It has been recognized that the work requirements of nurses and medical residents and students can leave them extremely tired. Surveys of nurses and physicians have found frankly scary rates of self-reported fatigue-related errors and falling asleep while driving home. A survey of over 1300 junior physicians in New Zealand found 24% reported falling asleep driving home since becoming a doctor, and 42% recalled a fatigue-related clinical error in the past 6 months (Gander et al., 2007). Similarly, a survey of 70 physicians in the United States who were sometimes on call found 49% reported falling asleep while driving, with 90% of these dangerous "naps" occurring post-call (Marcus & Loughlin, 1996). Physicians working traditional shifts of longer than 24 hours were more likely to make a serious medical error or be injured in a car accident than those working shorter shifts. Compared to residents working 16-hour shifts, physicians working traditional shifts made 36% more serious medical errors and 300% more fatal medical errors (Lockley et al., 2007). In short, overworked physicians are a danger to themselves and others. While shorter shifts are obviously necessary to fully ameliorate the effects of overwork-related fatigue, even a brief nap during the shift has been shown to have benefits. One study looked at physicians and nurses working 12-hour night shifts who either did or did not take a nap at 3AM. Clinicians who napped only slept about 25 minutes on average, but showed some improvements in performance at 7:30AM (Smith-Coggins et al., 2006). Specifically, they had significantly fewer performance lapses, more quickly performed an intravenous insertion, showed less dangerous driving in a driving simulator, and reported less fatigue and sleepiness and more vigor.

While a short rest cannot completely compensate for an excessive work schedule, it does produce substantial and measurable improvement in both emotional state and behavior. By incorporating this concept in your life by adding sufficient time for rest to your day, you may reduce stress and decrease high-risk habitual or unplanned behaviors.

To work on pacing and developing better rest patterns, try Exercise 3C (page 161), Exercise 3D (page 163) and Exercise 3E (pages 165).

Pre-planning and problem-solving
As we discussed, potential threats are only stressful if we feel like the outcome of the situation is out of our control. In contrast, encountering a problem for which we have a solution is not stressful because we know what to do to keep ourselves safe and healthy. In fact, encountering problems that we can solve is rewarding. Just the idea that you can find a new way to solve your problems can be a means of temporarily relieving stress.

While the threat of the problem may activate our stress systems and turn on our DRN neurons, our sense of control over the situation can activate our medial prefrontal cortex and help negate the effects of the stress. Solving the problem will provide relief that is not only reinforcing but will generally make us feel good about ourselves. Challenging situations are good to experience, so long as we have a solution to keep ourselves safe and in balance. Healthful stress is stress over which we have a good deal of control; however, it may still have a level of uncertainty regarding the outcome. Can I hike this mountain? Can I beat my best time? Can I solve this problem? Avoiding stress does not mean avoiding situations where we might fail. It means setting yourself up such that failure does not put you in serious danger. It is okay not to make it to the top of the mountain, as long as you have a back-up plan that leaves you safe come nightfall.

But how do we ensure that we only run into problems that we know how to solve? Obviously, this is not completely possible. However, in most cases our environments are predictable enough that we can make reasonable guesses about the types of problems that we may run into in the near future. By walking through scenarios in our heads, we can usually identify the majority of problems that we may encounter in our day-to-day lives. With a little practice, we can imagine possible impending problems before we experience them. If we can accurately predict and imagine the problems we might soon experience, we can start to figure out and plan solutions in advance to either avoid the problem in the first place or remedy it quickly when it occurs.

Some effective stress management programs include a problem-solving component. People with poor problem-solving skills often have more difficulty coping with life challenges, and training in problem-solving skills can reduce stress in individuals or families dealing with a life-threatening disease. For example, six sessions of problem-solving skills training reduced the number and severity of difficulties experienced by women with breast cancer, as long as they had at least average problem-solving skills (Allen et al., 2002). Presumably those with poor problem-solving skills required a more intensive training.

While there are many ways to solve problems, having a simple standard strategy for addressing everyday challenges may encourage more deliberate and rational decision-making. The structure provided by training may be particularly useful for people with severe mental illnesses such as schizophrenia, and has been shown to improve functioning and even reduce symptoms in these populations (Barbieri et al., 2006, Liberman et al., 2001). These studies trained clients to use a simple six-step strategy for solving their problems, focusing on individual goals that they identified in the training sessions. These steps were:

1. Identify the specific problem and goal.
2. List all possible solutions.
3. Highlight the advantages and disadvantages of each solution.
4. Choose the best solution.
5. Plan how to carry out the solution.
6. Review your progress and change plan as needed.

This simple strategy may be helpful to anyone. Running through these simple steps to pre-plan responses to problems we anticipate in our day-to-day life may help us feel more prepared and in control as we encounter life's inevitable challenges. That increased sense of control should reduce our stress response and further prevent us from making impulsive choices. Adding a pre-emptive problem-solving routine to your mornings may be a simple way to decrease stress. We will talk about problem-solving and pre-planning solutions more in Challenge #5.

To practice problem-solving and pre-planning solutions, see Exercise 5A (page 223).

Relaxation

Exercises that use breathing, imagery, focused attention on bodily sensation, or meditation to reduce stress are components of Western and Eastern wellness programs, including cognitive behavioral therapies, mindfulness-based interventions, and comprehensive yogic practices. Such practices have been demonstrated to reduce immediate stress and improve mood within weeks of regular practice. For example, participants who received a single session of abbreviated progressive muscle relaxation significantly reduced heart rate, subjective feelings of stress and anxiety, and cortisol levels after the intervention compared to participants who sat quietly in a room for the same period of time (Pawlow & Jones, 2002). Five weeks of daily practice using progressive muscle relaxation produced relaxation states and increased levels of mental quiet and joy (Matsumoto & Smith, 2001). Similarly, a pilot study found that six weeks of daily practice of Sudarshan Kriya, a form of yogic breathing exercises, reduced self-reported anxiety, depression and stress and increased optimism (Kjellgren et al., 2007). Small trials suggest that using relaxation techniques can help some people correct compulsive stress-related habits such as binge eating at night. Twenty minutes of progressive muscle relaxation practice for a week tended to help people with night eating syndrome - a condition where people have trouble eating in the morning, eat more than half their calories after 6 in the evening, and have trouble falling or staying asleep - eat less at night (Pawlow et al., 2003; Vander Wal et al., 2015). Larger studies emphasize the broad benefits of relaxation exercises. A metaanalysis of twelve studies of progressive muscle relaxation for patients with cancer-related symptoms found significant benefits for anxiety, depression, fatigue, and quality of sleep (Wang et al., 2024). Likewise, a metanalysis of four studies in patients with COVID-19 found that progressive muscle relaxation reduced anxiety, depression, quality of life and COVID disease severity scores and improved sleep quality (Seid et al., 2023). Relaxation exercises tend to be used in combination with other interventions in trials of chronic disease care, and therefore effects of using these exercises alone has not been investigated sufficiently to quantify expected benefits for specific chronic disease or mental health problems. However, cognitive behavioral therapy and mindfulness-based programs that often include these exercises have been shown to be effective and are recommended as first-line treatments for a wide variety of conditions, including depression, anxiety, substance use disorders, chronic pain, and insomnia (e.g., Trafton & Gordon, 2008a; Hoffman et al, 2012; Hoffman and Gomez, 2017).

While a variety of relaxation techniques exist, they all share a focus on ending or counteracting physical responses to stress. Stress can cause you to tighten up your body, causing tension in your muscles. Stress can shorten your breathing, making it inefficient. It can cause your heart to race, and your skin to prickle. These physical reactions can make you feel even more threatened and lead you to panic or have dark thoughts about catastrophic consequences. When repeated regularly, these feelings and thoughts of threat and stress can contribute to chronic pain, depression, anxiety, and other mood disorders. These feelings and thoughts can even worsen physical health; for example, potentially worsening the symptoms of heart disease and diabetes. Your physical and emotional responses to stress can become stressors themselves, leading to chronic stress-related problems. Relaxation exercises help people learn to control and limit these physical and emotional reactions to stress. By learning to notice your feelings of stress, and using techniques to dampen these responses, you may recover more quickly from short-term stressful situations and break the cycle of chronic stress response.

To practice using simple relaxation techniques, try Exercise 3F (page 167).

Adopt a healthful whole foods diet

Diet and other exposures (e.g., pesticides, antibiotics) can change the composition of the gut microbiome and increase risk for chronic gut inflammation. Gut inflammation activates interoceptive circuits (i.e., neuronal systems designed to monitor your internal state for signs of illness, danger, or other needs to adapt) and will trigger a stress response in the brain. As discussed in detail in Food for Thought: Changing How We Feel By Changing How We Eat (Goehler, 2022), many common components of processed food can generate signals that the immune system recognizes as a sign of damage or infection. In response, the immune system will turn on inflammatory responses and send signals to the brain indicating that the gut is under threat, triggering a stress response. As we've discussed, in the short-term, this stress response may encourage impulsive behaviors, favoring immediate rewards over potentially greater longer-term benefits. With chronic consumption of processed food, gut inflammation and stress can become chronic, contributing not only to impulsive behaviors, but also chronic stress-related disease.

Processed food components can produce these damage or infection signals, which are referred to in scientific literature as pathogen-associated molecular patterns (PAMPs) or damage-associated molecular patterns (DAMPs). For example, some fats and proteins can become oxidized when cooked at high temperature or processed in other ways. These oxidized fats and proteins act as DAMPs and trigger inflammation. Frying or eating oils in processed foods can increase consumption of oxidized fats and cause inflammation, particularly when one's diet is also low in antioxidants, such as those found in colorful fruits and vegetables. Likewise, sugars can bind to proteins during cooking or processing of foods. When sugar is eaten when blood glucose is high, the sugar may bind to proteins in the blood or body. These sugar-modified proteins are called Advanced Glycation End-Products (AGEs) and also act as DAMPs. Additionally, the herbicide glyphosate has been shown to act as a PAMP and trigger inflammation in both gut and brain. Glyphosate is used widely in agriculture and may be residually present on many foods. Glyphosate is applied to wheat crops before harvest to encourage ripening. It has been hypothesized that wheat products may therefore tend to contain glyphosate residue, and that gut inflammation caused by the glyphosate on the wheat may be responsible for apparent gluten-sensitivity in persons who do not have Celiac disease (Barnett and Gibson, 2020).

Early studies suggest that diet can have significant impact on reward-related choices and impulsivity. As described previously, people with obesity have been shown to have lower than normal D2 dopamine receptor expression in reward circuits, suggesting that dopamine or reward deficiency may contribute to over-eating and/or poor diet. More recent studies emphasize that this relationship is bidirectional; Low D2 dopamine receptor in reward circuits may contribute to impulsive choices, potentially encouraging consumption of immediately rewarding junk food options, and consumption of high-fat or high-sugar junk food may lower D2 dopamine receptor expression in reward-circuits. For example, in a large longitudinal study of older adults receiving supportive interventions to encourage a healthful Mediterranean diet, baseline impulsivity measures were positively associated with instead eating an unhealthful, processed-food heavy Western diet over the 3-year study period. Impulsivity at the start of the study was also associated with reduced likelihood of eating in a pattern consistent with a Mediterranean diet, a healthful plant-based diet, or the Dietary Approaches to Stop Hypertension (DASH) diet (Gomez-Martinez et al., 2022). Thus, tendency to make impulsive choices may encourage on-going consumption of an unhealthful processed food diet. Conversely, rats put on a high-fat diet showed down-regulation of D2 dopamine receptor expression within 2 weeks (Barry et al., 2018). Likewise, rats fed the same number of daily calories as a high-fat or high-sugar diet for 8 weeks made more impulsive choices in a food task than rats fed a healthy rat chow over the same period (Steele et al., 2017). Specifically, rats on the high-fat and high-sugar diet were more likely to choose an immediate reward of 1 pellet of food than a 30-second delayed reward of 2 pellets in a free-choice task. So, eating a high-fat or high-sugar diet causes the sort of impulsive choices that encourage an unhealthful Western diet, creating a vicious cycle.

Positively, the solution to this cycle of processed-food related stress and impulsivity is to shift to a healthful diet that reduces gut inflammation and stress responses, and resets reward circuits. The best studied healthful diets of this kind are the Mediterranean diet and plant-based diets that minimize processed food consumption. These diets are centered around whole grains, fruits, vegetables, beans, nuts, seeds, and uncooked oils such as olive oil, and avoid foods that are highly processed or that contain added sugar. Both the Mediterranean and healthful plant-based diets avoid red meat, but the Mediterranean diet includes consumption of dairy, poultry, and eggs in moderation. Avoidance of processed foods prevents activation of inflammatory responses by minimizing exposure to PAMPS and DAMPS, and consumption of high-fiber foods supports healthful gut bacteria that dampen inflammatory responses. Together, this reduces stress, enabling us to focus on long-term goals rather than short-term reward and relief.

Starting on a healthful Mediterranean or plant-based diet can be intimidating for many, but increasing interest in these diets is making it easier. Even a few weeks to a month of eating a whole foods diet can alter interoceptive and reward-circuits in ways that make it easier to continue to avoid choosing processed, high-sugar, or high-fat options. So, setting yourself up for short-term success supports long-term success, even if the short-term efforts aren't fully sustainable. For example, there are now many food delivery services that will provide curated kits to quickly make healthful meals consistent with a Mediterranean or plant-based diet. While these services may be too expensive long-term for most people, clearing one's kitchen of processed food and using a food delivery service for a couple of months might be helpful for learning how to prepare healthful food options and reshaping one's brain and gut to prefer them. Transitioning to shopping for components of those pricey delivered meals may make one's new cooking skills practically sustainable. Alternatively, support to adopt healthful diets is available on-line. For example, Veganuary, a non-profit movement to encourage and support people interested in trying a vegan diet for a month, provides free cookbooks, meal plans, and coaching emails at Veganuary.com to support attempts to shift to a more healthful and planet-friendly diet. Numerous health care systems, food bloggers, and for-profit companies offer free recipes and guidance to support cooking in adherence with principles of a Mediterranean diet. In Chapter 6, we review the 5 challenges and walk through examples of how to apply them to support weight management. These may provide other ideas to support transitioning to a healthful lifestyle fueled on nutritious whole foods.

Chapter 3.4: Recognizing habit cycles

What is a habit cycle?
Sometimes habits can string together to create a vicious and unending cycle. Consider the afterworld plight of the Greek mythological character Sisyphus. Sisyphus was compelled to try to roll a boulder up a hill, an odd, but potentially relatable habit for those of us driven to strive towards near-impossible goals. His labor invariably led to fatigue or error before he reached the top, leading him to drop the rock, which then would roll back to its starting point, and trigger him to start pushing it back up again. Those two linked habits of trying to reach an impossible peak and quitting or failing when the task got too hard, created a futile and miserable cycle that he was doomed to repeat forever. Whenever habits link together to make the outcome of the behaviors also the trigger of habit chain, one can get stuck in a potentially tortuous and pointless cycle.

Sisyphus' story is easily translated to American diet culture. To try to achieve unrealistic weight or appearance goals, people attempt extreme diets to rapidly lose weight. Those diets lead to malnutrition, exhaustion, and hunger, which eventually drive the dieter to quit and revert to prior eating habits, regaining the weight, potentially along with some extra as insurance against another period of starvation. But habit cycles can take on many forms, often preventing recovery and turning a challenge into a chronic disease.

Problematic cycles of reinforced behaviors have been recognized in multiple models of chronic behavioral health conditions. In these cycles, a habit behavior tends to produce an outcome that becomes a trigger for the habit behavior. These cycles are easiest to recognize when the habit behavior is active. For example, once someone is drug dependent, drug use behaviors cause a dopamine signal that reinforces the drug use, but then, as the drug levels in the brain start to decrease, drug use later leads to drug withdrawal symptoms. Those drug withdrawal symptoms can often become a trigger for drug use, closing the habit cycle and leading to a self-perpetuating repetition of the drug use behaviors. Likewise, self-stigma about eating in response to negative emotions can close a habit cycle. Eating comfort food when you are emotionally down activates reward circuits. This could be an infrequent behavior that makes you feel better, in which case, the comfort food indulgence could be an effective solution. But, if you judge and berate yourself for the eating behavior, that self-judgement may cause additional negative emotions, which can retrigger eating for comfort. In this case, you've created a habit cycle. Negative emotions cause eating for comfort, which causes self-judgment and more negative emotions.

Alternatively, the cyclic habit behaviors may be avoidant in nature. The Fear Avoidance Model of Chronic Pain is a well described habit cycle of this sort (Vlaeyen and Linton, 2000). In this model, pain causes a habitual fear of injury. The fear of injury drives avoidance behaviors that prevent exercise, work, and other recovery activities that would resolve the chronic pain condition. Moreover, fear and anxiety intensify the perceived severity of pain. The increased pain drives increased fear and more avoidance. The Fear Avoidance Model of Chronic Pain explains why efforts to reduce fear and catastrophizing about perceived pain, rather than efforts to make the pain go away (e.g., with analgesics or avoidance) are most likely to resolve the chronic pain. Successfully addressing the fear and catastrophizing breaks the habit cycle and enables effective recovery from injury and reduces pain.

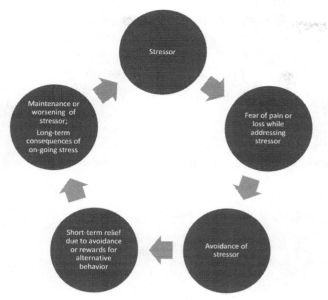

As illustrated above, responses that avoid rather than address a stressor in general can create a habit cycle. Fear of experiencing pain or loss of a comfort drives avoidant behavior that doesn't eliminate the problem or stressor. If that avoidant behavior is reinforced (e.g., by providing relief, eliminating challenging or anxiety-provoking situations, eliciting support from others) that will encourage repetition of that avoidant response. If the avoidant behavior or the lack of resolution of the stressor produces negative long-term consequences, the resulting negative consequences may lead to growing and increasingly severe disability.

Increasing severity of symptoms and dependence on the avoidant behavior may increase fear of engaging with recovery behaviors or trying something new. This can functionally leave patients stuck in harmful cycles, especially if making needed behavioral changes requires a period of experiencing pain, withdrawal, or loss of short-term reward on the path towards a much-improved state.

Learning to recognize and dissect habit cycles can help to identify the links that maintain the cycle. Once understood, it is often relatively easy to find and implement solutions that break the cycle. In the extreme dieting example, one simply needs to shift towards more realistic and incremental goals. For example, trying to eat more vegetables is likely to increase fiber intake and reduce daily calorie intake, supporting slow but progressive loss of weight. In the comfort food example, reducing self-stigma can help break the cycle. In the chronic pain example, reducing anxiety about anticipated or experienced pain can break the cycle. Guided and safe exposure to the feared experience could help with reducing the anticipatory anxiety. Supporting problem-solving and teaching active coping strategies may help a client address rather than avoid stressors. In each case, understanding the cycle can help to refocus behavior change efforts towards more realistic, achievable, and effective strategies.

Because there are so many possible drivers of habit cycles, there are not one size fits all approaches to resolving them. Reviewing the path of habit chains by breaking out both inherent and modifiable triggers and reinforcers can help to identify novel solutions to our own Sisyphean loops. Following, I've mapped out some examples of common stressors and avoidant responses and the sorts of modifiable psychosocial habits that might maintain them. Once identified, one may develop strategies to reduce the avoidant behavior itself, the psychosocial triggers, or the psychosocial reinforcers of the behaviors to try to break the cycle.

Examples of some common habit cycles and the psychosocial triggers and reinforcers that can maintain them:

Physical Stressor	Avoidant behavior	Potential reinforcers of avoidance behavior	Physiological effects of the avoidant behavior that can increase frequency of the stressor	Psychosocial triggers	Psychosocial reinforcers of the avoidant behavior
Pain from injury or disuse	Inactivity	Stops movement-related pain	Increasing deconditioning and weakness leads to greater pain with movement	Fear or stress related to the activity (e.g., concern regarding reinjury, anxiety regarding work or social responsibilities)	Reduced anticipatory pain related to feared/disliked activity.
				Dependence on social benefits of perceived disability (e.g., disability payments, social support, lower work expectations)	Doting, attention and support, financial support for disability.
				Acceptance and enabling of use of addictive medications	Social approval and encouragement of use of opioids, cannabis, and other reinforcing drugs.

Negative affect and stress	Comfort food	Activation of reward circuits by sugar and fat	Consumption of sugar and fat increases inflammation which activates stress and negative affect circuits	Self-stigma	Negative thoughts about ones eating or weight retrigger negative affect.
				Loneliness	Food provides bonding experiences and social opportunities.
				Boredom	Food provides novelty which enhances reinforcement.
Negative affect, stress, with-drawal	Addictive substance use	Activation of reward circuits by drug use	Drug dependence-related adaptations increase withdrawal symptoms with abstinence	Loneliness	Some social activities may center around alcohol or drug use.
				Anger	Drug use may be perceived as rebellion or revenge against someone you feel treated or judged you unfairly.
Feeling tired or exhausted	Late afternoon napping	Relief due to rest	Insomnia at bedtime or poor sleep during the night	Lack of pacing during daytime hours	Social reinforcement for over-working without breaks.
	Drinking caffeine to complete duties in the evening	Activation of reward circuits by caffeine use. Oxytocin-related reward from the warmth of the drink.	Caffeine dependence leads to withdrawal related headaches when caffeinated drinks are skipped. Contributes to poor sleep during the night.	Desire for connection	Social activities around sharing coffee, tea, or soda.
				Fear of failure	Sense of achievement when meeting personal or societal goals.
				Anxiety around asking for help	Relief from anticipated rejection or dependence on untrusted others.

Once you have mapped out the triggers and reinforcers of your own habit cycles, it is time to play creatively with ways of redirecting the pattern of behaviors. One approach could be to design and learn a new response to a trigger (i.e., develop an alternative response). Taking the example of feeling tired and exhausted due to caffeine consumption in the evening, one could explore herbal teas or sparkling water that one could drink as part of a break and refresh ritual with friends. Alternatively, one could try to find ways to remove exposure to a trigger. Taking the example of exhaustion due to overworking without breaks, one could work with one's colleagues, family, or supervisor to work out a schedule with set amounts of time for each daily job task and planned breaks. If the schedule is designed realistically, sticking to the schedule should prevent over-tiredness that leads to sleep-disrupting mid-day practices. Honestly considering your day-to-day practices to understand why you repeat things that aren't working for you can help you find different paths out of the loops that you hadn't noticed before. Engaging friends and family in the effort can be particularly helpful for both understanding the loops and generating ideas on how to break out of them. Paths that you may be blind to out of habit may be more obvious to those around you.

A Real-World Example of Habit Cycles: Creative Ways in which Narcotics are Used to Reduce Pain and/or Provide Reinforcement

Studies of animal models of habit cycles have painted a simplistic picture of how self-reinforcing behaviors lead to chronic repetition of unhealthful behavior patterns. But in the real-world, the reality of these cycles may be much more complex and nuanced. Deep diving into these patterns with patients may help to identify unexpected drivers of unhealthful behavior and point to novel strategies for healing.

This complexity was hammered home for me in the context of a qualitative study my team conducted to try to understand drivers and predictors of chronic opioid analgesic use (Lewis et al., 2014). We interviewed patients who had been receiving opioid analgesic medication from their providers for a prolonged period, expecting to find signs of classic addictive behavior, with opioid use producing rewarding feelings (e.g., pain or stress relief, euphoria) that drove on-going use despite negative consequences. We knew that medication diversion was a concern, with prevailing assumptions being that patients might sell their medication for profit. In extended interviews with patients however, we uncovered an exceptional diversity in drivers of on-going opioid analgesic-seeking and use, including rewarding effects through mechanisms we would have never imagined.

We saw many examples of patients repeatedly and effectively using their opioids to reduce their own pain though mechanisms that did NOT involve their taking the drug. For example, some patients used their analgesics to reduce pain in loved ones. Seeing loved ones in pain was distressing and caused empathic pain. Providing opioids to a loved one reduced the loved one's pain behaviors (e.g., grimacing, limping, emoting, etc.) and thereby eliminated empathic pain caused by the patient's viewing a loved one in distress. The patients shared their medications to avoid seeing someone they cared about experience pain. Others provided their opioids to community members to increase their contributions and perceived benefit to their social group. They found "playing doctor" for those around them increased their social status and inclusion and made them feel helpful and needed. Some used their opioids to reduce loneliness related to their disability. They found that sharing their opioids with others incentivized others to visit them, providing needed social contact, support, and entertainment. A particularly creative patient used their opioids to reduce environmental irritants while avoiding social conflict, by giving his opioid medication to the not-so-beloved, yippy, nervous dog of his beloved girlfriend. The sedating effects of the opioid subdued the dog's behavior, reducing the patient's irritation, and thereby decreasing his pain while he was alone at home with the dog during the day. Others reported needing the medications as a safety cue. Having the medication readily available provided these patients a sense of control over their pain. Knowing that they had a solution prevented them from catastrophizing when their pain flared. Staying calm minimized their pain and prevented them from needing to take the medication. Some simply found the prescriptions validating which reduced anxiety about their experience. When a doctor continued their opioid prescription, the patient felt that the physician believed their pain was real but didn't think it indicated other unknown threatening health conditions. This helped reduced the patient's health anxiety. It also made them feel that their clinician was committed to helping them and cared. This improved alliance with their health care provider. In all cases, the patients were not taking the opioid medication themselves but truthfully reporting to their doctor that the medication was effective for reducing their pain. Empathic experience of pain, loneliness, low social status, anger/irritation, catastrophizing, fear of an undiagnosed illness or injury, and lack of perceived support can all increase the experience or severity of pain, and patients came up with creative ways of using the medications they were provided "as needed" to reduce pain.

Effectiveness aside, each of these patterns involved completely unnecessary risks from unmonitored opioid use or dispersion of controlled substances across a community. In each case, other safer solutions could have addressed the same drivers of pain. Moreover, patients were remarkably self-aware and open about their behavior when asked, suggesting openness to alternative solutions. While helping a lonely disabled patient host a book club might not be among the guideline-recommended health care interventions for either chronic pain management or to reduce opioid overdose in the community, in an individual case, it may be a perfect solution for both. Recognizing that the reinforcement structures underlying habitual behaviors can be nuanced and complex and taking the time to listen to patients and explore the triggers and reasons for on-going harmful behaviors may help uncover unexpected solutions that enable change. Providing health care providers time to have these discussions with their patients may be crucial to cost-effective care.

Planning safe alternatives for relief

As is highlighted in the Fear Avoidance Model of Chronic Pain (Vlaeyen and Linton, 2000), catastrophizing can create a habit cycle. When catastrophizing, a person thinks about and responds to the worst imaginable outcome or cause of an experience. Catastrophizing increases stress and fear about an experience, amplifying feelings of anxiety, pain, and distress. Here, a person will now be particularly motivated to avoid the experience and will find quick fixes that provide relief to be both appealing and rewarding.

Just like addictive drug exposure creates opportunities for drug-seeking that can be hard to control if you have dopamine deficiency, catastrophizing creates opportunities for relief-seeking. If the same reward circuits control these relief-seeking behaviors, one would expect that persons with reward/dopamine deficiency would also have more trouble controlling maladaptive relief-seeking and avoidance behaviors. Interestingly, some of the same genetic variants of the D2 dopamine receptor that increase risk for developing substance use disorders also increase risk for disorders that involve avoidance or relief-seeking in response to catastrophizing. For example, genetic variants of the D2 dopamine receptor were found to be associated with risk of death by suicide (Kimbrel et al., 2022), a behavior that could be considered the most extreme example of a short-term relief-seeking behavior with negative long-term consequences.

Positively, interventions that help patients preplan responses for times when they find themselves desperately craving relief have been found to reduce catastrophizing, pain, and suicide behaviors. Specifically, a crisis-response or safety planning intervention, where patients work with a provider to develop a written action plan for how they will respond when experiencing suicidality, reduced suicidal behaviors among Army soldiers and Veterans treated for suicidality in emergency departments (Bryan et al., 2017; Stanley et al., 2018). Likewise, a single session treatment for chronic pain, entitled Empowered Relief, included development of a "self-soothing action plan" for use when pain experience becomes challenging. Empowered Relief was found to significantly reduce catastrophizing, pain severity and pain interference when conducted in-person versus health education or when conducted as group telehealth visit versus a wait-list control (Darnall et al., 2021; Ziadni et al., 2021). Importantly, the action plan must address what the patient will do during moments of crisis, rather than what they won't do. For example, developing a plan of what to do during a suicidal crisis was significantly more effective than planning not to resort to suicide behaviors in times of crisis (Bryan et al., 2017). The plan must provide alternative behaviors to achieve relief, rather than focus on withholding dangerous or unhelpful relief-seeking strategies when the need for relief is overwhelming.

Brain Challenge #3 Exercises

Exercise 3A: Identifying Stress Symptoms and Their Triggers

As we have noted, lack of control is a critical element in the stress response. We achieve greater control over the environment by being able to predict when stressors reach a critical mass and cause stress-related symptoms. I (W.G.) hypothesize that stress-related symptoms may be a kind of language that reflect the acute effects of distress and the chronic effects of stress.

Step 1: To help you identify stress-related symptoms, review the following checklist to see which apply to you during your typical stress experiences:

Musculoskeletal Symptoms
__ Tension headache
__ Orofacial pain: bruxism and TMJ
__ Upper back and shoulders (trapezius region)
__ Lower back (sacral region)

Cardiovascular/Cerebrovascular Symptoms
__ Hypertensive headache
__ Shortness of breath
__ Chest discomfort, angina
__ Dizziness, sweating

Immune System Symptoms
__ GI symptoms: e.g., IBS, colitis
__ Allergies: respiratory, bronchial, dermatological
__ Autoimmune symptoms: e.g., rheumatoid arthritis, lupus, thyroid
__ Immune-related fatigue: e.g., fibromyalgia

Sleep Symptoms
__ Difficulty falling asleep
__ Difficulty maintaining sleep
__ Difficulty feeling rested

Step 2: Can you identify situations that initiate stress-related symptoms?

Step 3: Can you identify resources that can help manage stress-related symptoms?

Step 4: Below is a list of health professionals that can help manage stress-related symptoms and help develop skills to assist in stress management. Consider these in addition to the resources you identified above.

Somatic Resources
Acupuncture
Athletic Trainer
Chiropractors
Health Coach
Massage
Physical Therapy
Tai Chi
Yoga

Mental Health Resources
Psychologist
Marriage and Family Therapist
Social Worker
School Psychologist
Psychiatrist
Mental Health Counselor
Pastoral Counselor
Human Resource Specialist

Medical Resources
Primary Care MD
Nurse Practitioner
Cardiologist
Pulmonologist
Allergist
Osteopath
Rheumatologist
Orthopedist

Exercise 3B: Do I Need Better Sleep Hygiene? Creating a Sleep Journal

Although it is difficult to know how many hours of actual sleep you obtained, it is not hard to tell how tired you feel and if you had difficulty falling asleep or remaining asleep. There are many different forms of sleep disorders. Problems with pain, discomfort, anxiety, altered sleep-wake schedules and interruptions can cause problems with initiating sleep. Difficulty in maintaining sleep can follow mood disorders such as low grade (dysthymic) or major depression or bipolar disorder. If a person (or spouse) discovers long respiratory pauses, loud snoring, and multiple brief awakenings – signs of sleep apnea – he or she should be referred to a sleep disorders clinic. Restless legs syndrome is another common cause of difficulty in maintaining sleep. The list goes on.

In most cases, there are environmental factors that worsen sleep quality and duration. Here we encourage you to identify these factors. By keeping records of sleep quality and duration, you can provide your primary care physician, psychiatrist, sleep specialist or other mental health professional with key information to diagnose and treat sleep problems. It is also possible it will help you see trends on your own. Perhaps you always have difficulty falling asleep when you consume caffeine after 6:00pm. Sometimes things can become so ingrained in our habits that we do not even realize the adverse consequences they may be having.

If you go online, you can find several different templates that can be downloaded without charge under the search terms "sleep journal" or "sleep diary".

Using your preferred form of documentation, each day when you get out of bed estimate and document the time you went to sleep, how long it took to fall asleep, how many times you remember awakening during the night, the time you woke up, your total sleep time, and the time you got out of bed. Keep notes about your emotional state, thoughts or environmental factors that may have altered your sleep.

There are some relatively simple rules, included in CBT-I manuals, that can help correct most insomnia problems. These focus on creating a regular pattern of sleep and associating your bedroom only with sleep. These rules include establishing and sticking to a regular bedtime (even on weekends), creating a relaxing routine before bed, finishing all eating, exercise, drinking and smoking at least 2-3 hours before your bedtime, avoiding caffeine within 6 hours of your bedtime, only using the bedroom for sleep and sex (no TV, computer, work desk, reading, etc.), exercising regularly and avoiding naps, and leaving your bed if you do not fall asleep within 10 minutes (e.g., go to another room and read and come back when you are sleepy). If you find you are not sleeping well, work on improving your sleep habits by following the rules above.

Exercise 3C: The Power of Structuring One's Life

Structuring your day-to-day life to ensure you get regular and adequate nutrition, exercise, and rest as you achieve your goals is key to minimizing stress in your life. The first step in setting up a healthful structure is becoming aware of your current patterns. An activity diary can help you identify areas and patterns in your life that may be stressful.

Use the Daily Activity Sheet on the next page to help you get started. Keep track of your diet, sleep, work, rest, exercise, and mood for a week. Review the diary to identify areas in which you are not getting what you need or where there is a lot of variation in whether or when you eat, rest, or exercise. If you are not sure what a healthful diet looks like, or how much sleep is enough, consult with a health professional. Once you have identified problem places in your schedule, make a plan to make one schedule change to improve your health.

WORKSHEET: Daily Activity Sheet

Date: _____

Hours of Day	Activity	Rest	Rec/Fun	Work	Exercise	Notes
		Type of Activity (check)				
Midnight – A.M. 12-1						
1-2						
2-3						
3-4						
4-5						
5-6						

Upon Awakening: Mood _____   Stress level (0-10 scale) _____

Hours of Day	Activity	Rest	Rec/Fun	Work	Exercise	Notes
		Type of Activity (check)				
Morning – Noon 6-7						
7-8						
8-9						
9-10						
10-11						
11-12						

At Noon: Mood _____   Stress level (0-10 scale) _____

Hours of Day	Activity	Rest	Rec/Fun	Work	Exercise	Notes
		Type of Activity (check)				
Noon – P.M. 12-1						
1-2						
2-3						
3-4						
4-5						
5-6						

At Dinner: Mood _____   Stress level (0-10 scale) _____

Hours of Day	Activity	Rest	Rec/Fun	Work	Exercise	Notes
		Type of Activity (check)				
Evening 6-7						
7-8						
8-9						
9-10						
10-11						
11-12						

At Bedtime: Mood _____   Stress level (0-10 scale) _____

Exercise 3D: Give Us This Day Our Daily Self-Monitoring

Having a schedule helps us plan out events and perform healthful behaviors each day. But even with a schedule, we may continue to make bad choices. Do you feel compelled to make the same mistakes day after day? Imagine if you had a way to record your mistakes and learn from them. Developing a system to learn from your own experience can increasingly improve your ability to cope with events and help you acquire ever-greater control. Any system to learn from experience starts with self-monitoring of daily events.

We modified the Daily Activity Sheet from Exercise 3C so you can use it as a structure to record problems or stressors you encounter each day. By reviewing this log of problems over a longer time period you can identify problems that repeat and start to experiment with different solutions. Note what you tried and notice the impact on your mood, stress level and resolution of the problem itself. If the new solution works, repeat it. If not, abandon that idea and try a new one. To the extent that you are able to dedicate five or ten minutes a day to this pursuit, it will give you an added sense of power to shape your life. Moreover, it will protect you from things that have gone wrong before by giving you the opportunity to develop a plan of action well in advance of the time you encounter the familiar threat. You can tailor the daily activity sheet to meet your needs. Most stationary stores have a variety of daily planners that can be adapted for personal use.

WORKSHEET: Daily Self-Monitoring Sheet   Date: _____

Hour of Day	Problems/Stressors	Mood (0-10 scale)	Stress (0-10 scale)	Resolution & Level of Success
Midnight – A.M. 12-1				
1-2				
2-3				
3-4				
4-5				
5-6				

Upon Awakening: Mood _____   Stress level (0-10 scale) _____

Hour of Day	Problems/Stressors	Mood (0-10 scale)	Stress (0-10 scale)	Resolution & Level of Success
Morning – Noon 6-7				
7-8				
8-9				
9-10				
10-11				
11-12				

At Noon: Mood _____   Stress level (0-10 scale) _____

Hour of Day	Problems/Stressors	Mood (0-10 scale)	Stress (0-10 scale)	Resolution & Level of Success
Noon – P.M. 12-1				
1-2				
2-3				
3-4				
4-5				
5-6				

At Dinner: Mood _____   Stress level (0-10 scale) _____

Hour of Day	Problems/Stressors	Mood (0-10 scale)	Stress (0-10 scale)	Resolution & Level of Success
Evening 6-7				
7-8				
8-9				
9-10				
10-11				
11-12				

Exercise 3E: Work/Rest Balance and Activity Pacing

As we have discussed, it is important to get enough rest and not overdo work or activities so you can reduce stress, prevent burnout, and avoid unhealthful decision-making. The first step to finding a proper work/rest balance is recognizing when you are pushing yourself too far. Consider the activity diary you kept in Exercise 3E. Is your level of activity fairly stable from day-to-day? Can you keep up that level of activity without becoming tired, depressed, or needing a day-off to sleep or escape from life? Do you feel like you are able to get enough done in the day to feel good about your life and your progress towards your goals and priorities? If so, congratulate yourself. You have done a reasonable job of balancing work and rest in your life and are likely already skilled at activity pacing.

Alternatively, do you find that you work really hard on one day (or a part of the day or week) and then become so tired, stressed, sore, sick or unmotivated that you cannot get anything done the next day? Do you work so hard during the week that you cannot get out of bed on the weekends, and feel like you are neglecting your family, friends, and personal goals? Do you exercise for hours on Monday, only to find yourself skipping your planned exercise for the rest of the week because you are just too sore to move? Do you sleep only four hours on Monday, but then require twelve hours on Tuesday to catch up? If you notice patterns like these in your life or activity diary, then you may benefit from improving your ability to pace yourself.

Pushing yourself too hard and maintaining inconsistent activity levels or schedules are stressful on your body and mind. Moreover, patterns of overwork followed by exhaustion tend to be inefficient. You get more done when you work at an even pace with rest and recovery time included than when you push until you cannot go any further and then crash from exhaustion. As the tortoise and the hare fable famously illustrates, the stress you endure from over-doing it does not even help you get ahead.

So, what can you do to help improve your pacing skills and improve your work/rest balance? The first step is to set yourself a plan describing a reasonable amount and duration of activity followed by a planned but time-limited rest period. You will likely find that you will need to set up these work/rest plans for various activities you do throughout the day and for various time scales.

For example, on workdays when I (J.T.) am expected to write for 8-10 hours per day, I have a set writing/rest plan. I attempt to write in a focused manner for 30-45 minutes and then give myself 5-10 minutes to distract myself and think about something completely different. While this may seem like a waste of time, this rest period not only invigorates my writing, but also breaks me away from what I am doing for just long enough that I am able to more objectively consider what I have written. It also makes me more able to see errors in my grammar and recognize badly written sentences. In short, these frequent breaks keep me writing efficiently and help me reengage my thinking skills so that I can persist without tiring over the course of the day. I also have plans for work/rest balance for the day; for example, a set wake-up goal and a set bedtime goal. Goals for balancing time for household chores versus playtime, and activity/rest goals for exercise sessions (note these are typically more on a seconds to minutes time scale) are also useful and helpful to plan. Setting these goals requires you not only to recognize your priorities, but also to be observant of your own abilities and limits. It may take multiple rounds of revising your activity/rest plan until you reach a proper balance that allows steady, gradual progress towards your goal and eliminates stressful work binges. It is helpful to continue with your activity diary as well as self-monitor your emotions/stress as you make these revisions so you can keep track of all the outcomes these changes influence.

Basic strategy for developing an optimal activity/rest plan
1. Set a goal in minutes for moderate activity.
2. Set a goal for a time-limited rest period.
3. Repeat the activity/rest cycle throughout the day.
4. Notice your energy and stress level at the end of the activity and rest periods. You should be ready for a rest, but not exhausted, at the end of the activity, and invigorated at the end of the rest.
5. Adjust your activity and rest goals as needed until you reach a pattern that allows for steady repetition of the activity pattern over the day or from day-to-day without need for catch-up activity or extra rest to prevent stress due to either overwork or underwork.

Exercise 3F: Relaxation

Here we describe some of the most common simple brief relaxation exercises and provide links to guided exercises where you can practice these techniques. Relaxation is a skill and requires lots of deliberate practice to master, so we encourage you or your clients to try a variety of exercises and then set a goal to practice the appealing versions at least several times per week. If you or a client wish to extend their relaxation practices beyond these brief exercises, classes in yogic practices, Tai Chi, Qi Gong, or mindfulness meditation provide more extensive practice in relaxation skills and can be found in most communities.

Breathing Exercises
Perhaps one of the simplest techniques for learning to relax involves practicing deep, controlled and intentional breathing. By bringing attention to your breathing, engaging your diaphragm, and taking long, deep, full, even and measured breaths, you will 1) stop the rapid, shallow and stressful breathing that enhances the feeling of stress, 2) reduce tension in your body, and 3) bring your mental focus to a calm place. As you attend to your deep, measured breathing, you eliminate negative thoughts by moving your attention away from them and toward the feelings of safety and calm that slow, full breathing induces. Notably, many yogic practices include breathing exercises as part of training in relaxation and health.

Progressive Muscle Relaxation
Progressive muscle relaxation adds a focus on muscle tension to the relaxation practice. Typically, this technique is used in conjunction with a focus on breathing. Like breathing exercises, progressive muscle relaxation encourages attention to your internal state and feelings. By intentionally correcting bodily responses triggered by stress, you help the feelings of stress fade. The general idea behind progressive muscle relaxation is simple. You work through the body, piece by piece, deliberately contracting each muscle to bring attention to it and then slowly releasing the muscle to relax it completely. For example, you may start with the right hand. Clench it tightly and slowly count to five, focusing on the feeling of tightness that flexing the muscle produces. Then slowly release the muscle, often in conjunction with release of your breath, noticing the difference in feeling and the relaxed sensation in the muscle. Repeat this sequence with your left hand, then your right forearm, then your left, and so forth until you have covered all the main muscle groups in the body. It can be helpful to focus some extra attention on muscles where people tend to become habitually tense with stress, such as neck and shoulder muscles, and even the muscles of the face and forehead. To ensure that progressive muscle relaxation is done safely and effectively, it is important to remember to breathe calmly and consistently throughout the exercise. It is good to remind clients or yourself to breathe at the outset, as the effort of tightening and focusing on muscles can make people forget to breathe or hold their breath. Not breathing can cause stress and reduce the impact of the exercise.

Guided Imagery
Guided imagery exercises encourage the participant to imagine that he is in a deeply relaxing, safe, and beautiful setting. Imagining the sights, sounds, smells, sensations, and feelings of the imaginary environment helps draw attention to the safe, comfortable

surroundings and induce feelings of relaxation and calm. Focusing on the sensory illusions of the imaginary setting can help the participant leave behind the physical, emotional, and cognitive feelings of stress built up in his or her day-to-day life. Incorporating breathing exercises can intensify the relaxation experience. Different imaginary settings may work best for different people. Everyone has his or her own special safe places, and these may work best for imagery exercises. The key is to be able to imagine the setting in enough detail to feel like you are there. Good examples could be warm, sandy beaches, a peaceful forest, a soft rug in front of a fireplace, or even a fresh snow on a mountain retreat, depending on your personal experiences and associations. Focusing simply on a sense of warmth and comfort in your body can work similarly.

Practice Exercises

There are a number of websites with scripts and exercises that you can use to practice or teach relaxation skills. Below are a few to get you started:

http://www.allaboutdepression.com/relax/

Provides written scripts and audio files with a variety of relaxation exercises led by clinical psychologists. The site includes all of the techniques mentioned above.

http://www.innerhealthstudio.com/relaxation-scripts.html

Provides a good number of written scripts for relaxation exercises that you can record for yourself or use with a client. The site also offers free audio recordings of relaxation exercises, a weekly podcast with relaxation exercises, and some video clips to help with relaxation exercises.

Brain Challenge #4
Training Your Reward Circuits To Make Healthy Behaviors Habitual

Challenge Introduction

My husband keeps nagging me (J.T.) to join him for morning workouts at the Master's swim team he joined last year. "It's so nice in the water," he says, "the rhythm of the swimming is so soothing, it's almost like you are still asleep but flying through the water". "You'll love it. It is such an energizing way to start a day." Always in need of energy but feeling nervous because I have never swum with a group before, I agree to come the next morning. That morning, I drag myself out of bed, scramble around the house looking for the things I need, go to the pool, bumble around the locker room trying to get my suit on and my goggles to stay on my face, and jump in the pool flustered and already tired just from trying to prepare. My husband is already there, looking calm, confident, eager, and ready to go. He gives me some quick pointers on how to follow the workout and I join the group. He moves gracefully, with long coordinated strokes propelling him smoothly forward. I, on the other hand, cannot get both arms to work evenly together, let alone synchronize them with what my legs are doing. Ugh, what are my legs doing? This is exhausting, I can hardly breathe, and as far as I can tell, I am at best getting in the way and probably likely to hit a team member with my flailing crooked attempts at swimming. Is my husband just a natural? Am I just uncoordinated? No, his one-year head start has completely transformed swimming for him, from a discombobulated, difficult, tiring exercise into an efficient, relaxing activity that he can do while he basks in the beauty of the sun rising over the warm pool. He has learned to swim properly and practiced regularly, and now can do it, nearly in his sleep, with his attention elsewhere. He has taken a difficult but healthful activity and made it easy. I have a lot of learning and practice ahead of me before swimming has a chance of becoming a personal morning meditation, but his example helps me see the great rewards such hard work can bring.

New and unpracticed behaviors require thought, effort and planning to carry out. With repetition, these behaviors become mastered and automatic. Different brain regions take over and can run through these behavioral programs without conscious thought and sometimes even without our awareness. This habit learning drives much of our behavior, from brushing our teeth and tying our shoelaces to binge eating and substance abuse. With training, it may be easier to do a behavior than to prevent yourself from doing it. That's why it is important to develop healthful habits. Once you develop habits to the point of becoming automatic they become really hard not to do. Whether they are good or bad behaviors, it is easier for you to do learned habits than less practiced behaviors. Too often this means doing learned bad habits over less practiced healthful behaviors. You will need to practice new health behaviors until they are as mastered and automatic as your old unhealthful behaviors to maintain meaningful behavior changes. In Challenge #4, we will discuss how our brains most efficiently learn new behaviors and turn them into habits. Then we discuss psychological techniques to help us make more attempts, repeatedly practice, and eventually master new behaviors. In Chapter 4.1, we describe what behaviors can become automatic, and what happens in the brain as behaviors become automatic. In Chapter 4.2, we discuss how we learn new behaviors and the importance of modeling, observation, and practice. In Chapter 4.3, we explain how to turn a new behavior into a habit through practice, support, monitoring, and rewards.

Chapter 4.1: The Abilities of the Human Autopilot

Skilled movements and even complex behaviors, although initially requiring effort and concentration, can become automatic through sufficient practice. These automatic behaviors are learned and performed using the basal ganglia, a brain region involved in habits and movement. The basal ganglia are critically involved in remembering automatic patterns of movement or habits, such as swimming, riding a bicycle, driving your car, brushing your teeth, washing your hands, or preparing your cereal for breakfast. Once learned by the basal ganglia, all can be performed with minimal awareness. In contrast, it is impossible to train the brain to automatically do something new, determine the fastest way home through traffic or rearrange your schedule to fit in a new exercise class because these are different skills that the basal ganglia is not equipped to learn. These behaviors require controlled processing. Behaviors that use controlled processing require focused attention to the task, and multitasking or stress will impair your ability to do them. The behaviors that the basal ganglia automatize as habits can be extremely complicated, but they must use specific learning and logic rules. You will never be able to count calories without deliberate thought nor will you be able to plan group meals without focused awareness. But you can learn the habit of drinking a full glass of water before starting dinner and of stopping eating when your stomach feels full. These habits are essential for maintaining stable health, particularly during busy or trying times.

It is important to understand the distinction between automatic processing and controlled processing (see Schneider & Chein, 2003) as we attempt to design and learn new health habits. Automatic processing is fast, more efficient, and accurate, occurs in parallel and does not require explicit attention. In other words, you can do tasks that require only automatic processing quickly and correctly, at the same time as you attend to other things in life, and without purposely paying attention to them. Riding a bike after you have already learned and practiced is an example of automatic processing. Controlled processing is slow, serial, and requires attention. In other words, you can only do tasks that require controlled processing if you take your time, only do one thing at a time, and pay attention to what you are doing. Composing new written text or doing long division are examples of tasks that always requires controlled processing.

Not all behaviors become effortless with practice. Consider long division, for example. While you can have some improvement in accuracy and speed through practice, new strategies, and some memorization, you can never do it automatically. Because there are infinite possibilities for numbers to divide, we cannot learn them all and must continue to rely on controlled processing to use multiple and variable cognitive strategies to determine the correct response. And when we use these processes, trying to do other things at the same time or getting stressed impairs our ability to do the behavior.

Automatic processing is less flexible but faster, and only develops with lots of practice. Importantly, it is less likely to be disrupted by stress, fatigue, or other distracters (Schneider & Chein, 2003). In other words, once a behavior is automatic, you can continue to do the behavior even when you have other things on your mind, are focused on doing something else, or are feeling too tired or out of sorts to focus on what you are doing. This feature of automatic processing is key for maintaining and consistently sticking to healthful behaviors. You cannot spend all your time thinking about eating right, getting exercise, and eschewing unhealthful options. But if you can make those behaviors automatic then you will do them preferentially as you go about your everyday life. Finding ways of making healthful behaviors automatic can improve your ability to adopt and maintain practices that keep you healthy over the long-term.

What behaviors can become automatic?

As we discussed, not all behaviors can be automatized, so what is the difference between behaviors that can versus cannot become automatic with practice? Research indicates one main requirement for behaviors that can become automatic is that there must be a consistent response to a consistent cue (Schneider & Chein, 2003). Automatic behaviors consist primarily of rules indicating, "when you encounter X, do Y". Whenever there is a given problem or set of inputs, there must be a consistent response that solves the problem. If you do the same thing every time, the problem will be solved. On the other hand, if the correct response varies or the situation requires using multiple or variable cognitive strategies to determine the correct response, then you will never be able to make that choice without paying some attention to it.

Automatic behavior can be something as simple as "notice the cue". For example, you might train your brain to notice signs for stairs when you enter buildings, which might cue you to think about using them instead of the elevator. Even if a health behavior involves a problem that will require multiple strategies (for example, taking pills while on vacation), you can still use automatic processing to consistently draw your attention to or away from a particular cue. For example, you might learn to habitually place your pills in a location that is conspicuous. This can help you notice specific opportunities or solvable problems in the environment that you might otherwise ignore. When decisions are more complex, it can still be extremely helpful to have trained yourself to notice opportunities to make a healthful choice or avoid an unhealthful one.

What happens to brain processing as behaviors become automatic?

All new behaviors require controlled processing to complete. You need to practice new behaviors repeatedly to make them automatic. You will not train automatic responses until you have tried them enough to figure out the constant relationships between cues or problems and solutions. Only with practice will you be able to do the new behavior without paying direct attention to the choice you are making. *In other words, practice and training is key for taking a new behavior that uses controlled processing and turning it into a habit that uses automatic processing.*

Repeating new behaviors via controlled processing strengthens brain connections that recognize the relevant situation and carry out the successful strategy. This strengthening of response behaviors becomes hardwired in brain regions outside the controlled processing system; in particular, the basal ganglia. With repeated strengthening, these behaviors will get triggered and performed as a sort of autopilot system run by brain circuits that are happy to do their work without your direct attention (Graybeil, 2008). Eventually, the controlled processing system may not even be engaged as you perform these well-trained solutions to your day-to-day problems.

To observe the difference between the brain processing required in early learning (i.e., using the controlled processing system) versus after practice (i.e., using the automatic processing system), researchers conducted a review of many imaging studies where brain activity was recorded 1) during early learning of an automatable behavior, and 2) after repeated practice of the behavior (Chein & Schneider, 2005). They looked across these studies to see what brain regions were highly active during early learning and much less active once the behavior was practiced, which would suggest where these "controlled processes" might take place. Because they were merging and averaging across studies, this provided a big but somewhat blurry picture. They found that in all these studies, activity in several areas of the brain (i.e., the lateral prefrontal cortex, medial frontal cortex including the anterior cingulate and pre-supplementary motor area, and the posterior parietal, occipitotemporal and cerebellar areas) showed consistent and significant decreases in activity over time as tasks were practiced and controlled processing diminished.

These brain regions, which are known to be involved in directing attention and motivation, problem-solving, and movement planning, were found to be active during early learning but much less so after practice. In other words, it takes many more areas of the brain when learning a new behavior but many less once the behavior is learned. A follow-up brain imaging study showed the same decreases in brain activity observed earlier. In particular, activity in prefrontal cortex areas such as the dorsolateral prefrontal cortex and anterior cingulate decreased to the point that activity in these areas when people were doing the well-practiced task looked the same as when they were just sitting around. Once the behavior had been practiced, the participants no longer needed the problem-solving abilities of the prefrontal cortex to correctly solve and answer the problems. This means that once you have learned how to do something, you can do so without any observable activity in the controlled processing areas.

Learning to ride a bike is a classic example of a task that requires attention, motivation and problem-solving when you first begin but becomes simple and effortless with practice (see the Figure on the next page). Just keeping the bike upright is a struggle at the start. Trying to do so while turning the pedals and manning the brake feels near impossible. But as we practice, riding the bike becomes easy. We can eventually maneuver the bike without even paying attention to the mechanics of the task. As you can imagine, if you are no longer thinking about the behavior when you perform it you will no longer be engaging the same brain regions. This automaticity of habits performed by deeper brain regions like the basal ganglia frees up our brain so we can complete multiple behaviors. On the bike, this means we can now talk to a friend, avoid traffic, or plan out a travel route.

FIGURE: Brain regions involved in controlled but not automatic processing

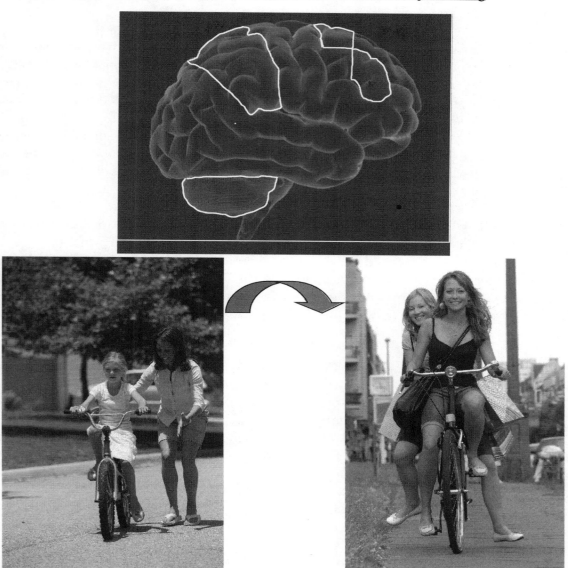

Legend: Learning a new behavior requires conscious effort and activity in brain regions involved in motor planning, problem-solving and coordinated action. Highlighted in white are some of the general brain regions that are highly active when learning a new behavior but show greatly decreased activity after the behavior has been practiced and becomes automatic (adapted and simplified based on Chein & Schneider, 2005). From right to left, these include the lateral prefrontal cortex, the pre-supplementary motor area, the posterior parietal cortex and the cerebellum. After behaviors become automatic, deeper brain structures (i.e., the basal ganglia, not pictured because it is not on the surface of the brain) can carry out the behavior without conscious attention and with little to no help from the cortical brain regions. When learning to bike (on the left), we would expect activity in these regions to be required to successfully ride the bike. When bike riding has been well-learned (on the right), substantially less activity must occur in these regions to successfully ride the bike, freeing up these higher processing areas to focus on other tasks, such as socializing with friends, shopping, or navigating busy city sidewalks.

Automatic behaviors can guide us as we focus on other things and deal with other stressors in our lives. But healthful behaviors can be pretty complicated. There is not always a single correct choice every time, which means we do need to use multiple strategies to make many health decisions. How can simple automatic rules help maintain healthful behaviors when the overall decisions and behaviors are complicated? To illustrate, I (J.T.) will give you an example from my own life: how I decide what to eat every day. By supplementing my detailed knowledge of nutrition with some simple automatic rules for noticing and picking foods, I do a decent job of maintaining my nutrition without having to obsess about it all day long.

While I personally have a pretty extensive knowledge of nutrition, food composition, metabolism, endocrinology, and the physiological consequences of food choice that I could and do use from time to time to make choices about what to eat, this knowledge is far too complicated to think about every time I need or want to eat. Instead, I will admit to relying fairly substantially on some very simple hardwired rules that I developed in my teenage years. These help me filter down my food choices and avoid making particularly bad decisions even when I am too stressed or tired to think about it.

My father's side of the family has a disturbing history of heart disease and truncal obesity. My grandfather and uncle died of heart attacks in their early 50's and 30's, respectively. So, when my dad had his first triple-bypass when I was a pre-teen, I concluded that products high in cholesterol and saturated animal fat were not options that should be a part of my future and switched to a vegetarian diet. With practice, I trained a couple of simple rules that are basically as follows:

1) When fresh vegetables and fruit are available, notice and eat them.
2) When meat or poultry are in or around food, ignore and avoid them.

I note that these rules are extremely simple and not very sophisticated. They also do not tell me what to do when exposed to a whole lot of foods, and there is still plenty of room for me to make bad decisions. For example, what do I do when I encounter a bran muffin or a Pop-Tart? I still need my controlled processing system to help me make those choices. Nevertheless, these two simple rules shape my perception of my environment to make it much more conducive to heart-healthy eating. By eating fresh vegetables and fruits when I find them, I keep myself from feeling hungry as often. This helps me make better choices when I need to think about them because I am not as stressed by hunger. And this, in turn, may make my controlled processing system do a better job when considering things like Pop-Tarts. By ignoring and not even considering products containing meat, I cut out many types of food that could worsen heart disease risk. My brain filters out whole restaurants, parts of menus, and sections of grocery stores that do not meet my criteria, protecting me from bad choices and drawing me towards good ones. On occasion, I have been rather shocked when a friend points out that certain meat-focused restaurants exist on main streets in downtown areas that I frequent to get other food. It may be years before I consciously attend to the fact that an Arby's or McDonald's opened a block away from my favorite falafel store. My brain automatically ignores such options, and I never have to waste my time considering whether a quarter-pounder and fries would be a good thing to eat right now.

With the help of these simple rules, I have never had a problem with my weight or my cholesterol and lipid levels, despite my family predispositions. But it only takes a few hours with my metabolic-syndrome-plagued father to realize that, although we live in the same environment, the food options that reach my awareness are vastly different than those that gain his attention. Because he lacks these simple trained rules, he is repeatedly faced with dangerous food choices every day and must struggle with each and every one of them. Add a little stress, and he is a dietitian's worst nightmare.

Training simple behavioral habits, particularly teaching yourself to notice and gravitate towards options for healthful thoughts and behaviors and ignore and avoid unhealthful thoughts and behaviors can set you on a path towards health that requires very little focus and effort. The environment we interact with consists more of what we attend to than to what actually exists in the whole of reality. Thus, training ourselves to habitually notice good choices and ignore bad ones can have a huge effect on our everyday behavior. By training ourselves to only attend to opportunities that align with our long-term goals and values, we can change the environment we experience without going anywhere.

Chapter 4.2: How We Learn New Behaviors

Imitation, mirror neurons, and the importance of modeling

If we consider the complex physics of getting a body to move in a coordinated, goal-directed fashion, it is frankly amazing any of us ever get up off the couch. So how do we learn complicated new behaviors every day without big struggles? We are extremely good at learning via imitation. While it is relatively rare for someone to develop a truly new behavior pattern, once one person has done it, it can spread through a population like wildfire. Theoretically, we can plan out new behaviors in our heads and enact the movements, but we are not all that great at doing so. But if we see it done, we can imitate it. Our brains allow us to imagine ourselves in other people's bodies, and the movements we observe activate the same neurons that plan our movements. When we see someone else move in a coordinated manner, we can relate their movements to moving our own bodies and record the movement pattern to try later.

Taking advantage of our human ability to mimic behaviors has been shown to be a crucial component of effective interventions to encourage health behaviors. Interventions that demonstrate and model health behaviors (i.e., let the trainee watch someone do the behavior and try it themselves) are much more likely to successfully train people to perform and adopt the health behavior (Trafton & Gordon, 2008a; Trafton & Gordon 2008b). Understanding how this system works can help us more efficiently learn new health behaviors on our own or design training programs for others that truly work.

Our ability to imitate other people and learn how to achieve goals through observation is facilitated by a group of neurons in the premotor cortex, the part of the brain that plans out actions prior to activating the neurons in the motor cortex that initiate muscle movement. These premotor cortex neurons are activated when you either 1) do something yourself, or 2) observe someone else doing that same thing (Joen & Lee, 2018; Iacoboni, 2008). These neurons are called mirror neurons, since their activity mirrors the activity of the same neurons in the person you are observing. Mirror neurons are specifically found in the inferior frontal gyrus and the rostral portion of the posterior parietal cortex. Mirror neurons fire when you plan to do something. They record and work out a behavior plan. Once the plan is finalized, mirror neurons can deliver the plan to the motor cortex, which instructs your body to carry out the behavior by sending signals to your muscles via the spinal cord. But mirror neurons also fire when they observe someone else doing a behavior, which means they can record any behavioral plan that they observe. Once that plan is recorded, it can also be sent to the motor cortex and acted upon. Monkey see, monkey do. Thanks to mirror neurons, we can learn new behaviors through imitation, rather than having to work out the whole movement on our own.

Studies that recorded the activity of these neurons in monkeys and imaged the activity of these brain regions in humans have provided us with an understanding of the general abilities and functions of these neurons. It turns out that a third of the mirror neurons act as described above. The monkey recording studies showed that these mirror neurons fire both when a monkey is doing a behavior or observing someone else doing a similar behavior (e.g., when picking up a pencil or watching someone else pick up a pencil). The other two-thirds of the mirror neurons are even more sophisticated than the description above suggests. Neuron recordings show these mirror neurons fire when observing behaviors that share a common goal (e.g., chopping food in preparation and actually cooking food). These neurons do not just mimic the movements they observe others make. They are sensitive to the intention of the actions as well.

A clever study in monkeys demonstrated that the activity of these mirror neurons depends crucially on the goal of the action rather than just the movements that were observed. In this study, a human researcher conducted various grasping actions in front of monkeys while recording the activity from their mirror neurons (Umilta et al., 2001). The monkey's neurons fired when the researcher grasped an object in front of them. But when the researcher made the same arm and hand motion without actually grasping an object, the neurons did not fire. This showed that the neurons did not respond to the motion of the arm and hand, but rather to the motion of the arm and hand in achieving a goal. The researchers then looked at how the monkey's mirror neurons would respond if part of the motion were hidden from the monkey. They first showed the monkey an object on the table and then put a screen between the monkey and the object. Then the researcher reached behind the screen and grasped the object. Surprisingly, half of the mirror neurons still fired when the researcher grasped the object behind the screen, even though the monkey could not actually see the grasping motion. They then repeated this set-up without the object. They first showed the monkey that there was no object on the table and replaced the screen. Then the researcher reached behind the screen and pretended to grasp an object. What the monkey saw was identical whether or not the object behind the screen. But when the object was not behind the screen, the mirror neurons did not fire. When the monkey knew there was no object to be grasped behind the screen, then there was no obvious goal to the observed movement and the mirror neurons were not activated. Thus, mirror neurons encode both what people are doing and why (e.g., what they achieve by doing it). These and similar studies have led to the hypothesis that mirror neurons help us to both recognize and imitate others goals, thus allowing us to understand others' actions, join them in collaborative work, and empathize with their feelings regarding a situation and its outcome (Iacoboni, 2008).

Understanding these properties of the mirror neuron system, we can make predictions about how people should learn new behaviors most efficiently. If we understand the purpose behind someone's actions, observe them doing the action, and have personal motivation to reach the same goal, then we should learn a new behavior relatively quickly. If we supply our mirror neuron system with the information it needs to record a movement plan to meet a goal, and have reason to try the behavior ourselves, we should be on our way to trying and eventually mastering a new behavior.

This system is likely involved in the social contagion of health behaviors we discussed previously. Mirror neurons help us mimic others, often without realizing it. Thus, this system may encourage us to learn the behaviors we observe others doing even if we have no intentions or goals of engaging in those behaviors. Such effects may, for example, encourage us to over-eat like those around us or like people shown in television commercials. This influence of our mirror neurons may contribute to the potent effects of our immediate social network and television viewing on weight gain (Cohen, 2008; Christakis & Fowler, 2007; Jason & O'Donnell, 2009). Watching people do healthful behaviors is important for ensuring that our mirror neurons drive us to mimic and learn healthful rather than harmful habits. Watching people or ourselves do healthful behaviors in our mind's eye (e.g., visualizing healthful behaviors) can also help us learn more quickly.

To practice using visualization to engage our mirror neurons in learning new habits, see Exercise 4A (page 196).

The importance of observation

The existence of this mirror neuron system helps explain a consistent finding in trials of interventions to promote health behavior change. Specifically, mirror neurons explain why interventions that include an element of modeling and practice of the new target behavior are much more effective than interventions that simply educate clients about what to do. People are much more likely to adopt a new behavior if they are shown the behavior. If they have a chance to try the behavior in a safe setting with an encouraging person, they are even more likely to adopt it. When people are only told what to do, no matter how compelling the reason given, they rarely take up the recommendation. Even when the behavior seems relatively simple, people generally need help translating what to do into how to do it. *Demonstrating the health behaviors that you wish a client to practice can greatly increase the chance that they do the behavior correctly and regularly. Didactic education alone (i.e., simply telling people what to do and why) has very little to no effect on changing people's health behaviors.* However, if you add a component where clients observe others doing a behavior and get a chance to try it themselves and receive feedback, much greater effects on behavior can be achieved. For example, programs to improve oral hygiene that demonstrate how to brush teeth have greater effects than those that simply explain what to do.

Without knowing much about mirror neurons, psychologists observed what worked for training people in new behaviors and described these strategies in their theories. One such theory that has received substantial empirical support is the theory of self-efficacy, which states that people who have observed, tried, been encouraged, and feel confident about doing a behavior are more likely to actually do it. I note that this is just what we would expect given what we know about mirror neurons. New behaviors are most efficiently learned when we can observe and receive coaching from another person who has mastered and can demonstrate the behavior. Next, we will discuss the theory of self-efficacy in more detail and explain how to use each piece in our efforts to learn and encourage new healthful behaviors.

Increasing your confidence to do a behavior: Practice, modeling, encouragement and anxiety-reduction

In his research on a concept he termed "self-efficacy", Albert Bandura, a professor of Psychology at Stanford University, identified several elements that facilitate behavior change (Bandura, 1997). These elements have been successfully used in programs to encourage health behavior change in a wide variety of domains, including encouraging physical activity, weight loss, pain management, smoking cessation, and chronic disease management (for a review of how the theory of self-efficacy has been used to change health behaviors, see McKellar, 2008). Self-efficacy refers to a person's belief about his or her ability to do a specific activity and has been shown to be highly predictive of actual behavior in many studies. Not surprisingly, if you are more confident that you can do a specific behavior, you are more likely to do it in general, and more likely to do it repeatedly in the future. According to Bandura's theory, there are four main ways you can increase your self-efficacy or confidence that you can do a behavior: (1) enactive attainments, (2) vicarious experience, (3) verbal persuasion, and (4) observation of your own physiological state.

1. *"Enactive attainments" refers to doing the behavior.* Not surprisingly, if you have tried and successfully accomplished a behavior, you will probably be more confident that you can do it in the future. Successfully achieving a behavior is probably the best way of increasing self-efficacy. This might explain the inherent appeal of the famous Nike ad campaign encouraging would-be athletes to "Just Do It". We all know that "doing it" would increase our confidence and help us see ourselves as competent and able. If we "just do it", then we know we are capable of the same things that we might otherwise idolize in others. But one concern is that trying and failing at a behavior can be counterproductive and discourage repetition of a behavior. That is why successful training of a health behavior often requires breaking down the complex behavior into simple steps, a process that is often complicated and not obvious. It can take an expert in the behavior to be able to parse a behavior into achievable pieces. When presenting new skills that clients need to master, such as the proper use of oxygen delivery devices, asthma inhalers, complex medication or rehabilitation regimes, or use of assistive devices, it may be necessary to break down the behavior into many small pieces to avoid failure and discouragement, rather than to try to teach the entire sequence all at once.

2. *"Vicarious experience" refers to watching someone else do the behavior.* Seeing someone else do something can increase our confidence that we can do it too. Watching someone else do something lets us know it is possible and provides us with an opportunity to develop a mental plan for how to do it. As we discussed, observing a behavior activates our mirror neurons and encodes the actions and motivations of the behavior in the part of our brain that plans movements. By seeing a behavior done, your brain wires in a plan of how to move your body to do that behavior or reach that same goal. Observation not only tells you that this behavior is achievable, but also provides you with enough information so you can probably roughly approximate that new behavior yourself by mimicking what you saw. Thus, by watching Michael Jordon dunk a basketball, I am convinced that people can dunk basketballs, and have a decent idea how it is done—however, jumping five feet above the ground is beyond what most of us can expect to attain. This highlights a major caveat of this type of learning. Observation teaches new behaviors better if the model is someone that the observer believes is "like them". As a 5'1" woman, I (J.T.) have trouble imagining myself as a 6'6" man, and thus watching NBA games has done little to teach me basketball skills. Having a model to whom you can relate is important for strengthening the effects of observation on learning.

This aspect of "vicarious experience" helps explain why mutual help groups are so effective for encouraging behavior change. Mutual help groups let you see and interact with people like you who are also learning and doing the behavior. They provide models for behaviors that you can do in your environment with things you know. People who are challenged by a condition can greatly benefit by finding mentors who have the same condition and have been successful in managing it. Examples where mutual help groups have been shown to benefit include children who have lost a loved one, preteens with depression, adolescents in residential settings, adults with HIV, survivors of sexual abuse, homeless women and children, people experiencing separation and divorce, parents with addictions, and elderly coping with bereavement (Gitterman & Schulman, 2005). Seeing my officemate lose all her baby weight by taking mid-day walks and making careful choices at the company cafeteria makes me confident that I can, within the realities of my world, really get back to my pre-pregnancy state. Interacting with and observing people like you doing the behaviors and reaching the goals that you wish to reach can greatly increase self-efficacy and encourage behavior change.

3. *"Verbal persuasion" refers to being encouraged to accomplish a behavior.* When someone tells me I can do it, I am more likely to believe I can and give it a try. Like we mentioned, simple verbal instruction is often insufficient for learning new behaviors, but verbal support can be an instigator for doing the behavior and motivating practice of a behavior. Encouragement, cheerleading, or expressed confidence in your abilities from another person can increase your belief that you can do a specific behavior. As with modeling, the impact of encouragement on your self-efficacy will depend on who is doing the encouraging. The person encouraging you needs to be knowledgeable and credible. You must believe that they know enough about how to do the behavior and enough about you and your abilities to make a decent judgment about your likelihood of success. Moreover, you need to respect their opinion.

4. *"Observation of your physiological state" refers to being aware of your fears and your stress level about trying something.* If you are terrified about doing a behavior, your self-efficacy will be lower. When you are anxious or think you could be hurt, you probably will not try the behavior. If you do try, you may quit partway through the behavior or only put a little bit of effort into it. You may be so focused on maintaining an escape in case something goes wrong that you wind up sabotaging your attempt. Gymnastics coaches warn their gymnasts against such fear-related half-attempts with the saying "when in doubt, don't kick-out". When you are upside down in the air, the last thing you want to do is quit and stop right there. Being aware of your fears and anxieties about a behavior and working to reduce them before you make an attempt can improve the chance that you really try, and thus have a chance at succeeding. And success or even surviving a feared behavior is good for your self-efficacy.

To walk through how Bandura's theory of self-efficacy can be used to increase the likelihood that someone develops and maintains a health behavior, let's consider the example of trying to get someone who has just been diagnosed with diabetes to test their blood sugar after meals. A brief visit with a nurse or educator who knows how to test blood sugar can be very helpful. The nurse or educator should demonstrate how to test blood sugar (vicarious experience), demonstrate that taking a blood sample is not very painful or dangerous (reducing the client's fear and anxiety about the needle stick), encourage the client to try and reassure them of their ability (verbal persuasion), and help them test their blood sugar themselves (enactive attainments). This simple visit uses all four of the elements to increase self-efficacy for testing blood sugar, and visits such as these are standard components of effective interventions to improve use of blood sugar testing to manage diabetes. The theory of self-efficacy and the effective interventions that use these elements highlight the importance of modeling and imitation, practice, encouragement, and support, and decreasing fear in encouraging new behaviors.

Chapter 4.3: Turning a New Behavior into an Old Habit

Practice, practice, practice: Getting yourself to train a new behavior

Once you are able to do a behavior and gain confidence in your abilities, you need to find ways to make the new healthful behavior habitual. If the behavior does not come automatically, you are not going to do it very often. What can you do to make a healthful behavior a habit? Well, we know you need to practice the behavior a lot.

But how do you get yourself to practice? For example, I (J.T.) have been taught how to swim, can swim laps reasonably well, and know that it would be good for my health to swim laps regularly. But I have not been in the pool for ages. How do I turn swimming laps into a regular part of my life? How do I get myself to practice and keep myself going day after day?

As we have spent a lot of time discussing, habits are generally maintained by rewards. We do things automatically when we repeatedly experience short-term benefits from doing them. While all healthful behaviors have long-term benefits, our reward system, which drives most of our habitual behavior, is only tuned into short-term ones. The effects of exercise on my bone density decades down the road are not inherently reinforcing and will not do a lot to encourage daily workouts on their own. Our brains simply are not set up to detect these long-term health benefits. Thus, to make a new behavior a habit you need to find or create ways of making that new behavior rewarding in an immediate sense. If you want to exercise consistently, you must make exercise benefit you right away.

The amount of practice that is sufficient to make something habitual will depend substantially on the complexity of the skills. Simple behaviors, such as "press this key when this message shows on the screen", can be learned and become automatic in less than an hour of practice. More complex, multi-step behaviors can take years to practice and automate. One study of new health behaviors found that depending on the complexity of the habit, daily repetitions for as little as 20 to over 250 days were required to make the new behavior automatic (Lally et al, 2010). Most importantly, however, all automatic behaviors require on-going reinforcement if they are to continue. Even after you train a behavior to the point that it is automatic, the behavior must continue to provide short-term benefits or it will slowly fade from your daily behavior. Finding ways of consistently rewarding our healthful behaviors is crucial to maintaining healthful habits over long periods.

Next, we will discuss some ways in which you can improve adherence to or maintenance of newly developed healthful behaviors to turn them from a skill into a habit.

Social support

For humans, the most powerful, readily available, and modifiable rewards are social. While you may not be able to afford to reward yourself with expensive gifts every time you do something healthful, with some purposeful effort you can almost always find a group of people who support your goals and will be pleased with your efforts towards them. The best way of turning a new behavior into a habit is to make it socially beneficial. If you get social approval and support for your new behavior, that behavior will now immediately improve your well-being and you will begin to favor it automatically. If you can find a social network that encourages and is impressed by your new behavior (or disapproves and is horrified when you do not do it), you are apt to continue it consistently over time. If the healthful behavior is normative in your social network, it will be maintained by the responses of those around you (see Brain Challenge #1).

As a simple example, let's consider a lunchtime workout program started by a co-worker at my office. A colleague who was very interested in yoga and practiced it regularly herself went to the trouble of finding a teacher willing to teach a low-cost yoga class in an open conference room during the lunch hour. At the start, it was primarily staff members who were already interested in yoga and had some yoga experience who attended the class. They loved having a new, convenient option where they could do their already learned behavior. Other staff members started to become more aware of the class as the initial attendees began scheduling their meetings around the class and talking about how great and important it was to them. A few brave yoga-naïve staff members decided to try it, and their positive reviews, as well as the subsequent cajoling of others, encouraged a few more to try. This eventually snowballed to the point that now, every Thursday at 11:50AM, an entire troupe of employees don exercise gear and start down the hall, collecting colleagues as they head to the yoga class. This healthy new habit has spread so effectively that finding staff members to cover the phones during the class is a substantial challenge.

For an excellent and amusing three-minute narrated video demonstrating the rapid spread of a new behavior through a social group, see "Leadership Lessons from Dancing Guy" on YouTube at the following link: http://www.youtube.com/watch?v=fW8amMCVAJQ.

Setting up social rewards for behaviors not only encourages them in individuals but can make healthful behaviors spread as if contagious. Reinforcing good behaviors in one group can set up social responses that reinforce that same behavior in other connected networks of people. Linking yourself to a network that already reinforces a behavior can help you make that behavior a regular everyday part of your life.

In the previous chapter, we mentioned how mutual help groups can assist in "vicarious experience" to visualize new behaviors. In addition to that, mutual help groups create a network of people with the same goals who provide support and social reward for maintaining the behavioral goal. Client support groups can be found for almost every major disease, and the World Health Organization and other major national and state organizations provide lists online. Moreover, health care providers can help their clients by providing names and contact information of support groups and individual members to encourage their clients to make use of this resource. For example, a study that linked new clients diagnosed with substance use disorder to volunteers from twelve-step-based support groups found that these efforts significantly increased both clients' use of these resources and abstinence rates a year later (Timko & DeBenedetti, 2007). Interventions like these can amplify the effects of "vicarious experience" as clients learn to master the key challenges they will need to confront.

Attendance at mutual help groups has been shown to be a strong predictor of long-term recovery from addictive disorders. This demonstrates the importance of a reinforcing social network for turning a new healthful behavior into a lifelong habit. Mutual help groups have been set up to help people with many different health and behavioral disorders. Mental Health America provides links to mutual help and peer-led organizations for mental health problems at: https://www.mhanational.org/find-support-groups. This directory can help people find networks of other people dealing with similar problems and with similar behavioral goals. Connecting with such organizations may be helpful, particularly when you are trying to incorporate a newly mastered behavior into your everyday life or are having trouble maintaining healthful behaviors in your current circumstances.

Including friends or family members in attempts to change behavior can also help reinforce the new behavior. For example, you may find it easier to make diet changes if everyone else in the house is supportive of the new diet and agrees to follow it as well. Not only does this help keep the home environment free of foods that the diet discourages, it also helps set up a home environment where healthful eating will be encouraged by those around you. Ideally, old unhealthful habits may be noticed and challenged by people close and important to you. Having the support of a group of people with shared goals encourages individuals to stick with their new behaviors, even though they may be time-consuming, tiring, inconvenient, or even painful or scary. A sense of obligation to the group members, the pleasure of shared effort toward a common goal, or simply knowing that other people will notice your behavior may encourage you to make the healthy choice in those moments when your old unhealthful habit sounds so much more comfortable and tempting. For example, a review of interventions to encourage people with serious chronic disease to exercise found that people more consistently stuck to their exercise regimens when programs used a group format rather than just targeting individuals (Buckworth & Sears, 2006). Studies of family involvement in weight control interventions suggest that spousal or parent involvement can improve effectiveness (McLean et al., 2003).

Behavioral Couples Therapy is an example of a therapy that specifically encourages social reinforcement of new healthful behaviors. Behavioral Couples Therapy for substance use disorders explicitly trains a significant other to reinforce and support healthful abstinence behaviors and avoid interactions that trigger or encourage old unhealthful substance or alcohol use patterns (O'Farrell, 1999). In this treatment, the therapist works with both the client and the significant other to help set up a pattern of social reinforcement that will encourage and maintain sobriety and healthful coping strategies. For example, the client and significant other may set up a contract where they agree not to bring up old substance-using behaviors or fears about future substance use outside the therapy session to discourage reminders and conflicts that may trigger relapse. Notably, Behavioral Couples Therapy reliably improves upon standard psychotherapies for substance use problems. The improvements are particularly obvious later in the attempt to change behavior (e.g., 6 months after a quit attempt) when people without this close social support start to slip back to their old habits. This approach also has a beneficial side-effect on relationships, further emphasizing the benefits of bringing those close to you on board during attempts to change behavior. Remarkably, this focus on encouraging supportive reinforcing behaviors within the family reduces domestic violence, child abuse, and martial separations, and increases happiness of relationships and success at sobriety (McCrady et al., 1991; O'Farrell et al., 1992). By reducing family conflicts during the difficult transition from a dangerous old habit to a new pattern of behavior and emotional response, Behavioral Couples Therapy not only increases the chance that the new behavior becomes normal and automatic but also improves relationships between family members. The success of interventions that purposely include a significant other or buddy to encourage, support and reinforce new healthful behaviors highlights the importance of consistent social reinforcement to make the new behavior a habit and maintain it once initial motivation has faded.

Note that unhealthful behaviors may also be learned and supported by our social networks. Results of the Framingham Heart Study found that both obesity and smoking were "contagious" and spread through social networks over time (Christakis & Fowler, 2007; Christakis & Fowler, 2008). Additional analysis of this same study found that happiness also spread through social networks over time (Fowler & Christakis, 2008). If the people in your social network were happy, you were more likely to be happy. If someone close to you became happy, you were more likely to become happy. Associating with a positive, healthy group of people can improve your health behaviors, and it can also improve your mood and happiness in life.

To practice in identifying and using social supports for your healthful behaviors, see Exercise 4B (page 198).

Monitoring and feedback
Setting up a whole network of people who support your behavior change or even finding a reliable buddy willing to help you learn can feel daunting. Instead, some of the same benefits of these social supports can be achieved just by knowing someone is watching and will evaluate your behavior. When interventions include a method to monitor behavior and provide periodic feedback about progress or success, people do a better job of following their behavioral plans. We have all seen people dutifully start driving the speed limit when they see a police car on the side of the freeway. Similarly, we are more likely to follow recommended health behaviors when we know someone is policing our behavior.

When we know that someone is watching, has a good and reliable way of measuring our behavior, and will respond with positive or negative feedback (in the case of highway patrol, mostly negative feedback in the form of scary intimidation and a big fine), we are much more likely to do the right thing. Thus, having someone monitor your behavior and provide feedback, even if it entails nothing more than an approving or disapproving word or look, can do wonders for changing a new behavior into an everyday one. The trick here is that the monitoring needs to be consistent. As the police example shows, a radar gun at one point on the freeway only slows down traffic for a mile or so at best. Once drivers know they are out of monitoring range, they may accelerate back up to their habitual excessively dangerous and wasteful driving speed. If we wanted people to consistently follow speed limits, we would need periodic vehicle checkpoints on the freeway where electronic monitors could track where a car was and how long it took them to get from the last checkpoint. This would allow monitoring of average speed over the whole distance, thereby catching (and potentially fining) those who drove above the speed limit consistently. While a single radar gun may slow drivers driving 90 mph down to 65 mph for maybe a mile, checkpoints would force them to keep their average speed to 65 mph, thus strictly limiting times they could drive 90 mph without punishment.

To illustrate another way, let's consider how monitoring and feedback have been used successfully to encourage other health behaviors. The effective weight loss program "Weight Watchers" uses monitoring of weight change at meetings to motivate people to stick to their diet plan, and bring attention to problems that might be stopping progress. They do not choose to take the police radar approach and watch people eat a single meal and rate them on their food choice. While this might be helpful for teaching people how to eat well in the first place, it probably would not do a lot to encourage consistent adherence. Most people would just wait for the person watching them to leave before having the big slice of pie and ice cream they were craving. Instead "Weight Watchers" chooses to monitor and reinforce a marker of average eating behavior, overall weight change. This makes sure that any pie and ice cream binges are identified, except in the rare instances that the dieter managed to eat nothing but undressed salad for their previous five meals.

Having a system where your behavior is consistently monitored and then rewarded or punished promptly after will reinforce target behaviors and encourage close adherence. Monitoring and feedback can be even more helpful if a problem-solving component is added to the feedback. Sometimes people do not stick to their target behaviors because they did not know how to do a behavior in a specific circumstance, or they encountered a stressful situation that disrupted their good intentions. While withholding rewards or punishing people in such circumstances may increase their desire to do the right thing the next time, if they do not know how to behave appropriately in that specific circumstance, they may fail again in similar situations. Instead, if failures to do the target behavior are treated as signals that the person needs additional training or help finding solutions to difficult situations, then they can be assisted with problem-solving in hopes of improving their chance of success the next time they encounter similar situations. Interventions that add a problem-solving and retraining component to the feedback can be very powerful in encouraging regular use of new target behaviors.

Let's go back to the "Weight Watchers" example. Let's say someone's goal was to lose two pounds over a week, but the weigh-in indicates that he gained two pounds instead. This obviously will not lead to approval from the counselor doing the monitoring, but it may provide useful information for problem-solving. The counselor might then ask the dieter about his eating patterns over the week and times he had trouble sticking to the planned diet. Perhaps the dieter reports that because of some impending work deadlines, he simply did not have time to grocery shop and make his lunch in the morning. Since most of the office cafeteria food was of highly questionable nutritional value, the dieter decided to skip lunch until he could get home and make something from his healthful cookbook. But then, three days this week, he got stuck at work late, and his boss bought thick-crust, greasy, meat pizza and sugary soda to keep the team focused on their work. By this point he was so hungry, tired, and stressed that he wound up eating five slices of pizza and drinking a lot of caffeinated soda as he worked. With this information, the counselor could help the dieter plan solutions to prevent this from happening again. The counselor could help the dieter go through the cafeteria options to identify things that would be consistent with his diet. Then when the dieter got busy, he could still eat lunch, preventing him from getting so hungry and tired that he made bad choices later. The counselor could also work with the dieter to practice polite but assertive ways of discussing his food needs with his boss. If the boss could be convinced to order some healthful food options or send employees home or out to eat before reconvening, then he would have a better chance of meeting his diet goals even when work deadlines made things more challenging. By using the monitoring to identify and address problems with adherence to planned healthful behaviors, you can make sure that your plans are not high-jacked repeatedly by problems you have not solved yet.

It is important to note that this monitoring, feedback, and problem-solving approach does not have to involve a second person. It is perfectly possible to set up a system where you monitor yourself, reward yourself for successes, and work on addressing problem situations you identify. Sticking with the dieting example, you could weigh yourself weekly and keep a food diary. Each week, you could allocate some time to evaluate your progress. When you meet your target goals, you could reward yourself with something you like. Maybe go see a movie in the theater, take off the afternoon to play soccer with your friends, treat yourself to a massage, or get yourself the really fancy loose-leaf tea you love. When you do not meet your targets, you could take an hour to problem-solve. Write down the problem(s) and brainstorm solutions. Look for information on the Internet. Call a friend for advice. Schedule an appointment with a professional for help. Not having an outside person to monitor you is not a reason to abandon this strategy.

Yet another option for improving adherence is remote monitoring. The use of telehealth for remote monitoring of biological data has been used to beneficially affect clients with hypertension, depression, asthma, and congestive heart failure (Trafton & Gordon, 2008b). For example, Robert DeBusk, MD, a Stanford cardiologist reported that simple telephone calls for monitoring people with congestive heart failure highly improved health outcomes (DeBusk, et al., 1994). Likewise, remotely collecting information on mood and pain symptoms and sharing it with nurses involved in treatment planning improved depression and pain management in patients with cancer (Kroenke et al., 2010). Even if you cannot find someone in your immediate community and do not feel like monitoring yourself will be sufficient, there are still opportunities to ensure your progress is tracked and evaluated. Numerous companies now offer on-line health coaching, in some cases in combination with self-management apps or on-line cognitive behavioral therapy programs. Joining an on-line health coaching program can provide useful and consistent monitoring and feedback. In some cases, these programs may be offered through your health insurer or workplace.

Typically, the hardest part of the monitoring and feedback approach is finding the right behavior or outcome to monitor. In the case of some behaviors, there are obvious things to monitor, like weight in our diet example. In other cases, it is harder to come up with something objective and measurable that is reliably associated with the behavior. For example, let's say someone wants to get his diabetes under control. He can monitor his blood glucose, but that is kind of like the police radar scenario. If he chooses to test himself only while he is following his diet and medication plan closely, then his blood glucose values will look much better than they are in reality. While selectively testing like this is obviously counter-productive in terms of meeting a goal, the reward of feeling good about oneself can sometimes favor this sort of "cheating". Just like we often want to fool the police officer who is trying to keep us safe, we often want to fool ourselves to avoid feeling bad about our failure. Thus, this individual needs a more stable marker of how well controlled his blood glucose is over a longer period.

Researchers have spent a lot of time trying to find good markers of recent blood glucose control that let you know how well blood sugar has been regulated in the last couple of weeks, rather than the last 30 minutes or 30 years. The best marker they have found is hemoglobin A1C. In this test, health professionals look at how much sugar has stuck to the proteins on your red blood cells. When you have higher concentrations of sugar in your blood, more sugar sticks to your red blood cell proteins. Since each red blood cell lives for about three months, the amount of sugar stuck to your red blood cell proteins provides a decent measure of your average blood glucose levels over the past three months. Thus, measuring hemoglobin A1C provides a longer-term measure of blood glucose control that cannot be fooled by selectively testing blood glucose levels only after appropriate meals. But three months is a long time to wait to get feedback. If you fix your behavior, you do not want to wait three months before anyone notices and rewards you for it. Conversely, if you do relapse to bad habits, you know that you have at least three months before your failure will be detected and you meet with disapproval. This time lag is terrible for encouraging adherence.

Thus, the best plan for monitoring blood glucose regulation involves using multiple methods. First, regular monitoring of hemoglobin A1C will provide a big picture of how well your blood glucose is regulated overall. Having a long-term outcome monitored will reduce the temptation to cheat on the short-term monitoring. Next, monitoring blood glucose levels in the morning and after meals will provide immediate feedback on how your diet and exercise choices affect your sugar levels. Lastly, monitoring when and how consistently you test your blood glucose will make sure that you stick with the monitoring plan such that you can catch behavioral problems. This is why blood glucose monitors record not only the blood glucose levels but also the time and date they are recorded. By monitoring and rewarding success on these three separate outcomes, you may encourage good diabetes care and not simply avoidance of criticism from your clinician or yourself.

In summary, for monitoring to be effective, it needs to catch behavior not just instantaneously, but also over time. Moreover, it must also be responsive to changes in behavior over relatively short time periods (e.g., days to weeks) so that rewards and punishments are associated with the behavior. In many cases, you may have to monitor multiple outcomes to meet all these criteria. Taking time to come up with a good monitoring system can make a huge difference in the success of using monitoring and feedback to encourage consistent behavior changes.

FIGURE: Examples of immediate and longer-term monitors for common health concerns

Health Concern	Short-Term Monitors (days to weeks)	Longer-Term Monitors (weeks to months)
Obesity	Calorie consumption	Body weight
Diabetes	Blood glucose level	Fructosamine, Hemoglobin A1C
Fitness	Minutes of exercise	Maximum aerobic capacity (VO2max)
Alcohol use	Breathalyzer, Standard drinks per sitting	Carbohydrate-deficient transferrin test
Smoking	Carbon monoxide breath test	Cotinine urine drug test (only 2-4 days)
Substance use	Urine drug screening	Hair sample drug screening
Dental hygiene	Flossing frequency	Plaque levels
Risky sex	Consistency of condom use	STD and pregnancy testing
Heart health	Cholesterol blood test (HDL and LDL levels)	High sensitivity C-reactive protein test

EXAMPLE: Health success based on a self-monitoring program

In 2007, I (W.G.) was diagnosed with Grave's disease, an autoimmune thyroid disorder. I was producing five times the normal amount of thyroid hormone. In addition to extreme fatigue, a racing heart rate, and weight loss, I also found myself having difficulty concentrating. In the 19th century, 50% of people with this disorder died of it. But now, advances in medicine have made it possible to radioactively ablate the thyroid gland and then pharmacologically replace the correct amount of thyroid hormone needed for proper brain and body function. With this treatment, my symptoms went away and I expected to return to normal except for one troubling statistic.

I had read that a typical client after being treated for Grave's disease gains 20-30 pounds in several years. I was determined not to let this happen. My father, his brothers, my mother's brother, and both grandfathers had heart disease; both grandfathers and two of my uncles developed type II diabetes. With a resting metabolic rate of less than 1500 Kcal/day, I knew I had to carefully monitor my weight, restrict calories, and have sufficient physical activity to protect myself against the risks of hypertension, heart disease, diabetes, and stroke.

The first thing I did was to develop a way to monitor my weight on a daily basis. I created a daily diary in which I recorded my weight, body fat, duration and type of physical activity, and daily hints that could help me maintain this program over the long-term. I noted situations when I would overeat or forget to exercise. I kept the notebook in a location where I could not fail to notice it before going to bed.

In the first few months, despite my best efforts at self-restraint, I gained close to ten pounds. I realized this was going to be a lifelong challenge and I needed to improve upon my strategy. I began to identify triggers and emotional situations that led me to overeat. I learned to avoid my favorite Indian buffet. I practiced refusing seconds and stopping eating before I felt full. It was and remains trial and error. I cannot tell you my efforts have led to a permanent cure; but for the three years following thyroid surgery, my weight and body fat percent are well below what they were prior to developing the thyroid disorder.

If I gain a pound, I make extra effort to lose it and change my eating and physical activity patterns until this achieved. I've discovered this kind of feedback is what works for me—not the kind of feedback I get from the hunger centers of my brain, which would tell me that I could be starving. If I pay careful attention to the "fullness" in my stomach, I can use that kind of feedback to indicate when I am full, even if not fulfilled. It took a year to realize that I could keep my weight constant if I either went to sleep with an appetite equal to about 200 calories, or if I exercised such that I burned an extra couple hundred of calories. My wife has been very supportive of my efforts and continues to prepare original creations that manage to remain healthy within the portion size I have requested.

Another thing I learned is that it is necessary to discover what kinds of exercise I really enjoy, and then to continuously vary them so that no one set of muscles is apt to get sore. For me, moderately-paced walking, swimming, and Hatha Yoga are the most enjoyable and relaxing, but I will use interval training to get my pulse up when running around the park or on a treadmill. I have not reached my goals, but am far closer than would be the case if I had not developed this self-monitoring. Each person needs to discover, on a trial and error basis, what works best for them. I have no idea if this will work for you.

Below is an example of what I recorded in the daily diary of weight, body fat, and other concerns that I made for myself using a simple college-ruled spiral-bound notebook.

Month: July
Goals: weight <160, body fat <20%

Date	Day	Weight	Body Fat	Duration & Physical Activity	Insights
6/20	M	164.5	22%	45 min. moderate walking	

Creating immediate contingencies for health behavior

As we mentioned above, monitoring and feedback can be helpful even when you do not have someone else to monitor your behavior and provide reinforcers. When shaping your social situation is not feasible, you can reinforce new behaviors by setting up rewards for yourself. While social reinforcement is a cheap and powerful source of reward, any sort of reward will work for encouraging your new behavior. If you get something nice or get relief from something unpleasant shortly after you complete a healthful behavior, you will be encouraged to keep doing that behavior. You can set up rules or systems so that you are quickly rewarded for doing something healthful. This method to reinforce behaviors can be helpful when a person is not particularly responsive to social cues or rewards. For example, some people with autism or psychopathy may not respond to or may have unpredictable responses to social reinforcers. These individuals may find that using other non-social rewards may more effectively train in new target behaviors.

Monitoring and feedback interventions that use short-term rewards contingent on completing a pre-defined target behavior are often called contingency management programs. These programs have been very well-tested, particularly for treating substance use disorders. There are many variations on contingency management programs that have been shown to be effective for reducing substance use, but the typical program works something like this: Clients are put on a frequent periodic urine drug screen schedule to monitor their drug use. When they provide drug-free urine samples, demonstrating that they did not use drugs in the last few days, they receive a reward, most commonly a gift card or a ticket for a lottery of goods and services held periodically at the clinic. A large number of studies have shown that contingency management programs such as these reduce substance use or increase other target behaviors, at least during the period in which the program is in place (see Stitzer & Petry, 2006 for a review). However, unsurprisingly, if reinforcement of the target behaviors ends then people start slipping into old habits over time. As such, an important element of reward-based programs should be for participants to learn how to develop ways to continue providing rewards to themselves after the program ends.

While contingency management programs have been most commonly studied for reducing substance use behaviors, this strategy can be used to encourage all sorts of behaviors and has been shown to be successful when tested for other behaviors. Notably, these interventions can be used progressively. Not only can they successfully increase the practice of a single behavior, they can also encourage practice of increasingly more difficult or complicated behaviors by adding to the behavioral goals as the original goal becomes mastered. This is referred to as behavioral shaping, and can be particularly helpful when the targeted behavior is complex or multi-part (refer the example about progressive behavioral shaping on page 105). To use our diabetes example, you could first reinforce regular glucose monitoring regardless of the result of the testing. Then you could reinforce adherence to the individual's daily insulin or medication regimen. Once this is done correctly and consistently, you could train and reinforce good breakfast eating habits and reward these. Then lunch behaviors, or exercise, or food choice at restaurants, or so forth could be used as targets. Eventually, combined together, this collection of behaviors should lead to the final outcome of stable blood glucose control, which could then be monitored and rewarded as the longer-term endpoint.

Research on contingency management programs has identified a number of elements that are crucial to the success of this strategy (Petry, 2000; Higgins & Petry, 1999):

1. *The target behavior has to be doable.* In other words, this is a program for reinforcing a new behavior that you have already learned but do not do consistently. A contingency management program will not help if you have yet learned to do the behavior. Strategies such as those discussed earlier on confidence and self-efficacy can help you learn a new behavior. Contingency management can only help you use it more consistently.

2. Rewards need to be provided as soon as possible following completion of the behavior. Remember, our reward circuits are not very good at associating behaviors with rewards in the distant future. The more concurrently the target behavior and the reward are tied together, the more effective the reward will be in reinforcing the behavior.

3. Bigger rewards are more reinforcing than smaller ones. This observation is pretty self-explanatory. Nevertheless, even very small or probabilistic rewards (e.g., lottery tickets) have been shown to effectively shape behavior.

4. Rewards for good behavior are more effective than punishments for failure for encouraging good behaviors. Punishments for failure tend to primarily encourage people to avoid whomever or whatever is monitoring the behavior. If a client were getting monitored in a substance use disorder treatment program, he may stop coming to treatment when he has a lapse and used drugs. If he had diabetes and wrongfully ate a box of cookies, he may conveniently forget to test his glucose after that meal. Rather than encouraging people to do the healthful behavior more frequently, punishments encourage them to avoid the systems and people who are trying to help them become healthier. Thus, punishments are not recommended, as they are just as likely to lead the person to stop trying to get better as they are to encourage better behaviors.

An additional helpful element of contingency management programs is that it sets up a pre-planned alternative to the habit behavior you are trying to avoid. This encourages your brain to consciously consider and make a decision between the two options, which may increase control over automatic behaviors (Regier & Redish, 2015). In addition to reinforcing good choices, having an alternative behavior formally planned can help shape the decision-making process to slow habit choices and increase behavioral flexibility.

The contingency management concept can be used to encourage consistent uptake of new behaviors in a range of contexts. For example, self-guided smoking cessation programs encourage individual smokers to use self-rewards. Smokers making a quit attempt are encouraged to stow away the money they would have otherwise spent on cigarettes that week and get themselves something nice with the money they saved from not smoking. Some health plans offer incentives to people who take part in preventative health programs (Marosits, 1997). The government has offered tax breaks to people who purchase certain fuel-efficient vehicles (Internal Revenue Service, 2024). Some companies encourage people to bike or take public transit to work by providing incentives or bonuses for not driving (Wikipedia, 2010). The simple concept of providing immediate rewards to encourage consistent use of behaviors that naturally have long-term benefits (e.g., reduced risk of disease for smokers and people following preventive health regimens, and fuel savings and better air quality for people driving more efficiently or not at all), is effective for increasing and maintaining goal behaviors regardless of whether the concept is applied to individuals, programs, or even whole communities.

These contingency management programs can be effective when they are as simple as the tax break programs described above but they can also be more complicated. For example, a fairly complicated contingency contract and lottery system was used to elicit substantial weight loss in a study where clients with a goal to lose 16 pounds were randomly placed into one of three groups: (1) a control condition consisting of only a weight-monitoring program with monthly weigh-ins and a home scale for daily self-monitoring, (2) the weigh-ins plus a lottery component where participants could win daily prizes of varying value (averaging $3.00/day, and reported to the clients daily by text-message) but these clients would only receive the prizes if they achieved the monthly weight loss goal, or (3) the weigh-ins plus a deposit contract system where participants could contribute $0.01 to $3.00 per day which would be matched plus $3.00/day. They received daily feedback on the amount they had accumulated but would only receive the funds if they met the monthly weight loss goal. Forfeited money was split among participants who lost more than 20 pounds over the trial. While only 10% of controls were able to reach the weight loss goal, about 50% of those in the lottery and deposit contract groups successfully lost 16 pounds. Control participants lost an average of about 3 pounds, but in the deposit contract and lottery conditions, the participants lost an average of about 13 -14 pounds (Volpp et al., 2008).

Setting up artificial systems to reward target behaviors is a consistently effective strategy for achieving goals, even those as difficult as losing a substantial amount of weight or quitting a long-term substance addiction. Designing such a program for yourself can be a helpful tool. The main challenge for people using this method is maintaining the behaviors after the end the contingency management program. Ultimately, you want to set up some other type of consistent reward that exists outside the program. One of the most reliable ways to ensured continued practice of your desired behavior is to get involved in a community that supports the behavior during the time you are being rewarded through the program. Self-monitoring, and the satisfaction associated with achievement, may also effectively support maintenance of behaviors trained using contingency management approaches (Regnier et al., 2022).

Immediate awards may also be highly valuable for helping children learn a new habit. Using a calendar, you can place a star on each day of the week your child washes her hands before dinner or remembers to brush his teeth before bedtime. Once these early habits are engrained and lifelong, their persistence is probably as valuable in preventing disease and improving wellness as more difficult-to-implement habits in adulthood.

Another framing of this approach is called temptation bundling. Here one attempts to link short-term rewards with behaviors needed for long-term goals in daily practice. This is framed as connecting short-term "wants" with long-term "shoulds" to reinforce doing the "should" behavior. Conceptually, one is encouraged to intentionally pair a pleasurable indulgence with a behavior that provides long-term benefits but is painful or unpleasant in the short-term. In essence, pairing the want and should behaviors creates a mini-contingency management program, adding immediate reinforcement to the "should" behavior.

As a close-to-home example, my husband rather possessively volunteers to fold the laundry as one of his regular family chores. He saves up the laundry and folds the clothes in front of the television while watching a "guilty-pleasure" television series, temptation bundling his watching the show he wants to watch with the family chore that he should do. My personal inability to find anything I "want" to do to pair with my "should clean the bathroom" chore leaves my cleaning motivation tied to my need to relieve disgust, a reinforcement strategy that admittedly does not lend itself to prompt, proactive, bathroom cleaning. Designing a temptation bundling approach to keeping my bathroom shiny and fresh, I might consider making cleaning the bathroom the initial steps of a soothing warm-bath ritual and encourage myself to self-indulge in a bath a couple of times a week.

A clinical trial tested whether a temptation bundling approach could increase participants success at exercising regularly (Kirgios et al., 2020). The trial randomized participants in an exercise program to either receive an audiobook of their choice and encouragement to temptation-bundle listening to the book only when working out at the gym or the audiobook alone. The audiobook plus encouragement increased the likelihood that the participant would work out at least once per week by 10-14% for at least 17 weeks. Adding a small temptation to the long-term goal behavior increased the likelihood of initiating the behavior.

For help in designing your own contingency management program, try Exercise 4C (page 199).

Brain Challenge #4 Exercises

Exercise 4A: Using Your Mirror Neurons to Master a New Behavior

Our mirror neurons provide a powerful system for rapidly learning ways to meet our goals through imitation. As you may remember, they are activated by what they observe and can help teach our brains how to do behaviors or solve problems to achieve goals. We can activate our mirror neurons by actively observing others solving problems or achieving goals that we wish to achieve, but also by visualizing ourselves or others solving problems or achieving goals in our imagination or mind's eye.

Visualizing yourself doing behaviors can help train in these behaviors even before you have the opportunity to try them in real life. Visualization can also allow you to practice and to try out variations without actually doing them. For example, studies have shown that not only does mentally imagining oneself practicing a behavior improve performance on the task, but it also reshapes the brain in similar ways as does real practice (Blakeslee & Blakeslee, 2007). Real repetitive practice playing the piano increased the area of the motor cortex that was devoted to representing the fingers; one week of mentally imagining oneself practicing the piano two hours per day caused the same changes in motor cortex representation of the fingers. Visualization activates many of the same circuits as real practice of a behavior and produces learning and brain changes that help you do the real behavior later.

This can be particularly helpful when the goal you are trying to reach involves substantial risk, extreme effort, or rare circumstances to try. Giving yourself time and space to relax, think about your goal, and imagine your way through attempts to achieve it, can be a powerful method for learning and practicing a new behavior in a safe environment.

Using visualization to learn and practice behaviors is a skill in itself and you will become better at it as you use and practice it more. There is no one correct way to use visualization, and it can be done alone or with others to good effect. Group imagination exercises can be fun, and adding others to the creative process can provide you with possible solutions that you would not have imagined on your own. It can take some added practice to be able to "see" or imagine other people's stories. But since it is generally an entertaining practice, most will find this an exercise that reinforces itself.

To get you started, let's go over the basics of individual and group visualization exercises. Then find a quiet space and give visualization a try.

1. Find a space where you feel safe and not distracted by things going on around you. Closing your eyes is helpful for most people.
2. Think about your goal or the problem you want to solve. Imagine achieving that goal. What would it be like to have already solved the problem? What would that look and feel like?
3. Think about ways that you could reach that goal. Be creative and let yourself try out ideas that may seem a bit ridiculous. Imagine yourself trying ideas you think might work. What happens as you work towards your goal? Are there other problems that come up? Are there places you get stuck? If so, step back and think about other ways

of reaching your goal or imagine solutions to the new problems that arose in your imaginary simulation.

4. If you can imagine a story in which you achieve the goal, run through it several times. Can you see yourself actually doing the behavior? Does it come out the same way when you think through it again? Are there other stories in which you also achieve the goal? Is one more appealing to you than another?
5. Let your mind wander and give yourself time to play in your imagination.
6. If you find yourself in a bad place, feeling negative, and failing repeatedly in your imagination, take a break and try again later when you are in a better mood.

Repeatedly imagining failure can train you to fail in real life. In my experience, when I (J.T.) fail in my imagination it is because there is some part of the behavior or situation that I fear. Recognizing and acknowledging my fear, taking time to assess whether my fear is valid, and finding ways of being or feeling more safe in that situation can make it easier to get past such imaginary and real life setbacks.

If you want to practice visualization with another person or a group, the basic steps are similar but you need to find a way to share what you are imagining or seeing among the group. This typically involves people narrating the story in their heads out loud. Describing what you are seeing, doing, and experiencing can bring the group together into a shared visualization. The trick here is finding ways of letting everyone participate in the story-making. Sometimes, a single individual can wind up dominating the talking and crowd out others' contributions. If this is agreed upon beforehand, that can be fine. Letting a single person guide others through a visualization can be a powerful way of sharing a solution. But if the goal is for the group to create a shared experience from their collective imagination then it is important for everyone to be able to participate. Encouraging people to talk slowly and pause after sharing an observation can help in this process. Ultimately, once you have visualized the behavior or goal you wish to achieve, either by yourself or with others, you will need to implement it in real life to determine whether your visualization was successful in preparing you for the task.

Exercise 4B: Finding Social Supports for Practice

Having social support for your health behavior can greatly increase your motivation and consistency in sticking to your new behavior. But finding friends and colleagues that are expert at or committed to your new goal behavior can be difficult. It is likely that you will have to specifically search out the social support you need. Below are some suggestions to help you find or develop a supportive social group to encourage your health improvements and focus on your goal behavior.

For nearly all but the simplest health behaviors, you can find <u>classes</u> that will teach you about a health issue or train you in new health behaviors. These will range from a simple 30-minute lecture to months of hands-on training and practice in a new behavior. Regardless, such classes are a great place to meet at least one expert in the new behavior as well as other people interested in the health issue. Classes may be offered by a variety of organizations in your local area. Good places to look for classes include local community colleges, hospitals and health care systems, athletic clubs, community centers, and after-school programs. You can find a listing of community colleges in the US with links to their websites at: <u>http://www.a2zcolleges.com/Comm/</u> You can also ask your health provider for the names of groups in your area that offer support for your area of interest.

Exercise 4C: Creating Your Own Contingency Management Program

New behaviors must be rewarded consistently if they are to be learned and used habitually. Sometime new behaviors are naturally reinforcing, such as eating more fruit or practicing relaxation exercises. In other cases, artificial rewards may be needed to train and maintain a new habit. In this exercise, we will help you develop a system of artificial rewards (i.e., a contingency management program) to keep you practicing a new health behavior.

Part 1: What health behavior do you want to learn to practice regularly?

_____

Part 2: To develop a contingency management plan, you will need to define the following elements. We will walk you through each of these decisions to help you design your own program.
1. What specific behavior will be rewarded?
2. How will it be objectively assessed whether the behavior was done?
3. Who will provide the rewards?
4. How and when will the behavior be monitored?
5. What will the reward be?
6. How often will the reward be available?
7. How quickly will the reward be provided?

1&2. What specific behavior will be rewarded? How will it be objectively assessed whether the behavior was done?

In order to consistently and correctly provide rewards, you must clearly define what is to be monitored and rewarded. First, consider whether you will reward a marker of the behavior or observation of the behavior itself.

If you plan to use a marker, it is useful to consider the following:
a. How accurate is the marker? Can it reliably tell if a behavior was done or not done?
b. How often is the marker wrong?
c. For how long can the marker detect a behavior?
d. Are there ways to fool the marker? In other words, are there ways to cheat on the test?

If you plan to use the behavior itself, you will need to clarify all the parts of the behavior that must be done in order to count as successfully completed. For example, if your target health goal is to exercise, does it count if you put on your walking sneakers and walk around your house, or do you have to walk at least thirty minutes without pause to call your exercise attempt successful?

Describe the marker or the criteria for successful completion of the behavior here:

_____

_____

3. Who will provide the rewards?

There are only a few key criteria that the person who will provide the rewards must meet. First, they must have some objective way of assessing whether the behavior was done. If you happen to have a clear marker of whether the behavior was completed that can be observed after completion of a behavior, then anyone who you see periodically could provide the rewards. For example, a breath test on a carbon monoxide meter can be used by anyone to tell if someone recently smoked. This means a health professional, co-worker, friend, or family member could do carbon monoxide testing on a regular schedule and reward non-smoking. Likewise, it would be easy for someone to check whether you consistently monitored your diet over the week by reviewing your logbook. However, sometimes it is hard to find a reliable marker of a behavior after the fact. If this is true of your health behavior, then the person who provides the rewards must be present while you are doing the behavior to verify that you did the behavior. In this case, the person providing the rewards will have to be someone close to you, such as a spouse, friend or even yourself.

Second, the person providing the rewards must be invested enough in encouraging your new health behavior to consistently monitor and reward it. When considering who could realistically monitor whether you did your health behavior, pick the person you can rely on to pay attention to your behavior and reward it. It is absolutely fine if you yourself are the only person who meets these criteria.

Enter the name of the person who will provide the rewards here: _____

4. How and when will the behavior be monitored?

It is good to consider how and when the behavior will be monitored. Is the person who is doing the monitoring and providing the rewards always around when the behavior is done? Will you need to make special efforts to have them present? Do you need to schedule special times or events to verify the behavior?

It is also important to consider the times when your behavior will not be monitored. Is there a risk that you will sabotage your health efforts during the times you are not being monitored? Are there safeguards you can put in place to prevent unhealthful behaviors while you are not being watched? For example, if your spouse is monitoring your saturated fat intake but cannot tell what you are eating for lunch at work, could you get your office-mate to monitor you at work?

Describe the times when your behavior will be monitored:
_____
_____

5. What will the reward be?

It is important to decide beforehand what the reward for the behavior will be. Rewards must be meaningful to you but may or may not be expensive. If you are creating self-rewards, you might consider determining your play budget based on your success at your health behavior. Such a plan may be easiest if you happen to be giving up an expensive habit like smoking or frequently eating out at unhealthful restaurants. If someone close to you is providing rewards, there are many options for free rewards. A spouse might agree to do the dishes for each day you meet your behavior goal. Your kids might agree to give you fifteen minutes of quiet time. A friend might give you stickers to save up towards a massage. If you prefer monetary rewards but do not have a lot of money to spare, you might consider state lottery scratch cards as rewards. We tend to overvalue probabilistic rewards, so even though it is rare that these provide a substantial reward, the anticipation of the possibility can be reinforcing.

Consider your options and enter your planned reward here: _____

6. How often will the reward be available?

Depending on the behavior and the reward, there may be few or many opportunities to successfully complete the behavior. Thus, it is important to define how often the reward will be available. For example, if I wanted to encourage proper dental hygiene, I might consider providing rewards each time I successfully brushed and flossed my teeth after a meal. Alternatively, I could provide rewards only for each day I successfully brushed and flossed after every meal. I probably would not want to make rewards available for brushing and flossing anytime because I might encourage brushing teeth ten times before going to bed or some other strange pattern of behavior. Defining the schedule on which rewards can be obtained can help to pattern the behavior and prevent your plan from failing because rewards become too expensive or time-consuming to provide.

Enter the frequency at which rewards can be obtained here: _____

7. How quickly will the reward be provided?

Rewards are better at reinforcing behaviors when they are received as soon as possible after the behavior. Consider your reward plan. Is there a way to provide the reward in close proximity to completion of the behavior? Define when the reward will be delivered to prevent discouragement due to delayed rewards.

Define when rewards will be delivered here: _____

Now, pull all these pieces together to describe your contingency plan in full! For example: My goal is to walk 3 miles per day. I will wear a pedometer daily to track my behavior. My spouse will monitor my success by checking the pedometer before bed each day. Each day that I meet the 3-mile goal, I will put $5 in a fund towards the weekend yoga and spa retreat that I have wanted to do for years. My spouse will tell me the balance I have saved at the end of each week. Once I have saved the $700 I need for the trip, I will schedule the weekend and go.

Describe your full contingency management plan here:

_____
_____
_____
_____

Brain Challenge #5
Making Flexible Decisions to Empower Your Brain to Make Healthful Choices

Challenge Introduction

I get home from work, unlock the door, and walk inside my house. I am tired, hungry, and really need to think about something other than work. I start to think about what I need to do. I need to call my friend with whom I promised to exercise, and I need to make something decent for dinner. I head to the kitchen to look in my pantry. There are some beans, onions, broccoli, pasta, chips…. Next thing I know, I have the chips open and the TV on. An hour later, I remember I was going to make myself some real dinner and go out with a friend. But now I have already eaten about 800 calories worth of chips and my friend has probably already gone to the gym without me. I meant so well. Why do I always do this, day after day?

Our health-related habits set in motion a chain of behaviors, some conscious and some below our level of awareness. Certain brain centers have their own priorities, setting in motion actions that may surprise us. Long-term survival of our species over thousands upon thousands of years has relied on us storing sufficient fat to outlast long periods of scarcity. No wonder those chips are so appealing. There is now convincing evidence that "will power" may be no match for tempting but unhealthy foods that we encounter. In some cases, making healthful choices may require us to ban these temptations from our immediate environment.

Optimal health requires the ability to make creative, flexible decisions based upon your current condition and the local environment. To be able to adapt to the unexpected, you need to be able to problem-solve and implement novel solutions. As humans, we have impressive and rare brain circuits that can solve complex problems. However, these circuits are the last to develop, require training to become efficient processors, and are the most vulnerable to damage and dysfunction with age. Moreover, they are slow. These circuits must stall behaviors long enough to give themselves the opportunity to decide upon and plan a new behavior. In Challenge #5, we discuss how these circuits work and techniques for improving their function. In Chapter 5.1, we explain the limitations of trying to use willpower to stop unhealthy habits. In Chapter 5.2, we describe the process by which problem-solving skills develop and disappear including the role of new neuron growth. In Chapter 5.3, we provide techniques for improving problem-solving and cognitive skills so that you will be able to successfully engage in healthful behaviors.

Chapter 5.1: Delaying Automatic Unhealthy Habits to Try Something New

To give ourselves enough time to come up with a new plan for how to respond in a familiar circumstance, we need to be able to postpone doing our habitual response long enough to enact the new plan. The dorsolateral and orbitofrontal cortex circuits can stall impulsive habits, giving the prefrontal cortex circuits time to consider options and come up with new plans.

This ability to develop flexible thinking has been extensively studied by psychologists using behavioral tasks such as Go-NoGo tasks. A simple example of a Go-NoGo task is the game, "Simon Says", where one is supposed to carry out commands except when the command does not include the words, "Simon Says." In these tasks, participants are tested to see how well they can stop themselves from doing a well-practiced, automatic response.

These tasks have shown that there is considerable variation from person to person in how well they can stop a habitual behavior. Clients with impairments in part of the prefrontal cortex, specifically the dorsolateral area, do very poorly at Go-NoGo and similar tasks, as do children whose prefrontal cortices have yet to develop. Notably, even in a single person, this ability varies depending on what other things the person is trying to do at the same time. It turns out that, at least when it comes to stopping us from doing habits, our prefrontal cortex is not a very good multi-tasker.

But before we continue, let's remind ourselves what the prefrontal cortex is trying to do and why. We know from Challenge #1 that our limbic reward circuit holds learned patterns. The limbic reward circuit can identify situations where a habitual response is likely to result in short-term gain and can initiate that habitual behavior if it seems worth the effort. Importantly, the limbic reward circuit can do this without the conscious approval of prefrontal cortex circuits. Also, the limbic reward circuits can make decisions to do a habitual behavior very quickly because they use efficient but relatively simple and pre-defined decision rules (Saling & Phillips, 2007). Meanwhile, the prefrontal cortex circuits can often take longer because the decisions they are making are relatively complex and require use of a variety of multi-stage logic processes. The prefrontal cortex circuits can calculate and weigh difficult multi-stage decisions that include consideration not only of short-term gains, but also long-term consequences, our goals and values, and special circumstances of the current situation. The more complicated the decision and the more things that need to be considered, the longer it will take the prefrontal cortex to finish processing the decision. Thus, for anything other than simple decisions, the prefrontal cortex will come up with its plan for behavior much later than the limbic reward circuit. But our prefrontal cortex's decision will be useless if our limbic reward circuit has already started our habitual response. Therefore, it is crucial that our prefrontal cortex can stop the limbic system from carrying out the habit until it has had time to finish its own analysis.

Luckily, we know that, with conscious effort, our dorsolateral and orbitofrontal circuits can work together to stall or stop the limbic reward circuit from carrying out the habitual behavior. To successfully guide our behavior, our prefrontal cortex must stall the limbic reward circuit from carrying out our habitual response long enough to finish its calculations. The more complicated the decision, the longer the prefrontal cortex must stall. In some of the examples we will present next, you can observe this stalling. You can see that most people slow down their decision-making when the instruction or task is harder to follow. Some people appear to be better at slowing down their decisions than others, and this may explain differences in people's ability to successfully overcome old habits and try new behaviors.

Why willpower is not enough
Willpower can be very helpful for getting people through a difficult task. Motivation and determination to do something can help someone keep going through an uncomfortable situation and persist through a grueling undertaking. Like "The Little Engine That Could" who said "I think I can" over and over to get over the hill, willpower can help you make that deadline, cope through a painful event, or sprint the last mile of a run.

However, willpower is not effective for getting people NOT to do something. Trying to use willpower to stop you from eating the chocolate that you love is not likely to work, and might even lead to your eating more than normal. There are clear biological and psychological reasons for this rooted in the design of your prefrontal cortex circuits.

Your prefrontal cortex has the ability to prevent or stop you from doing habitual behaviors. For example, your prefrontal cortex can stop you from eating the chocolate sitting in front of you, or keep you from pulling your arm away from the poor phlebotomist drawing blood from your needle-phobic veins. However, your prefrontal cortex can only do this with conscious effort. For your prefrontal cortex to inhibit a behavior, you first must be aware of the behavior you are trying to inhibit! This is where the problem lies. Part of the process of stopping habits involves remembering that you want to avoid that behavior. Your prefrontal cortex has an ability, called working memory, to keep thoughts that it intends to use during upcoming decisions ready to access on a moment-to-moment basis. To delay a habit, you have to keep that behavior or thought in your working memory so your prefrontal cortex has access to that information when a situation presents itself. When the time comes to make a quick decision, your prefrontal cortex will include that working memory information about the habit in its rapid calculation. If your brain had to go rummaging through your long-term files to try to dig up the information about what you intended to do, your limbic system would have already carried out the habit before your prefrontal cortex figured out what to do.

The problem with keeping the thought of an undesirable habit in your working memory is two-fold. The first problem is that if you keep a thought in your working memory then your prefrontal cortex will tend to include that thought in all of its decision-making and not just for decisions related to the habit. For example, if I put chocolate in my working memory, then my prefrontal cortex will tend to include chocolate when considering all of its decisions. This may help me stick to my intended decision not to eat the chocolate that my well-meaning office-mates have left in our shared area. However, it also means my prefrontal cortex will consider chocolate in other decisions it's making. When I start feeling a bit hungry or when a work deadline stresses me out, my prefrontal cortex will at least consider chocolate as a possible solution. When I think about what I should get my friend for her upcoming birthday, chocolate is apt to come to mind. With chocolate in my working memory, I will now problem-solve with chocolate on the short-list of all solutions. This may lead me to expose myself to more opportunities where I could eat chocolate, or even make me decide to go out and buy chocolate on my own. In most cases, trying to use willpower to avoid eating chocolate leads people to eat more chocolate than they would have if they never tried to stop themselves. (Note: For those who want to read more, this concept has been termed the "White Bear Effect" by David Schneider. He described and studied it by instructing people not to think of a white bear, which, of course, they were compelled to think about thereafter.)

The second problem with using working memory to inhibit an undesirable habit is that this system gets slow and inefficient as working memory gets cluttered. The more thoughts you put in your working memory, the slower your prefrontal cortex is at remembering what to do with them. If your prefrontal cortex gets too slow, it may not remember what habit you were trying to block until after you have already done the habit. When I get busy and have a lot on my mind, I may already have the chocolate in my mouth before I remember that I was not going to eat any.

The limits of willpower in overcoming habits
In one brain imaging study, participants were asked to try to inhibit a habit using a version of the Go-NoGo tasks we described earlier (Hester & Garavan, 2004). Specifically, the researchers flashed letters on a screen and asked the participants to press a key every time a letter appeared. Once that task was learned, they showed the participants a letter and told them to remember it (i.e., put it in working memory) and not to press the key when that particular letter was flashed on the screen. Because the vast majority of the letters shown were not that particular letter, the participants were quickly trained in a habit of pressing the key whenever something flashed on the screen. This forced the prefrontal cortex to try to use the specific letter in working memory to inhibit the key-pressing habit when that letter appeared. Most people could do this very well. Then the researchers made it harder. Instead of just one letter, they gave the participants five letters to remember and asked them not to press the button when any of these were presented. These extra letters cluttered up participants' working memory, and most people got much worse, often pressing the button before they recognized that the letter was one they were trying to remember. Notably, most people realized shortly after pressing the key that they had messed up, but the prefrontal cortex was now too late to actually inhibit the key-pressing habit.

The corresponding brain activity may help explain what happens. Looking only at the times when people correctly inhibited their key-pressing response, increasing the number of letters to remember increased activation in parts of the prefrontal cortex (the left medial frontal cortex, and anterior and posterior cingulate cortex). Additionally, the amount of activity in the anterior cingulate was associated with doing the task correctly in the five-letter version, suggesting that activity in this region is important for overcoming the increase in working memory demand. Supporting this further, typical people increased their anterior cingulate activity as more letters were added to the task, but regular cocaine users, who have difficulty inhibiting the key-pressing, did not increase their anterior cingulate activity as more letters were added. We know the anterior cingulate is required to monitor for and assess errors in learned behavior (e.g., Weinberg et al., 2015). Thus, this study suggests that as we start to multitask and hold more things in our working memory, our brains must work harder and harder to identify mistakes in our planned behavior. If we try to multitask too much, this will lead to mistakes in our planned behavior even if we have a very healthy anterior cingulate and prefrontal cortex. We will start to do our habitual behaviors despite intentions otherwise.

Damage to the anterior cingulate and other associated regions of the prefrontal cortex, such as that caused by years of cocaine or other stimulant abuse, can make it very difficult to intentionally inhibit habits (Thompson et al., 2004). Further, people with obsessive-compulsive disorders, who feel as though they are constantly required to be on alert to solve working memory-types of problems, have been found to have abnormalities with the anterior cingulate. Moreover, response to behavioral treatments for obsessive compulsive disorder has been associated with cortical volume change in anterior cingulate over the course of treatment (Fullana et al., 2014). In contrast, damage to the anterior cingulate can induce a state of lethargy and motivational inertia known as akinetic mutism. Even the healthy aging brain, experiencing typical mild cognitive impairments, is more likely to have working memory problems. In other words, trying not to eat a tempting piece of chocolate may become even more difficult as we age.

Alternatives to willpower

These studies highlight the need to use other strategies beyond willpower to keep us from carrying out our bad habits over the long-term. We are going to have other things to think about in life. We will get busy and clutter up our working memory. Moreover, there is great individual variation in ability to inhibit habits while multi-tasking, which means it will take different people differing amounts of clutter before they can no long inhibit their habits. Some can handle thinking about many things at once without making too many mistakes, but others start to revert to habits pretty quickly. While our ability to inhibit a habit may be crucial for preventing us from reverting to bad behavior patterns in the occasional, unavoidable, high-risk situation, relying on this system alone during attempts to unlearn bad habits is certain to fail.

Using problem-solving strategies to reduce exposure to situations where we do bad habits, as well as using the strategies discussed in previous chapters, is key to long-term success in quitting bad habits. We are much more likely to achieve success in changing our bad habits if we problem-solve before we are faced with an opportunity to do the bad habit, rather than waiting until we are in a high-risk situation and then trying to stop our habit and do something else. If I really do not want to eat chocolate, I should do my problem-solving before I am in the common room with the chocolate in front of me. Knowing that there is often chocolate in the common room, I could decide to always walk down a different hall or make sure that I never got very hungry at work by keeping lots of salad and vegetables in my office and snacking all day long. If I am forced to sit in the same room as some tempting dark chocolate, I can move it far enough away to keep it out of reach.

Problem-solving ahead of time takes the pressure off your prefrontal cortex. Without the urgency of a situation where you could get immediate rewards for doing your bad habit, your prefrontal cortex can focus on coming up with a solution without fighting to hold off your limbic reward circuit while it searches for alternatives. I am much better at figuring out how not to eat chocolate when it is not sitting in front of me, teasing my nucleus accumbens and begging to be consumed.

Chapter 5.2: How Do Our Problem-Solving Skills Develop and Fade?

Developmental stages and cognitive decline

The prefrontal cortex is a highly complex and evolutionarily recent feature found only in a small number of mammal species. It is substantially larger in humans than other primates and constitutes about 40% of the entire cerebral cortex. As noted, the prefrontal cortex is extremely slow to complete development. Cortex development involves a process where neurons insulate the connections between each other with specialized fat cells called myelin. This myelin increases the chance that a signal sent by a neuron gets successfully delivered to the next neuron, just like putting insulation on a wire makes it conduct electricity more efficiently. Additionally, cortex development starts by making lots of interconnections between the neurons until the neurons learn which connections will be useful. As cortex matures, these neurons start to get more selective about their connections. They start to eliminate connections that do not contribute to successful signal transmission or problem-solving. This pruning makes the cortex more efficient and consistent in its decisions. While some parts of cortex finish this myelination and pruning process during the toddler years or very early childhood, the prefrontal cortex continues to add myelin and prune connectivity substantially through at least adolescence. Consistent with this late anatomical development, performance on tasks that make use of prefrontal circuits improves up until one's early twenties.

For example, the Stroop task is commonly used to assess how successfully one can inhibit a well-trained behavior. Like the Go-NoGo tasks described earlier, this task requires the participants to inhibit their habitual response. This task makes use of the fact that, at least among literate people, reading is a habitual behavior triggered by the presence of words. That is, when we see a word, the first thing we do is read it, not notice the font, or the type size, or the color. We can obviously do all those things as well, but our first instinct is to read the word. The Stroop task looks at how well a person can block this reading habit in order to report other characteristics of a word. First, the Stroop task asks people to read a number of color words, printed in black text (e.g., "red", "blue", "yellow") to get a measure of reading speed. Next, the task asks people to identify the color of a series of "XXXXX" printed in various colors to get a measure of how quickly they can identify colors. Finally, the person is asked to inhibit their reading habit. The person is asked to identify the color of the type in which a color word has been printed (e.g., "red" written in blue ink should elicit a response of "blue", "yellow" written in red ink should elicit a response of "red"). The number of incorrect responses and the change in speed in the person's ability to identify colors is an indicator of how much trouble the person has inhibiting their reading behavior to successfully name the colors (Stroop, 1935). To try the task yourself, go to: http://faculty.washington.edu/chudler/java/ready.html

As we might expect given the slow development of the prefrontal cortex, people get better at the Stroop task during late childhood, and continue to improve during adolescence, reaching a relatively stable level of their personal best performance in late adolescence. This level of performance is on average maintained until about age 65, when performance on a population level starts to decline (Comalli et al., 1962). Notably, not all older adults show large declines in executive function as measured by Stroop. Researchers found that although Stroop performance generally declined with advancing age, the declines in performance were substantially greater in individuals with a lower level of education (Van der Elst et al., 2006). This emphasizes the importance of training and practice for development and maintenance of executive function. Education early in life may provide extra training of prefrontal circuits that buffers the effects of aging-related decreases in prefrontal abilities. We will discuss this more in the next section.

Risk aversion and risky decision-making

The slow development of the prefrontal cortex can lead to more impulsive and risky behavior in children and teenagers compared to adults. Prefrontal cortex function has been associated with "risk aversion", which refers to the idea that people are generally very careful not to lose things they have obtained or to subject themselves to even small risks. This trait is less pronounced in children and adolescents, as well as people with damage to ventromedial region of the orbitofrontal cortex circuits, people with psychopathy and substance use disorders, or people who have been deprived of sleep.

In his excellent book *Descartes' Error* (1994), the eminent neurologist Antonio Damasio describes a client, initialed EVR, with ventromedial prefrontal cortex damage. EVR had a meningioma tumor growing in the midline area just above his nasal cavities that compressed both frontal lobes upward. Although EVR scored in the superior range on tests of intelligence, his ability to make decisions was impaired, especially in social situations. He could sense that topics that used to evoke emotion, no longer did so. Although he had social knowledge, he now lacked feelings of embarrassment. Like other clients with lesions in this region, he no longer avoided risky behavior, despite threats of loss of social standing, or other unpleasant consequences. EVR did not show risk aversion, nor the emotional responses that generally accompany it.

Deficits in risk aversion can be studied with behavioral tasks. The Iowa Gambling task has been used to characterize problems with decision-making, particularly in one's ability to learn and adapt their choices based on punishments or rewards. Participants are presented with four card decks from which they must choose cards. The goal of the task is to try to win as much money as possible, and typically participants are given a portion of their earnings at the end as a motivator. Participants are told that some decks are better than others and asked to make 100 card choices. Two of the decks have cards indicating a relatively large gain of money, but also occasional cards that provide an extremely large penalty loss. Consistently choosing from these decks leads to a net loss of money. The other two decks have cards with generally lower gains than the other decks, but also much lower penalties. Consistently choosing from these two decks leads to a net gain of money. The average person with high risk aversion will relatively quickly learn to avoid the decks with the extremely large losses out of fear of a future large loss. However, people who are very driven by opportunities for big immediate rewards will tend to choose more from the decks with the higher wins, even though this is a poor long-term strategy that leads to loss of money.

Individuals with ventromedial prefrontal cortex damage like EVR consistently make decisions guided by immediate possibilities rather than longer-term rewards or consequences (Bechara et al., 2000). This may be in part because they cannot use emotions associated with past losses to adjust future behavior. They will consistently pick from the high win/high loss deck, tempted by the bigger gains even though it is an overall losing deck. Children and adolescents tend to show more of this pattern of choosing than adults, and slowly improve over time as their prefrontal cortex develops. As children age, they slowly make more complex decisions in the Iowa Gambling task (Huizenga et al., 2007). First, they start to consider the frequency of loss. Only later can they consider both the amount and frequency of losses in their choices.

In healthy adults, sleep deprivation leads people to choose more frequently from the high gain/high loss money-losing deck than they do when they are well rested (Killgore et al., 2006). Notably, this effect of sleep deprivation cannot be reversed by caffeine consumption (Killgore et al., 2007)! This same study observed that although age did not predict performance on the Iowa Gambling task when people were well rested, age did predict performance when people were sleep deprived, with older adults showing more immediate reward-driven choices than younger people. This suggests that older people are more sensitive to sleep deprivation than younger people and show more risky reward-driven behavior when poorly rested.

Taken together, these studies indicate that a fully functioning ventromedial prefrontal cortex is needed to learn and follow good strategies to maximize long-term benefit. When the ventromedial prefrontal cortex is not working well, that person will tend to make risky choices that put their longer-term well-being in jeopardy for a chance at a big immediate reward. Moreover, it is not particularly rare for someone to have only a partially functioning ventromedial cortex, either because it has not developed yet (e.g., teenagers) or because it is not rested enough to work correctly (e.g., following sleep deprivation). This could lead to all sort of risky behaviors. For example, teenagers might drive dangerously fast just to experience the thrill, even though they are risking devastating injury or even death by doing so. A sleep-deprived adult might eat a whole box of cookies just because they taste good, even though they know they need to get their weight down to keep their diabetes under control or else risk heart disease or foot amputation. Thus, fostering development, training, and good up-keep of one's ventromedial prefrontal cortex is crucial for encouraging healthful behavior.

Making good long-term decisions also relies on having a well-functioning orbitofrontal cortex, and people show abnormal behavior on the Iowa Gambling task when their orbitofrontal cortex is damaged. But in this case, they demonstrate a lack of punishment learning. They do not switch to the more conservative decks after experiencing huge losses on the high gain/high loss decks. Individuals with sub-clinical psychopathy symptoms also show this pattern of decisions on this task (van Honk et al., 2002). This finding is consistent with anti-social behaviors that individuals with psychopathy display. Basically, their brains do not modify their behavior when they do something that upsets other people or even causes them immediate harm. Their choices are driven only by the chance of being rewarded and not by the risk of punishment. Thus, if you want to make good long-term choices, you need both the ventromedial prefrontal cortex to help you consider the long-term consequences of your decision and your other portions of the orbitofrontal cortex to help you avoid choices that lead to immediately damaging results.

Use it or lose it: The effect of novelty and activity on lifelong cognitive function
Knowing how important our prefrontal cortex is for making good long-term decisions for our health, how do we help our prefrontal cortex become strong and sophisticated? First off, it appears that the prefrontal cortex is a bit like our muscles. If you want your prefrontal cortex to work optimally, you need to work it out regularly. You need to train it, and then provide it with regular challenges to maintain its fitness. But what constitutes a good workout for your prefrontal cortex?

Since your prefrontal cortex generates alternatives, solves problems, and makes decisions, a good workout for your prefrontal cortex is anything that presents you with a lot of problems. More complicated and novel problems are even better for building up the prefrontal cortex. Since school is generally designed to help you identify problems you do not know how to solve and help you work toward a solution, education would be expected to strengthen your prefrontal cortex. As expected, education tends to be associated with improvements in decision-making skills. The importance of education becomes more obvious during old age when brain function starts to decline. As they age, people who received less education tend to show greater losses of problem-solving skills than more educated people. Researchers have argued that education when you are young helps create a "functional reserve" of brainpower. If you train your brain exceptionally well when you are young, your prefrontal cortex will have so much extra strength that your problem-solving skills will still be up to par when your prefrontal cortex starts to deteriorate (Fillit et al., 2002). Studies have also shown that continuing to train the prefrontal cortex can keep it "in shape" and maintain problem-solving skills. Older people who remain engaged socially and challenge themselves with new problems on a regular basis show less loss of problem-solving skills over time. For example, playing cognitively challenging games, be they videogames or board games, has been found to improve cognitive performance not only on the games themselves, but also on general neuropsychological tests and function, and prevent cognitive decline with age (Fissler et al., 2015). Overall, these findings are consistent with the view that continuing education throughout life is good for your brain, good for your health, and enlightening too.

While we generally lose brain cells and function as we age, this does not mean that our prefrontal cortex slows down over time. However, it may be working harder than before. Brain imaging studies have demonstrated reliable increases in prefrontal activation in older adults, indicating increased blood flow to this region that suggests the cortex may in fact work harder as we get older. Older adults who had the largest tissue losses in the hippocampus over a ten-year period showed the greatest additional activation in the right dorsolateral prefrontal cortex (Park & Reuter-Lorenz, 2009). The right dorsolateral prefrontal cortex is implicated in executive control, mental flexibility, and problem-solving. People with damage to this region demonstrate some of the following impairments: perseveration (i.e., sticking with the same strategy even when it ceases to be rewarding), impaired divergent thinking, impaired retrieval, and distress intolerance (see Millder & Cummings, 2006).

Since the dorsolateral prefrontal cortex is substantially more active for older adults with greater degeneration in the hippocampus compared to younger people and older adults with less degeneration in the hippocampus, it is reasonable to assume that the additional activity contributes to compensatory processing. When the parts of the brain that normally help with memory begin to fail, other parts are recruited to help. When we start to lose brain resources, we put more pressure on the parts that remain to solve problems. These back-up systems that rely on alternative brain pathways allow us to continue achieving our goals so we may continue to function normally even as we lose neurons with age. Ongoing challenges that require flexible thinking and exercise can help build and maintain these back-up problem-solving systems and help prevent declines in our abilities as we grow older.

How does training strengthen the prefrontal cortex's ability to problem-solve? This probably occurs through a few mechanisms, such as strengthening connections and adding new neurons. First, practicing problem-solving appears to strengthen neuronal connections in the prefrontal cortex. This practice probably teaches the prefrontal cortex specific strategies for tackling a problem. As these strategies are practiced, the connections between neurons needed to implement this strategy will be strengthened. This will make it easier to try this strategy in the future. Second, adding new neurons and support cells (glia) to the prefrontal cortex appears to strengthen it. This process is called neurogenesis (for neurons) and gliogenesis (for glia). For years neuroscience lore suggested that your brain does not make new neurons after early development, but neuroscientists have now shown that this is not true. The brain can and does make new neurons throughout adulthood, particularly in the hippocampus. New neurons, but more commonly new glia, are also generated in the prefrontal cortex. Neuroscience lore also suggested that glia have little to do with cognitive processing, but it is now increasingly clear that these cells, in addition to their role in providing nutrients and related functions, also have their own signaling system that can influence the function of neurons during learning and memory. Albert Einstein's brain was found to have exceptionally high volumes of glia, suggesting they are important for high cognitive functioning.

While it is still not known exactly how adding new cells strengthens the prefrontal cortex, birth of new brain cells has been suggested to help maintain good prefrontal cortex function and prevent mood disorders. Perhaps the new cells replace ones that get damaged with aging, or perhaps they are needed to make or strengthen new circuits that address new problems. Encouraging glia to multiply or become more effective in their supportive roles may improve cognitive function. Further research is needed to figure out how neurogenesis and gliogenesis improve prefrontal cortex function, but until then we can still encourage the birth of new cells in our brain and reap the benefits in our prefrontal cortex.

Doing your part to keep up the birthrate in your neural neighborhood

Birth of new brain cells does not appear to occur at a consistent stable pace. Rather neurogenesis and gliogenesis appear to be triggered or increased in response to environmental interactions. We have learned a substantial amount about when birth of new brain cells occurs and what prevents it from occurring by studying animal models.

The first finding regarding growth and death of new brain cells was that chronic stress is doubly problematic for keeping brains healthy and functioning. Chronic stress makes neurons vulnerable to damage, loss of connections, atrophy, and cell death, particularly in the hippocampus (Sapolsky, 1999; McEwen, 1999). On top of this, chronic stress, including chronic social stress, reduces or prevents birth of new brain cells in limbic brain regions and the prefrontal cortex (Czéh et al., 2007). Thus, chronic stress makes you more likely to lose brain cells and less likely to replace them, a combination that is obviously not good for keeping your brain connections intact and functioning. This means that steps to reduce stress in your life, such as those we discussed in Challenge #3, should help you keep your neuron numbers up and maintain your problem-solving functions.

Next, poor diet has been found to contribute to brain deterioration and cognitive decline (Freeman et al., 2014). Rats only developed deterioration in the hippocampus (e.g., retraction of apical dendrites) when they were exposed to stressful social events (e.g., unstable housing and viewing a cat daily) if they were also fed a diet high in animal and saturated fat (Baran et al., 2005). A fatty diet has been associated with chronic stress and both have been linked to increased risk of cardiovascular disease, dementia, and depression. The gut microbiome seems to be important for shaping neurogenesis and related health effects, most likely by regulating neuroinflammation. For example, transplanting gut microbes from a stressed mouse into a non-stressed mouse is sufficient to reduce neurogenesis in the recipient mouse's hippocampus and cause depression behaviors (Alonso et al., 2024). In contrast, adherence to a low fat, Mediterranean diet has been linked to a lower risk of age-related cognitive impairment (Féart et al., 2009). Further, adherence to a Mediterranean diet, alone or in combination with regular physical activity, reduced the risk of Alzheimer's disease (Scarmeas et al., 2009).

Long-term caloric restriction also has been shown to protect the hippocampus of aging rats (Mladenovic Djordjevic et al. 2010). In rhesus monkeys, caloric restriction by 10-20% extended longevity by about 10-20%, prevented Type II diabetes, and reduced the risk of stroke and age-related cognitive impairment (Colman et al., 2009). Caloric restriction seems to be a daunting idea for most adults, and it remains unclear whether it is possible for more than a small percentage of people to exercise this kind of restraint. Intermittent fasting, where eating is limited to a time-restricted portion of the day, induces hippocampal neurogenesis similarly to caloric restriction (Melgar-Locatelli et al., 2023). As this is a more practical alternative to caloric restriction, additional research in this area is underway. Notably, in encouraging healthful dietary patterns, the cells in the prefrontal cortex that make informed decisions and protect us from unhealthy temptations would be preserving their own existence by reducing the risk of hypertensive stroke or age-related cognitive impairments from a diet that promotes diabetes, a key risk factor for Alzheimer's disease.

While the idea of reducing caloric intake, cutting fat from your diet, or damping down your stressful life commitments may seem like signing up for a life of perpetual sacrifice, there are an increasing number of people shifting to a more relaxed, minimalist lifestyle that embraces these goals. For example, the "Slow Movement" encourages people to "downshift" their lives, reducing time pressure and commitments and connecting in more meaningful ways with the people in their communities, the food they eat, and the work or services they provide (http://www.slowmovement.com/). Reframing stress reduction and lower caloric intake into terms of reducing time pressure to allow yourself to become more engaged in the core things you do and to savor the things you eat more deeply, can make these same behavioral changes seem highly appealing and even downright indulgent. For maintaining neurons, less is more, at least when it comes to social pressure and food consumption. And less social pressure and food consumption can be torture or paradise, depending on how you approach it.

In addition, exposure to enriched and novel environments, depression treatments, and voluntary exercise has all been shown to increase neurogenesis in the hippocampus and/or gliogenesis in the prefrontal cortex (Banasr & Duman, 2007; Mandyam et al., 2007; Olson et al., 2006). For example, old rats that lived in cages where there was plenty of visual stimulation and the opportunity to play generated more new hippocampus neurons than rats living in ordinary cages. Further, rats living in complex environments showed greater ability to learn and solve problems. Extrapolating to humans, there are good reasons to maintain a complex and stimulating environment, one that engages your mind and body.

It has been suggested that the effects of antidepressants on the birth of new brain cells is actually responsible for the reduction in depressive and posttraumatic stress symptoms that the medications produce (i.e., the ultimate effect of changing serotonin levels is to increase the birth rates of new brain cells), and researchers are now looking for new medications that increase cell birth rates in hopes of finding new treatments for depression and anxiety disorders (Banasr & Duman, 2007; Bremner et al., 2008). The birth of new neurons in the hippocampus is thought to be mediated by a growth factor known as Brain Derived Nerve Growth Factor (BDNF), which can be stimulated by antidepressants, electroconvulsive shock treatment used to treat depression, and moderate physical exercise (Castrén & Rantamäki, 2010). Notably, voluntary exercise not only stimulates the birth of new brain cells but also tends to reduce depression (Daley, 2008). This is consistent with the idea that birth and development of new brain cells causes reductions in mood disorders.

Recent models suggest that new neurons in the hippocampus may be important for pattern separation or learning how to differentiate new context or situations from previously learned ones (Oomen et al., 2014). Generally, pattern separation helps make similar patterns of brain activity more distinct, improving identification of people, items, new situations, cues and so forth. Oversimplified, this pattern separation may help old dogs recognize contexts for trying new tricks and sort out new situations where an old habit isn't appropriate.

Overall, these studies suggest that maintaining exposure to new environments and challenges, having a rich diverse lifestyle, proactively treating mood disorders, and exercising regularly should improve and maintain cognitive abilities and problem-solving skills late in life. These predictions are supportive of a growing body of human research that suggests that social engagement, intellectual stimulation, and physical activity all contribute to maintenance of cognitive ability in older age (Butler et al., 2004).

Lastly, one of the best ways to maintain cognitive performance is to not damage your brain cells in the first place. Recent studies of the effects of concussion and traumatic brain injury emphasize the damage to brain structure and neurons that these injuries can cause, and suggest that these injuries can make the brain more vulnerable to cognitive decline with age and other insults (e.g., poor diet, lack of exercise, stress) (Moretti et al., 2012). The protective helmet you wear when you ride a bicycle or the safety belt that keeps your head from striking the windshield are important for preventing damage to neural circuits. Taking precautions can meaningfully reduce head injuries in sports, occupational injuries, from firearms and from falls.

In addition to traumatic brain injury, there are many insidious causes of brain injury resulting from toxic, behavioral and neurodegenerative causes. These include diabetes, hypertension and vascular disease, sleep disorders, depression, alcohol, and substance and medication misuse. The benefits of regular screening for these causes of neuron loss cannot be underestimated. Daily adherence to medically-prescribed exercise and drug regimens can be life- and cognition-saving. For example, hypertensive stroke can be prevented in a majority of people through adequate monitoring and treatment of high blood pressure. Likewise, minimizing use of alcohol and other recreational drugs can prevent cognitive decline. For example, a longitudinal study of a birth cohort examined the cognitive effects of persistent use of marijuana during young adulthood, assessing neurocognitive function at age 13, before cannabis use, and at age 38 (Meier et al., 2012). While those that did not use cannabis showed small increases in IQ from age 13 to 38, those with chronic marijuana use showed significant declines in IQ over this period. This effect was still evident after controlling for education, alcohol, tobacco, and other drug use, though the decline in IQ over time was even greater for those with less education. Managing sleep disorders can also be helpful. In a sample of over 2000 community-dwelling older adults, sleep disordered breathing predicted an earlier onset of mild cognitive decline; But, persons with sleep disordered breathing who were treated with continuous positive airway pressure devices (CPAP) had a similar age of onset of mild cognitive impairment as those without sleep-disordered breathing, suggesting that treatment prevents the effect of sleep disorders on cognitive decline (Osorio et al., 2015). Addressing common insults that can damage brain circuits, from metabolic disease, to substance use and sleep deprivation can help preserve cognitive function over the life-span.

Chapter 5.3: Improving Problem-Solving and Cognitive Skills

What prevents problem-solving?
Assuming your prefrontal cortex is well-trained, well-rested, and healthy, is there anything that would make your prefrontal cortex make short-sighted decisions? As we discussed in Challenge #1, our thoughts, expectations, and learned associations about the value of immediate rewards can make our brains, including our prefrontal cortex, believe that these rewards are more important than their objective value. For example, if we are convinced that eating a gallon of ice cream will make us feel better, or expect that drinking a six-pack of beer will make us more attractive and socially adept, then our prefrontal cortex will include those assumptions in making its decisions. We will be more likely to eat the gallon of ice cream or drink that six-pack of beer if we hold those beliefs. Correcting these beliefs by consciously observing that we feel sick to our stomach after eating that much ice cream or that we wound up embarrassing ourselves while drunk can shift the decisions our prefrontal cortex makes. To make good decisions, our prefrontal cortex not only needs to know how to solve problems and make good choices but also needs accurate information about the choices it is considering.

In Thomas Jefferson's Declaration of Independence, he wrote about self-evident truths, justifying the rights of life, liberty, and the pursuit of happiness. For some, it is "self-evident" that the freedom to make self-destructive choices is an inalienable right for the pursuit of happiness. As a society, we have chosen to put few rules around the marketing and promotion of products, such as sugar-filled food products and alcoholic beverages that provide a quick transient pleasure but ultimately make us feel worse. Many marketing dollars are put into efforts to encourage us to attend to the quick "happiness" associated with the most common self-destructive habits. With personal effort, we can train ourselves to attend to the delayed effects of our choices. Listen to your body, and practice connecting the longer-term feelings produced by a choice to the choice itself. Remember the hangover instead of the intoxication, and beer will not be as appealing.

Our bodies communicate a kind of truth through these delayed somatic symptoms (e.g., a hangover) that should help us to protect our life and liberty against the indiscriminate pursuit of happiness. However, the time delay prevents our limbic circuits from recognizing the connection between these bad feelings and the choices that caused them. It takes conscious attention to link these later consequences and unhappiness to the choices that caused them. Only your prefrontal cortex can link the hangover to the beer. *Be aware of over-valuation of rewards. Your prefrontal cortex cannot make good choices if it is starting with inaccurate information.* Pay attention and consider the longer-term consequences of choices. This will provide the prefrontal cortex with the more accurate information it needs to make decisions that lead to lasting happiness, rather than the futile pursuit of quick pleasures that ultimately make us unhealthy and sick.

Tricks for helping your prefrontal cortex
1. Be prepared. Problem-solve possible problems before the situation occurs.
Knowing that problem-solving is a relatively slow process, you can improve the chance that you make good long-term choices by pre-planning responses to situations that you

expect to encounter. If you already have a solution to a problem figured out beforehand, you will not have to do the problem-solving during the situation. This will not only speed up your problem-solving, but also help ensure that the stress of the moment does not bias your decisions towards things that produce immediate relief rather than long-term benefit. Having predetermined solutions to situations that you expect to encounter can help your prefrontal cortex make up for its slow processing time. This helps ensure that you do not fall back on your habitual behaviors just because you did not have time to come up with a better response.

To practice pre-planning solutions, try Exercise 5A (page 223).

2. Ask or observe respected role models.
Although planning solutions beforehand can greatly increase your ability to make good long-term choices, this trick is still restricted by the limits of your own creativity. Pre-planning will only help you come up with solutions that you can think of based on your own problem-solving skills, knowledge, and past experience. Moreover, you can only come up with solutions for situations that you can anticipate. If you are not happy with your solutions, want to come up with new ones, or feel like you are often confronted by problematic surprises, you may want to either ask others what they would do or watch people respond to similar situations.

Obviously, the new solutions that asking or observing others provide will tend to be better when the person you are asking or watching is highly skilled at solving that particular problem. Thus, finding experts or role models who have mastered the behaviors you are interested in is key to making the most of the learning opportunity. If you are trying to learn to better control your anger, talk to a person who is particularly skilled in mediation. If you want to learn how to keep your diabetes under control, talk to a nutritionist or a person with well-controlled diabetes. If you want to learn how to swim for fitness, get advice from someone who has swum regularly for many years. Networking with friends, coworkers and teachers can provide powerful new solutions to stubborn problems.

If you want to observe others solving a similar problem, you will likely need to find a high-risk environment so that you can readily observe people being challenged. The difficulty with this strategy is that you will likely need to be in this high-risk environment yourself to do the observing. Thus, this is only a good idea if you can find a way to protect yourself while you are doing the observing. For example, if I wanted to observe strategies people use not to overeat when provided an excess of food, going to an all-you-can-eat buffet could provide a good opportunity to watch people's behavior and see who successfully eats in moderation and who eats more than necessary. However, I do not want to wind up over-eating myself. Making sure I am protected from eating too much, by not purchasing the buffet, going at a time when I am not hungry, or finding a restaurant where I do not like the food, is key to giving me space to observe behavior without getting into trouble myself.

Many successful therapies and interventions include a component where people are encouraged to learn from and observe experienced others. For example, therapists may rehearse new solutions with their clients and model new behaviors. Mutual help groups such as Alcoholics Anonymous encourage people in stable recovery to come to meetings and mentor people who are still having trouble initiating behavior change. At these meetings they can provide suggestions regarding ways that they successfully navigated difficult situations or solved problems.

To learn some prefrontal mnemonics for questions to ask yourself or your role models, see Exercise 5B (page 226).

3. Play! Logic problems, games, sports, and exploration.
Finding fun and challenging pastimes is very important for ensuring that your prefrontal cortex gets regular workouts. The more practice your brain gets solving problems, the stronger and faster your prefrontal circuits will become. Since you cannot solve problems unless you have problems, this means that you need to find ways of exposing yourself to challenges. However, as we mentioned before, stress, especially chronic stress, weakens the prefrontal cortex. Thus, the trick is to expose yourself to problems without getting stressed.

This is where the fun comes in. You need to give yourself time to play. By play, we mean you need to give yourself challenges where your success or failure is of little consequence to your actual well-being. For example, I could try to master a new videogame. If it is a decent game, I will have to learn a number of new strategies to progress through the game and will likely learn to enact them quickly. This is a good prefrontal cortex workout. At the same time, it does not really matter if I fail at the game repeatedly. I can always just restart and try it again. Thus, the problems the videogame provides should not be stressful. I suppose I could get all worked up and stressed about the game if I tried, but with any amount of perspective, I would see that I was being silly. These are the sorts of challenges you need to create.

To really strengthen the prefrontal cortex, it is also important to make sure that you get a lot of variety in the challenges you create. Otherwise, your prefrontal cortex will get really good at solving one type of problem but be terrible at others. Diversity in your games is important! Playing a single videogame all day long will not make you a great overall problem-solver, it will just make you great at the skills needed for that videogame. So, mix it up! Try some crossword puzzles. Take piano lessons. Master Sudoku. Learn a new language. Join a debate club. Study organic chemistry. Play basketball. Attend cooking classes. Practice yoga. Immerse yourself in a new culture. Try some logic problems. Do a jigsaw puzzle. Take a multivariate calculus class. Learn to knit. Join a creative-writing group. Garden. Test out investing strategies by tracking simulated trading practices. Train to run a marathon. Teach a child to read. Figure out how to get the stains out of your living room carpet. All of these will force you to address new problems and situations that you have not encountered before. Figuring out how to successfully solve those problems will teach you how to respond when you encounter similar or analogous problems later. And in all of these cases, who cares if you fail 27 times before you get even close to a workable solution. Half-finished crossword puzzles, missed free throws, a sweater with two different length arms, the wrong answers on some math problems, and a burnt dinner are not the end of the world. Get out there and try the things that interest you. You almost certainly will not be good at them for a while after you start, but that is a good sign that you picked something you need work on. Each try on a new problem helps train your prefrontal cortex, regardless of whether you succeed or fail.

Lastly, the fun part is also important for encouraging practice and persistence. Becoming a good problem-solver takes work and repetition. If you give yourself challenging play that you do not enjoy, you will not keep at it and you will not develop your problem-solving skills. For example, I (J.T.) once decided I wanted to learn to wind-surf and signed up for lessons, thinking it would be a fabulous way to spend spring afternoons. But a couple of lessons in, I was forced to admit that I hated it. The water was freezing cold, and the lake we were learning in had big yucky weeds that got tangled in your legs and shifting gusty winds that knocked you over almost every time you started going. I am not very cold tolerant and found the whole experience miserable. Rather than ensure that I never tried the sport again in my life, I stopped going to those lessons and took up water polo instead. I was equally bad at water polo, but the pool was reasonably warm, the coach had a sense of humor (which he needed to put up with my lack of talent), and there was so much to learn that I could not help but get substantially better relatively quickly. It provided a much better environment for learning and practicing. My failures did not involve a torturous dunk in ice-cold, muddy, slimy water, and my successes were so unexpected that they excited both my supportive coach and myself. Even though the water polo lessons were exceedingly challenging for me, and I was by far the worst person in the class, I looked forward to the class and made sure to never miss one. It was fun. So, follow your interests, do not be afraid to look foolish or fail, but do find challenges and a learning environment that you honestly enjoy. Otherwise, you will never practice long enough to learn anything.

To practice building problem-skills by playing games and doing physical activities, see Exercise 5C (page 227) and Exercise 5D (page 229).

<u>EXAMPLE:</u> The value of expanding your horizons and trying new things

I (W.G.) took up yoga despite (or perhaps because of) substantial inflexibility. At first, I felt hopelessly overmatched by the capabilities of the students who had learned these skills and made them seem easy, while I found the poses beyond my capabilities. Although I did not "believe" yoga would do me any good, I initially persevered because my aching neck and shoulders felt much better every time after I exercised. My teacher gently reminded me, "you don't have to believe in it to benefit." Several weeks later, I quit, felt worse, returned, felt better, quit again for a shorter duration, felt much better when I returned, and soon the habit stuck. For the last couple of years, I have attended a yoga class two to three times a week and I always look forward to it.

The challenge is not only in doing the poses, which, for the most part, I am still much more deficient in performing than most of the other students, but in paying absolute attention to the constantly changing instructions. These 90-minute sessions are sufficiently focused so that there is no time to worry about the usual things on which my wandering mind usually perseverates. This experience is more than doing, but one of being. It occupies my nervous system intensively to stay focused and balanced.

My experience has been duplicated by investigators who have studied the health benefits of Hatha yoga and found that it is associated with a reduction of stress hormones such as noradrenaline and cortisol in practitioners (Ross & Thomas, 2010). Taking up a new activity can be healthy for your brain and body. Explore your choices and expand your brain.

Brain Challenge #5 Exercises

Exercise 5A: Pre-Planning Solutions to Situations Where You Have Difficulty Acting Healthfully

There are many high-risk situations that trigger learned bad habits; for example, to drink excessively or use drugs, to eat too much, to eat non-nutritious food, or to express oneself inappropriately. Identifying high-risk situations that tend to initiate your bad habits is a first step towards pre-planning new solutions to these challenges. For example, this list describes high-risk situations for drinking that are common to many people with drinking problems:

When I pass a bar
When I am with other people who are drinking
When I feel tense
When I have to meet people
When I think that just one drink would cause no harm
When I am feeling depressed
When I am not at work that day
When I am happy
When I have money to spend
When I feel myself getting angry
When I feel frustrated with my life
When I feel tired
When I feel disappointed that other people have let me down
When I remember the good times I was having
When I have already had a drink

Now it is your turn to generate a personal list of high-risk situations for the bad habit that you wish to change.

Step 1: Select a bad habit you would like to change:

_____

Step 2: Brainstorm situations where you tend to do the habit. These are your high-risk situations:
*
*
*
*
*
*
*
*
*
*
*

Step 3: Develop a plan for dealing with a situation.

Now that you have identified the situations that tend to trigger your bad habit, you can begin to problem-solve new ways of preventing or responding to these risky situations.

Often preventing exposure to the high-risk situation is the simplest and most effective solution. For example, if I have trouble not drinking when I pass by a bar on my way home from work, I might simply change the route that I take to get home to one that did not pass by a bar. After getting used to taking the new route, I would be able to avoid that high-risk situation with little effort.

Pick one of the situations you listed above: _____

Consider the situation you picked. Is there a way that you could prevent or limit your exposure to the situation? If so, write it here:

_____

_____

Sometimes, high-risk situations are unavoidable or should not be avoided. For example, if I have trouble not drinking when I am happy or have something to celebrate, it would not make sense to try to avoid being happy or successful. Here, it is important to find alternative behaviors that would be better to do in these situations. If these alternative behaviors can only be done instead of the bad habit, rather than in addition to the bad habit, the new solution may provide more protection from the high-risk situation. For example, instead of a bottle of wine, I might decide to treat myself with a massage, invite friends over to play board games, or go to a social dance event (one where alcohol is not served).

Consider the situation you picked. Is there something you could do other than the bad habit which would serve the same purpose? Write down ideas for alternative behaviors here:
*
*
*
*
*

Consider the list you just generated. Of those ideas, which can only be done instead of the bad habit?

_____

_____

Step 4: Practice the new solution.

Now that you have some ideas of new ways that you could handle high-risk situations, it is important to practice them a bit so that you are ready to use them.

Choose a solution that you think would work for you: _____

In your head, or role-playing with a trusted friend or close relation, walk through the situation as you carry out your new solution. Did the solution work out the way you thought it would? Practice walking through the situation a few times, ideally varying the context and responses of those around you, to help solidify the plan in your head and work out difficult areas where it might be easy to slip back into habit rather than continuing with your new solution.

Did you come up with any changes or revisions? If so, make note of them here:

_____

_____

Exercise 5B: Four Forms of Forethought for Your Prefrontal Brain

Some find mnemonics to be extremely helpful tools to remember complicated information and encourage its use in everyday life. I (W.G.) remember both key strategies for encouraging behavior change and key areas of the prefrontal cortex involved in those behavior changes through the use of some simple mnemonics:

1. Daily Life Planning (DLP, DorsoLateral Prefrontal cortex): Consider your choices. Am I making the same mistake repeatedly? What can I do that I have not tried before? What new behaviors have a reasonable chance of working?
2. Action Control Guide (ACG, Anterior Cingulate Gyrus): Consider your motivation. How motivated am I to manage the problem? Do my goals and values favor my behavior? Have I consistently tried to deal with this issue in a meaningful way? If I am not motivated, what might motivate me?
3. Valued Momentary Pleasures (VMP, VentroMedial Prefrontal cortex): Consider your impulsivity. Are you taking big risks in hopes of a big, but maybe not likely, reward? Is your excitement about what you could have jeopardizing what you have already achieved? Are you valuing momentary pleasures more than achievement of your long-term goals and maintenance of health and happiness?
4. One's Friends and Confidants (OFC, OrbitoFrontal Cortex): Consider the social context of your behavior. How does my behavior affect the feelings of other people involved in this issue? Have I obtained sufficient social support to achieve my goal? Who can help me? Have I communicated my concerns in a way that resonates with the feelings of others?

Try using these mnemonics to guide you through your assessment of a health behavior problem. Considering your choices, your motivation, your impulsivity, and the social context involved in your health behavior problem will help you identify areas where focused attention or problem-solving may improve your chances of successful behavior change.

A more comprehensive discussion of the way these prefrontal areas work together and separately as cortical-subcortical loops to create and maintain habits is described in Appendix 3.

Exercise 5C: Building Problem-Solving Skills By Playing Games

There are hoards of games, puzzles and riddles that challenge problem-solving skills and creativity. All of these can strengthen your problem-solving skills and create new options in everyday life. Adding some of these games or puzzles to your daily or weekly routine can improve your ability to find answers to seemingly complicated problems you encounter. Remember, solving a problem is a reward and a problem with no solution is a stressor.

<u>Some tips</u>
First, do not get upset if the puzzles seem hard or impossible when you start. That is a good sign. It suggests that these puzzles use skills you have not learned yet or are difficult for you. There is a lot to be gained by playing with a type of puzzle that completely stumps you. Problem-solving skills grow by practice, so you will get better at them if you just keep trying.

Second, when you are stuck on a problem or a new type of puzzle, it is OK to "cheat" and look at the answer, so long as you go back and work out how to get from where you were stuck to the answer. Working backwards from the answer to figure out the strategy for solving the problem still teaches you the problem-solving strategy and can sometimes be the only way to figure out new types of problems. So, when you get stuck, do not give up. Look at the answer and figure out where it came from. You will be better at the next problem.

Third, do not be shy about asking others for advice or help if you get stuck. Sometimes other people notice things that you have not seen. It is always nice to have someone who is really good at a particular type of puzzle around to ask for advice or walk you through a complicated bit of logic. If you do not have such a person handy nearby, I note that many of the puzzle websites on-line include forums for people to post-questions and comments to one another. With an internet connection you should never find yourself lacking assistance and guidance from others.

<u>Links to puzzles and games</u>
There are many websites that provide brainteasers and puzzles that can be done online or printed and completed. To get you started, try the sites below. Most break the different types of puzzles into varying levels of difficulty. Start with the easier ones to help you figure out the general puzzle strategy and then work your way to harder ones!

www.brainbashers.com

www.brainden.com

www.braingle.com

http://www.rinkworks.com/brainfood/

<u>For the brilliant among us</u>
http://www.mensa.org.uk/puzzles/
Mensa, a society "for people with IQ's in the top 2%" includes weekly brainteasers on their website and sells games and puzzles which challenge problem-solving skills.

<u>Designed for kids</u>
https://kids.niehs.nih.gov
National Institute of Environmental Health Sciences (part of the National Institutes of Health (NIH)) has a page of puzzles, riddles and brainteasers meant for kids, but which is fun for adults too!

http://www.hoagiesgifted.org/brain_teasers.htm
This page, intended to provide stimulating activities for gifted children, includes lots of links to sites with games, puzzles, and brainteasers. There are hours and hours of fun problems to solve here that would be enjoyable for anyone.

<u>Designed for pairs or groups</u>
Many board and card games include substantial problem-solving challenges and test your skills. Any of these can be great ways of learning and practicing new strategies in the context of fun with friends. The key here is to be deliberate as you play. Think out your options and their immediate and longer-term consequences. Deliberately choose a strategy and observe the outcome over several plays or games. This will not only develop your frontal cortex, but also make you a better, more successful game player! There are lots of games to choose from and playing a variety is probably a good idea. Some suggestions include Mastermind, Chess, Checkers, Card Games (e.g., Bridge, Cribbage, Hearts), Scrabble, The Game of Go, and Mahjong, but there are many, many great others.

Exercise 5D: Mixing Physical Activity with Problem-Solving Skills Development

For those of you who already spend enough time sitting, additional quiet time spent doing puzzles may not be very attractive. There are plenty of options for mixing problem-solving skill development with physical activity, although in most cases it may require that you pay deliberate attention to focusing on problem-solving during the activity.

Below are some activities that can be used to develop problem-solving skills. These are only examples; if none of them are appealing, use your creativity to come up with ways to exercise your prefrontal cortex and body at the same time.

Orienteering
Orienteering is both a sport and a pastime basically consisting of a race to an endpoint or endpoints over unmarked terrain guided by only a map and a compass. It is most commonly done on foot, but can be done in combination with just about any form of locomotion (e.g., mountain biking, skiing, canoeing, horseback riding, or a mix). The main problem to be solved is how to reach the target destinations most quickly. Solving this overall problem will require solving many smaller problems and considering your options, strengths and weaknesses, and ability to pass obstacles, as well as those of your competitors. It also requires developing navigation skills. Where are you on the map? What do your compass readings tell you about where you are and where you are headed? Should you take the shorter route up the hill or go around? Should you run up this trail or will that only tire you out and slow you down for the subsequent six-mile trek? What is the best way around or through this stream?

A nice thing about orienteering is that it gets you outside in new and often very pretty places. It can be done competitively or casually, independently or in groups, and by young and old. It can be a great activity for a family, group, or class. Adding a group dynamic brings in all sorts of additional social interactions and decisions that must be solved. What do you do when people disagree about strategy? There are associations with national and local groups and teams where you can learn more about orienteering and find other interested people to share the fun. See the US Orienteering Federation at: http://www.us.orienteering.org/

A variant on the "get outside and test your navigation skills" concept is "Geocaching". In this game, people hide small "treasures" all over the world in outdoor spaces and then provide clues and latitude and longitude markers online for other treasure seekers. You can look up treasure clues in your area and head out with a GPS device to try to find them. A website provides space to log your successes. For anyone who has ever had pirate treasure hunting fantasies, everything you need to get started can be found at: http://www.geocaching.com/

Bouldering
Bouldering is a variant of rock climbing where the object is to figure out and execute a climbing strategy for a specific route. Because no ropes are used, the endpoint is typically not far off the ground. Otherwise, the inevitable failures involved in problem-solving

would be too painful. Bouldering can be done wherever there are things to climb, assuming you can get a mat or crash pad underneath. It is most commonly done at rock climbing gyms, outside on the base of rock faces or large boulders, or even on roughly textured buildings or other architecture (although this can sometimes anger the owners, especially if you get chalk marks and shoe smudges all over the structure). Solving a bouldering problem involves figuring out a pattern of movements that will get you up a challenging route. Importantly, there is no one solution to any boulder problem, and your personal solution will require considering both the specifics of the problem and your own height, weight, reach and balance, and strengths and weaknesses. Watching others can give you ideas, but what works for another person may not work for you. Because the route is short, you have the opportunity to try out lots and lots of potential solutions. With each try, you not only sharpen your problem-solving skills, but also improve your strength and coordination.

Indoor rock climbing gyms are a great place to get started, learn skills and meet other people with whom to practice and share ideas. They also tend to be staffed by rock climbers and bouldering enthusiasts who can direct you to good places to boulder outdoors. A directory of indoor rock climbing gyms can be found at:
http://www.indoorclimbing.com/worldgyms.html

Team Sports
Team sports offer a variety of physical challenges catering to people with different body types. Most share some general problem-solving challenges. How can we best organize, focus, and motivate a group of people to meet a goal? For example, how do I organize a group of people with varying abilities and skills to most consistently get a ball into a goal? There are questions of overall game strategy. For example, should we play all our best players hard at the start of the game or save some until later so they are fresh and energetic at the end of the game? There are questions about immediate game strategy. How should the team move the ball (or whatever) to best score or prevent the other team from scoring in the next thirty seconds? There are questions about interpersonal dynamics and motivation. How do we keep our star player from getting frustrated and quitting while he is being guarded by a much larger and very aggressive defense? The fact that team sports are almost universally played against a second team which changes from game to game means that the most effective strategy and organization is apt to change from game to game based upon the skills, strengths and weaknesses of the challenging team. In short, there are endless opportunities to practice problem-solving skills in team sports.

The big problem with trying to use team sports as a way to practice problem-solving skills is that coaches typically do 95% of the problem-solving. Thus, with normal team sport dynamics, the coach practices his problem-solving skills and the players practice carrying out his instructions in the immediate setting. Thus, while players may have to do a lot of quick, reflexive, improvised problem-solving on the field, the coach does nearly all of the deliberate planning and strategizing that challenges the frontal cortex. Notably, a coach's abilities at general problem-solving seem to be related to the success of the team. For example, a study in Germany found that national top-league basketball and team handball coaches out performed local-league coaches in problem-solving challenges unrelated to their sport (Hagemann et al., 2008). Finding ways of sharing in the coaching duties can turn team sport participation into a great problem-solving exercise. You may find that taking over the role of coach may be easier to do in small pick-up games with friends than in actual organized leagues.

Chapter 6: Surmounting the Challenges: The Example of Achieving a Healthful Diet and Body Weight

Example Introduction

Even when you know things, it takes practice to understand how to apply them. To help illustrate how the concepts we discussed in the five brain challenges can be put to practical use, we now go back through each process and consider how it might be used to target a common problem; specifically, how to eat healthfully and maintain a healthful weight. We hope you will not only find these tips helpful for managing diet and weight, but also better understand how seemingly unrelated or small behavior or environment changes can have a big impact on achieving a large, long-term health goal. What may initially seem like overwhelming or intractable problems are often best solved by constantly doing the little things you can do right now rather than feeling like you must run at the whole problem head-on.

Challenge #1: Valuing Health

Social reinforcement and peer pressure

Misconceptions and biases about healthful and unhealthful foods are substantial barriers to healthful eating. People often do not know what is and is not healthful to eat. And even when they do, they often have biases and expectations that discourage eating well. Healthful foods are often assumed to taste bad or be unsatisfying while unhealthful foods are assumed to be delicious and rewarding to eat. In reality, this is not true. Healthful food can be amazingly delicious, tempting, and satisfying, particularly when you know how to prepare it well. For example, my husband and I (J.T.) eagerly await fresh fig season every year, when we tend to gorge ourselves on giant arugula and fresh fig salads to the exclusion of the rest of our planned meal. Having spent years trying healthful vegetable-focused recipes out of cookbooks and off the Internet, I now view fresh produce as a wondrous treat that offers up numerous options for combining and cooking into joyous meals.

To make meaningful changes in your diet that will encourage weight loss and long-term weight maintenance, it can be helpful to challenge your beliefs about healthful and unhealthful foods. First, there are many cultural misperceptions about what constitutes healthful food. It may be helpful to take a nutrition course to learn to think about food from a more objective perspective. Next, challenge ideas that healthful food will taste bad or be torture to eat all the time. If you do not know how to prepare tasty dishes made with healthful foods, consider taking a cooking class or asking a healthy friend to share recipes. Whenever you eat a healthy meal you enjoy, learn the recipe so you can replicate it yourself. Find food apps or blogs that focus on healthful recipes, and flip through recipes and pictures to find and try ones you find interesting. Some of my (JT's) personal favorites include the Food Monster app, connoisseurusveg.com, minimalistbaker.com, and ohsheglows.com. Search the Internet for healthful versions of recipes for your favorite but unhealthful meals, by adding in search terms like "low calorie", "vegan", "whole food", "plant-based", or "Mediterranean" to the recipe you want to find. For example, by searching for "vegan cheese sauce", I found a wonderful recipe to make a flavorful, cheese-like sauce for nachos, casseroles, macaroni and cheese, etc. made primarily from boiled potatoes and carrots ("vegan cheese" at veggieonapenny.com). Now I can eat my veggies while my brain thinks I'm indulging in cheesy comfort food. Conversely, challenge ideas that unhealthful foods are truly flavorful and make you feel good. Reflecting on how you feel 30 minutes after eating unhealthful foods can help to correct beliefs that eating unhealthful foods will make you happy, content, or satisfied.

The power of suggestion: Placebo and nocebo effects

Food as medicine

Food is often presented as a "cure all" for problems of all sorts. "Eat this, it will make you feel better." Some suggestions for foods that will make you feel better are so frequently repeated that they may be considered American cultural clichés or even alternative medicine. Examples include eating chicken noodle soup for colds and flu, indulging in ice cream when you have a sore throat or relationship problems, or having a glass of warm milk to help you sleep. Generally, these expectations are helpful lore, providing harmless interventions that, via placebo, will make people feel better and give concerned loved ones something to do to help. However, when the occasional use of food as medicine transforms into a habit of eating to feel better, this helpful placebo effect can become a significant driver of obesity. Expectations that food will elevate your mood, when combined with frequent experiences of negative moods, can lead to chronic overeating. If you find you yourself eating to feed your feelings rather than true hunger, you may benefit from learning and practicing new strategies for managing mood or stress. A psychologist or other health professional may be helpful here. Simple mindfulness techniques can provide an opening to avoid eating to cope. Pause, recognize what you are feeling or what is bothering you, and then consider other options that will solve the problem or make you feel better. Examples might include meditation on a nice place, a walk, cuddling with a pet, calling a friend, or spending a few minutes with a favorite activity, such as coloring, solitary card games or puzzles, or even dancing in your kitchen.

Weight loss panaceas

The American advertising landscape is littered with products promising to solve all weight problems with little effort in a short period of time. Driven by great hope that these miracle cures will work, people may achieve rapid initial weight loss with these diets, pills, and services, but this rarely lasts and can lead to rebound weight gain. While great expectations may allow us to persevere through unhealthful treatments or behavioral plans to drop a few pounds quickly, these stressful attempts at a quick fix tend to encourage binge or over-eating. The typical person who tries these crash diet plans will, after losing a few pounds in the short-term, regain the weight plus a bit not long thereafter. Do not be fooled by the hype and avoid these placebos. Only patience and true stable changes of behavior and diet will take off a substantial amount of weight over the long-term.

Marketing your own expectations and rewards

As we discussed, advertising is extremely effective for increasing consumption, thus justifying the billions of dollars spent by corporations to encourage consumption of their products. Cutting back on exposure to TV and thus advertising has been shown to reduce weight gain in numerous studies in children (Jason & O'Donnell, 2008). Direct food cues (images of food) and the positive cues (happy families, sex, fun, success, plenty) that have been linked to food by advertisers are everywhere. Once these associations have been created, it will be difficult to avoid exposure to cues. But if we become more aware of the associations that are presented to us, we may be able to reduce our exposure and challenge the assumptions underlying the associations. Will eating a hamburger make me sexy? Will my family get along better if we eat at a particular restaurant? Will drinking a soda lead to world peace? Casting doubt on these associations may help to devalue some of the cues that advertising has encouraged us to overvalue.

Work to create cues to encourage healthful eating. Put a refillable water pitcher in the front of your refrigerator so that you always have cold water as an option. Make sure your kitchen is filled with healthful snacks so that you eat these before you get too hungry. Put cookbooks with healthful options on your bookshelves, or a list of quick healthy meals on your refrigerator door, so that you do not fall into bad habits or go out to eat just because it is too hard to think of something healthful to prepare. Plan your menus in advance so you can get the fresh ingredients you need. Think about positive associations you have with healthful foods. Link good times you have had with positive eating habits. Barbecues can be fun, but it is not the over consumption of beer and beef that makes them so. Focus on the fun you had with friends, or the naturally sweet fresh corn on the cob that you grilled, or the amazing pitcher of fresh iced peppermint tea that you shared. Go beyond the standard stereotypes to create associations that help drive you toward healthful eating habits.

When helpful is hurtful: Rescuing, doting, and enabling

Do loved ones in your life feed you to soothe your emotions? Do others "give you a cookie" when you are upset? For example, my (J.T.) sweet Italian grandmother found it hard to see family members upset and loved to cook and feed people. When anyone showed signs of negative emotion around her, she was likely to have their favorite food ready and waiting shortly thereafter. My two cousins, whom she cared for frequently, developed significant obesity problems as kids as her treats trained their reward circuits. They would get upset, she would feed them in response, and that would encourage them to get upset again, creating an unpleasant cycle for all. The combination of my grandmother's discomfort in seeing loved ones upset, her tendency to dote, and my cousins' poor emotional regulation, fueled my cousins' weight gain.

Because patterns like these are driven by the reward systems of both the person doing the doting and the person being doted upon, they are automatic rather than conscious responses. Thus, they can often continue unacknowledged and unaddressed for years or even decades. In trying to achieve and maintain a healthy weight, it is important to recognize these patterns and discuss them with those who tend to feed you when they are uncomfortable with the emotions you are experiencing. Help them come up with more helpful responses to your bad moods. Might they give you a hug instead? Maybe they could walk you through some breathing exercises? Perhaps they could help you problem-solve or reframe your situation? Work with them to help them respond to you better. Then work with yourself to try to come up with better ways of expressing your emotions to others. Are you catastrophizing or exaggerating how upset you are? Are you getting upset around your loved ones to get sympathy, attention, special treatment, or food? Try to tone down the cues you present to others that lead to their attempts to feed you into sedation or contentment. As you work with your loved ones to try to address these patterns (if they exist), be wary of your own tendencies toward extinction bursts. Work with your loved ones when they try responding to you in a new way. Do not escalate your bad mood or emotion-fueled behavior.

These sorts of interacting habits can be difficult to break. Sometimes, altering the context of your interactions with doters and rescuers can be more effective. For example, my grandmother was more likely to overfeed people when she had her own kitchen available. Spending time with her in settings other than her home would be another way of reducing the impact of her tendency to dote on others'. While other people's behavior is not usually in your control, creating or choosing the situations in which you interact with them can allow you to reduce the likelihood of certain unhelpful and unhealthful behaviors.

Comparing against others: Correcting perceptions through normative feedback
As we discussed in Challenge #1, weight gain is contagious. We pick up the habits that lead to weight gain from the loved and respected people in our social networks. Our social circles can normalize unhealthful eating patterns and encourage us to conform to these local norms, leading to weight gain. Being aware of these social influences is an important first step to preventing the spread of obesity. Even simple awareness that bad eating habits within one's immediate social circle are not shared by the broader community can help counteract some of this social pressure. For example, as a teenager, the "cool kids" in my (J.T.'s) neighborhood used to meet at the local convenience store on the way to the bus before school, where they would purchase and consume big bags of chips and bottles of soda for breakfast. I was thankfully buffered from this rather unappealing routine by the fact that I spent much of my free time outside of my neighborhood with a group of gymnasts from all over the region, who I knew would be horrified by this choice of breakfast fare. My exposure to a broader sampling of social norms protected me from more local pressure to adopt poor dietary habits. Aware that not all my peers ate this way, I felt confident in my choice not to join this group practice, and simply ate my bran flakes and fruit before leaving the house. Taking a hard and critical look at your everyday behaviors, especially those that "everyone does", may help you identify and correct bad habits that you picked up from those around you.

As you begin to make healthful changes to your diet and eating practices, be prepared for the near inevitable discouragement that you will receive from your peers. Your successes at improving your diet will almost certainly be punished by some members of your inner network. "You always used to eat the triple burger with cheese. Why not now?" "If you are going to insist on eating your home-cooked food, maybe you shouldn't join us for lunch anymore. It's embarrassing having you eating that with our group." In responding to these challenges, we have found some strategies to be helpful and others problematic. On the helpful side, explaining your deviance from the normative eating practices of the group as a response to a personal problem, rather than a decision that the normative behavior is wrong, can help diffuse others' anger about your choices. For example, I have had many people get upset when I insist on sticking to a plant-based diet. Explaining that my choice is in response to a terrible family history of heart disease and that I understand that others may have different dietary needs tends to quell the anger. Conversely, relating the data on the consequences of a meat- versus plant-based diet tends to start a long, protracted argument. As we discussed in Chapter 1.3, while it can be tempting to extol the virtues of your new healthful habits and point out others' unhealthful habits, this is sure to lead to battles that may make it difficult to maintain your new practices. Admitting that you are different but not attempting to challenge or judge the group can help minimize social punishment.

The special case of drugs of abuse

Drug use and dependence can lead to weight gain and may underlie some people's weight problems or sabotage their attempts to lose weight. Substance use is one of the largest risk factors for eating disorders, including problems with binge eating. People with eating disorders have higher rates of substance use and substance use problems than matched individuals without these disorders (e.g., Krug et al., 2008), and it is likely that the substance use contributes to disordered eating behaviors. Moreover, there is growing evidence that substance use disorders and binge eating problems stem from shared underlying biology (e.g., Serafine et al., 2021; Kessler et al., 2016; Davis & Carter, 2009). Substance use problems can lead to weight gain or and may contribute to the maintenance of unhealthful habits and impulsivity. As you work to achieve and maintain a healthful weight, it can be useful to assess your use of alcohol and other illicit drugs, and to get help if you need it.

Alcohol is calorie-rich and drinking may simply add to caloric intake. Moreover, it may encourage other reward-seeking, and lead you to overeat when you drink. It may also lead to negative mood states that some may manage with food consumption.

Similarly, marijuana is one of the best-known appetite stimulants. People (and laboratory animals) really do "get the munchies" after using marijuana. Chronic marijuana use can lead to weight gain and hurt efforts to lose weight. For example, a student of mine told me about a psychiatry client they were seeing who had been treated for nearly a decade for a binge eating disorder and had tried about every diet, medication, and behavioral treatment available, before it was discovered that she used marijuana four times per day. She and her doctor had never considered that her binge-eating problem might be caused by the fact that she was smoking a powerful appetite stimulant multiple times per day. Addressing the drug use helped her gain control of her eating patterns again.

Additionally, while quitting use of cigarettes has huge health benefits, smoking cessation does tend to result in weight gain. Still, those benefits far outweigh (no pun intended) the negative effects on weight. A recent study suggested that smoking cessation increased weight gain by 21 pounds over 5 years, once analyses controlled for differences between people who were successful versus unsuccessful in quitting smoking in clinical trials (Eisenberg & Quinn, 2006). Concerns about weight gain can be a problematic barrier to attempts to quit smoking, and thus a significant amount of research has been conducted to find ways of minimizing weight gain during smoking cessation attempts. Individualized interventions, very low-calorie diets, cognitive behavioral therapy, and pharmacotherapies including bupropion, nicotine replacement therapy or fluoxetine may reduce weight gain during smoking cessation (Parsons et al., 2009). Proactively addressing the likelihood of weight gain during smoking cessation attempts can have significant benefits for long-term maintenance of a healthy weight.

Challenge #2: Enriching Your Life

Are you an ant or a grasshopper?

Realistically assess your biological drive for immediate gratification from food. Can you have dessert around without eating it? Can you fill your plate with yummy food and leave half of it there? Can you have a bad day and not empty the freezer of ice cream? If you find you are more like Aesop's fabled ant and cannot help but store up all the food you encounter, a first step is to recognize this tendency and adjust your environment such that you encounter calorie-dense or excessive portions of food less often.

Shaping your environment to fit your biology
Portion control

Studies have confirmed that the more food someone is served the more they will eat (Rolls et al., 2002). For example, when researchers manipulated the amount of pasta served at a restaurant, without changing the price or the food itself, they found that customers ate 25% more calories during their meals but did not report any difference in the appropriateness of the portion size or notice any difference in the portion size as compared to the amount they normally ate during a meal (Diliberti et al., 2004). This general effect of eating more when portions are larger without consciously being aware of the increased consumption is easy to replicate. With larger portions people of all sorts reliably serve and consume between 20-50% more (Wansink & van Ittersum, 2007). Problematically, the concept of a standard portion has grown considerably in the last century. The surface area of the average dinner plate has increased 36% since 1960, and cookbooks have increased serving sizes. For example, entrée portions in the current *Joy of Cooking* are as much as 42% greater than the 1931 edition, and over-sized options at restaurants provide 2.5 times the portions of the standard meal. Knowing this, there are a few simple things you can do to improve your portion control and eat less without noticing:

1. Use smaller plates and dishware. When plates are smaller, people will put less on them. If you serve yourself food on a smaller plate, chances are you will eat less over time. Replacing large dishware with smaller versions can be a helpful weight loss intervention.

2. Do not even consider "all you can eat" options, "supersizing", or buying the "large" because it is cheaper by volume. (Note: If you are used to "supersizing", consider keeping track of the money you save by not buying the larger version, and save it up for a non-food treat for yourself). Only expose yourself to meals or snacks that are appropriately sized. Select restaurants that provide reasonable portion sizes and do not go to ones that offer over-sized portions. As you start, you may need to look at the nutritional information sheets available at most restaurant chains to distinguish between those with reasonable versus excessive portion size. But once you become aware of the problematic restaurants and filter them from your list of possible meal sources, you will find it easier to lose weight.

3. Stock your kitchen only with healthful options in reasonable quantities. The garbage-bag-sized package of corn chips from the wholesale store may be a great deal if you happen

to run a taco truck, but it is a terrible thing to have in your personal kitchen. Purchase products in packages that provide appropriately small servings.

Reduce exposure to unhealthful food cues
While it is important to try to prevent yourself from learning false associations between food cues and other pleasures, most of us have already learned many associations that now overvalue and drive us to eat specific foods. Since these associations are difficult to unlearn, it can be extremely helpful to reduce your exposure to these cues and thereby avoid this habit-driven eating. While you will likely benefit from developing plans to steer clear of food cues that cause you the most difficulty, there are a few techniques for avoiding food cues that help most people:

1. Turn off your TV and limit screen time. Reduce your exposure to advertising. Many of the most effective interventions to prevent weight gain or encourage weight loss in children involve reducing screen time. As we have described, the prefrontal brain regions take longer to develop. Children, like the "ants" among us, tend to have stronger drive for immediate gratification than the average adult because of their continuing brain development. If you tend to eat when food is offered, exposing yourself to the most persuasive food ads that high-paid advertising experts can devise to lure you to their product is not a good idea. If stepping away from screens is unthinkable to you, at least consider watching media where commercials are limited or somewhat more controllable. The internet offers suggestions for ways of limiting ad exposure on various platforms.

2. Do not go to the grocery store without a clear plan. Letting yourself impulse shop can leave you with a kitchen full of calorie-rich treats. Grocery stores have learned to carefully place and highlight impulse items to encourage you to purchase them in times of weakness. For example, it is no coincidence that the candy is right beside the news and tabloids. With media headlines to arouse or stress you while you are captive in line, you are much more likely to reach for the chocolate bar. If it is available in your area, consider local produce delivery. Having a big box of vegetables show up on your doorstep can help you feel compelled to eat them and discourage trips to the grocery store. Write yourself a clear and complete shopping list before you go to the store, and search only for those items on the list. Withdraw only as much cash as will cover the items on the list and leave your credit cards at home. Do not let any additional items sneak into your cart.

How can I enrich my life? Increasing healthful opportunities.
Improving social skills and social engagement and adding enrichment activities
Not all weight management efforts need to be focused on food and exercise. The more that we find approval, relief, and solutions to our stressors from those around us, the less we will turn to food for pleasure and consolation. Making general efforts to increase access to rewarding opportunities in your life should reduce impulsive eating and help you lose weight. Honestly take stock of your social abilities. Are you able to elicit help from others when you need it? When you interact with others, is everyone generally satisfied with the outcome or do some win and others lose? Use the social skills exercises in Chapter 2.2 to find ways of having more positive interactions with people. Then get out and interact! Use your new social skills as you add new hobbies or activities to your life. Join an interest

group, an exercise group, a support group, a volunteer or religious community, or a learning group such as a class or book club. Volunteer on community projects. This can be a great way to both practice positive social skills and benefit from the immediate gratification of doing something that solves a community problem. While these activities may not seem directly related to a weight loss goal, social engagement and support has been shown to be related to recovery from all sorts of addictive behaviors and mood disorders. Being a valued part of a local community may dampen your need for immediate gratification and allow you to think twice before eating a whole bag of cookies.

Progressive behavioral shaping

When you set a goal for yourself, how often do you fail? If you fail frequently, there is a good chance that your goals themselves may be the problem. They may be too big, too vague, or too difficult to put into action, or too far in the future to be achievable. As an extreme example, while working with homeless poly-substance users, I had multiple clients state that their plan to improve their life was to "get on Oprah" and in doing so immediately become famous and rich. While saying you want to lose 15 pounds may sound a bit more realistic than the "get discovered by Oprah" plan, these goals are similar in that they are very long-term and require a wide variety of behaviors over a long period of time to achieve. Learning to break down your long-term goals into small doable steps can greatly increase your success and move you forward toward your bigger life goals. To lose weight, you will need to break your end goal into achievable pieces. If you want to make it formal, get a small notebook and a stopwatch. Write yourself a doable goal for the next four-hour period. For example, an initial goal could be to have a small bowl of whole grain oats for breakfast. This is much more immediate and achievable than losing 15 pounds and is a helpful first step along the way. If you eat the oats, you can note your success, and then come up with a new goal for later in the day. For a second goal, you could ask your scheduled lunch date if she would be willing to walk to the café down the road instead of driving. For your third goal, you could try cooking up the dino kale you made yourself buy at the grocery store and resolve to eat it even if you think it tastes funny at first. As a last goal for the day, you could plan to reconnect with a good friend that you have not talked to in a while instead of turning on the TV after dinner. If you manage to complete each of these, you will have successfully achieved four goals in one day, each of which involves doing a behavior that fosters a lifestyle where you could reasonably lose 15 pounds and keep it off. If it helps you recognize your success, chart your achievements with gold stars in your notebook. While you may feel a little silly, it may help keep you going and remind you of all the progress you have made toward your long-term goal. If you are not completing your four-hour goals, do not quit or give up hope. Instead, make your immediate goals easier so that you can achieve them. Reaching your long-term goals requires completing lots of little behaviors in the right direction, not a few big ones. Keep trying until you find the little behaviors that work for you.

Plan healthful responses to your inevitable exposure to "opportunities for relief"

For many of us, eating can become an automatic response to unpleasant feelings or distress. For example, you may eat when you are tired, hurt, angry, stressed, or nervous. When you feel bad you create an opportunity for immediate relief, and food is immediately rewarding. Consider the situations where you tend to eat in response to negative feelings. Is there another way to find quick relief that would be more in line with your weight loss goal? For some, practicing other ways of responding to distress can have a huge impact on food consumption. Sit down and pre-plan a healthful way of finding relief and then set yourself up so that alternative is consistently available to you.

As an example, I (J.T.) will start searching for food when I am anxious, tired, and overwhelmed, and this can be problematic at work and at home. I find warm tea at least as soothing as food, and it has no calories. So, I keep an electric teapot in my office and another in my home kitchen along with a large and varied stock of tea. I can make myself a cup within three minutes without leaving my desk, and the warm, fragrant liquid makes me feel better when things get a little crazy. Another response that makes me feel better without consuming additional calories is fidgeting. A brief burst of movement can help me shed my anxious energy and feel like I am escaping from my overwhelming situation. At work, this may just consist of running down the hall to check my mail, talking with a colleague, or using the restroom. If I am stuck on a conference call in my office, I might shuffle through the paper on my desk or clean things during the discussion, or turn off the video and bounce, do some squats, or play with the free weights I leave under my desk. Having released some stress through movement, I can turn the camera back on and/or unmute my phone and contribute much more thoughtfully to problem-solving without having eaten an extra meal.

Notably, letting myself fidget is not only a helpful diversion to keep me from running to the refrigerator when stressed, it may also encourage weight loss in its own right. One study compared the non-exercise-related movement patterns of lean versus mildly overweight self-described "couch potatoes" and found that the lean group spent a full 152 minutes per day longer upright, while the overweight group sat more consistently (Levine et al., 2005). The differences in holding still accounted for a 350 calorie difference each day! Another study looked at daily energy expenditure in 177 people while they were confined in a small, office-like, chamber. They found huge variation in the amount of energy individuals used, with fidgeting, or spontaneous physical activity, accounting for most of the difference, a full 100-800 calories/day! (Ravussin et al., 1986).

Other ideas for providing quick relief include breathing practices, snuggling with a pet, or a short diversion, like checking e-mail or reading a quote from a humor book. If chewing on something is a hard-wired response to distress, you could make sure you have consistent access to sugar-free gum, celery, or another safe option. We are all driven to make ourselves feel better during difficult moments. Making sure you can find relief in something other than cookies or chips can make a big difference for long-term weight loss.

Imagine how your ideal future self would feel and behave
Vividly imaging how you would think, feel, and react in a future where you have adopted and love healthful eating habits and regular exercise can help reduce delay discounting and help you avoid short-term temptations that sabotage your long-term goals. Run through future scenarios in your head. For example, if your ideal future-self packed a lunch, what would that look like? What would you think as you picked what to pack? What would be in your ideal refrigerator and pantry? What would you include in your lunch? What would

the healthful food smell like to your ideal you? What memories would it trigger? Would you be excited for lunch time? How much would you pack? Would you log what you packed? This sort of vivid future-thinking can help you orient towards your long-term goals, and practice being your ideal you. By setting your brain up to value your ideal future more than your immediate gratification, you set yourself up for success in your day-to-day decisions. We all tend to discount rewards that come later, but spending time imaging the future can decrease that tendency. Additionally, running through future situations can help you pre-plan your ideal response. If you have already imagined how your ideal self has felt, thought, and reacted, you have a model for acting like you wish you would. So, day-dream your ideal self in key situations. What would ideal future you do at your favorite restaurant? What would your ideal self feel like and do at the gym? What would your ideal self do to unwind after a stressful day at work?

Challenge #3: Stress Resiliency

Chronic stress is a substantial contributor to obesity, making stress resiliency a key skill for preventing obesity and maintaining weight loss. For example, the Whitehall study looked at the impact of stress at work at four time points during a 19-year longitudinal study of nearly 6900 men and 3500 women on subsequent obesity. They found that work stress independently predicted later obesity, with those reporting stress at three time points having 173% the chance of becoming obese as those who reported stress at no time points (Brunner et al., 2007). Learning strategies for preventing stress and relaxing when you start to get tense is important for weight loss as well as mental health. Physical health and emotional health are interlinked in endless ways. Getting formal or informal help when you are having trouble emotionally is an important starting point when you are trying to improve your physical health.

Pacing, scheduling, and self-care
Maintaining a regular eating schedule is crucial for keeping caloric intake stable and appropriate. Skipping meals is physically stressful. This stress, combined with true hunger, tends to lead to binge-eating and caloric consumption well beyond that skipped in the last meal. Meal skipping can have substantial negative effects on weight gain over time. For example, middle-aged American men who consistently ate breakfast were nearly 25% less likely to gain eleven or more pounds over the next ten years than their breakfast-skipping peers (van der Heijden et al., 2007). Likewise, getting enough rest is crucial for preventing obesity. Short sleep duration has been associated with current and future obesity in both cross-sectional and longitudinal studies (Patel & Hu, 2008; Knowlden et al., 2023, Miller 2023). In a population-based study, women who got less than six hours of sleep per night were nearly twice as likely to be obese and over three times as likely to be extremely obese as compared to women who slept between 7 and 8 hours per night (Anic et al., 2010). Additionally, stress-response, blood-glucose regulation, and circadian rhythm systems all signal using cortisol. Eating right before bed-time can prevent reductions in cortisol that are supposed to occur during sleep to enable recovery and repair of cells and organ systems, and has been associated with obesity (Goehler, 2022). Time-restricted eating, where food consumption is restricted to a specific window of time during the day, has been associated with improved weight and blood-glucose control, particularly when eating was restricted

to earlier in the day (Chambers et al., 2023). An important first step toward a healthful weight is to work out a consistent schedule with regular meal-times and adequate sleep and then stick to it.

Pre-planning and problem-solving

It is important to identify your stress triggers and plan solutions to them in advance of their occurrence so that you can prevent yourself from responding immediately to instant gratification (e.g., eating food) and can instead implement your pre-planned responses (e.g., tea and fidgeting). Make note of situations in which you tend to eat in response to stress and preplan what you will do instead. If you tend to eat available snacks in high-stress meetings, you might plan on eating something healthful immediately beforehand. If you tend to eat your pushy mother-in-law's high-caloric meals to appease her, you may offer to cook a meal for her to both offer her a rest and provide a healthful alternative.

Relaxation

Exercise may be particularly promising for both reducing stress and increasing stress management and helping to increase metabolism and weight loss. Yoga, Tai Chi, and similar wellness-focused exercise programs directly target stress management and may be ideal for those trying to improve stress resiliency and increase activity levels. Take a few classes and see if they work for you. If you have already learned physical activities or sports that helped you manage stress in the past, adding these to your daily or weekly plans can be useful. For example, maybe a run helps you clear your head or thirty minutes of gardening helps you forget the stress of the day. Give yourself time and permission to do these activities.

Challenge #4: Training Good Habits

Identifying and mastering your new behaviors

As we keep mentioning, losing weight requires consistent repetition of a lot of small pro-weight-loss behaviors. Identify these small behaviors. Learn, practice, and become confident in your ability to do them and then keep at them until they become old habits. Observe and talk to others who do these behaviors, visualize and role-play, get a mentor or coach, and address your fears or concerns about a behavior by talking to someone with experience or a health professional.

Some habits that may help you lose or maintain weight:
1) Drink water before you start your meal.
2) Chew slowly and fully before swallowing.
3) Eat your vegetables first.
4) Add fiber to your meals (e.g., put your food on a bed of greens to help fill you up)
4) Park at the back of the parking lot.
5) Include the stairs in your normal travel routes.
6) Pack healthful snacks and a lunch in the morning.
7) Eat something healthful every 3-4 hours.
8) Rest when you are tired.

9) Ask food-preparers to skip or put dressing, butter, mayonnaise, excessive cheese, or red meat on the side.

10) Eat breakfast.

11) Change positions regularly or stand at your desk.

12) Go for a walk after meals.

13) Skip the processed food aisles at the grocery store.

14) Practice saying "no thank you" when others offer you food.

15) Drink water or tea instead of soda or juice.

16) Associate unhealthful food with things you find disgusting or non-appealing (e.g., notice that sausage and candy bars can look like dog poop).

17) Serve yourself an appropriately sized portion of food, and then put the rest away for tomorrow before you sit down to eat.

18) Rinse out your mouth and/or brush your teeth right after eating to discourage going back for more.

19) Schedule regular activities that get you moving (e.g., an exercise class, a walk with a friend,

These are just some examples to get you started. Brainstorm ideas that might work for you, and practice until they become automatic!

Reinforcing your new behaviors

Social reinforcement

Having someone to praise or share your successes and help catch you when you are having trouble can be extremely helpful for reinforcing new habits and preventing relapse to old ones. Try recruiting a friend or family member to join you in your attempt to change your habits to manage weight. If that does not work, consider joining a group that shares your goal, such as a Weight Watchers or Overeaters Anonymous group. Time spent with a community of people working on the same problems is extremely valuable for weight management efforts.

Monitoring and feedback

As we mentioned before, people who have had long-term success with weight loss tend to track what they eat and how much they weigh daily. This regular monitoring and feedback can help correct problems quickly and reinforce good behaviors. Weight Watchers, one of the few weight loss programs that has data to back up its effectiveness (Truby et al., 2006), has formalized this monitoring and feedback strategy. But anyone can follow this same strategy through judicious use of (1) measuring cups or a postage scale and (2) the calorie and food content information on food labels or available in calorie tables for standard ingredients available online.

Digital apps have made it much easier to monitor what you eat and even provide regular automated feedback. For example, I (J.T.) found the MyFitnessPal app helpful for losing 10 pounds of stubborn weight from my third pregnancy. This and similar apps make it easy to track what you eat and how much you exercise. You can search their database for the food, scan the bar code, or even upload recipes from the Internet. Enter how much you ate, and it will track not only the calories consumed but also the nutritional content (e.g., fat, salt, sugar, vitamins) of your diet, along with how much you exercise. Moreover, they provide praise for meeting your goals, help with guiding portion size decisions, and give warnings when your choices do not align with your goals. Even if you only track what you eat for a short period, it can help to shape your understanding of how much and what types of choices align with your idealized diet.

Creating immediate contingencies for health behavior
Finding natural rewards in some behaviors can be difficult, at least at the start. Turning down dessert or opting for water at dinner can be hard to reframe in a positive light when everyone else is indulging. In these cases, it may be helpful to set up plans to reward yourself for your good work. For example, you could keep a log of the costs saved on all the desserts and drinks you did not buy and let yourself spend it on a non-caloric treat at the end of the week or month. The thought of the new clothes, a massage, book, artwork, trip to the new science museum, night of babysitting, or whatever treat you had in mind may make the dessert or drinks easier to avoid.

Challenge #5: Improving Problem-Solving

Novelty and new experiences
Most people approach dieting by trying to restrict themselves to eating less of their normal diet, or only a subset of the foods that they currently eat. This can leave you feeling deprived, and feeling deprived can lead you to relapse back to your old eating patterns. Choosing instead to adopt a new novel diet including different ingredients, different recipes, and different restaurants than those in your normal diet can be an easier way to improve your nutrition and reduce your calorie intake. Novelty has many benefits. First, novelty increases the brain's valuation of a reward; in this case, reminding your brain that this is good food and you should eat it again if you can, thus increasing your estimation of how good it is. Next, novelty challenges your brain to learn something new and will encourage growth of your cortical and limbic brain circuits. This may improve your general ability to problem-solve and hold back a habit, which will be helpful the next time you are tempted by a treat. Lastly, by eating something new, you avoid the need to stop your old habits before making decisions about what to eat. If I have eaten at McDonald's for years, it will take some mental effort not to order a burger before I remember my weight loss goal and consider a salad. If I try the new restaurant down the street, I will at least have to read the menu and consider my options before I am drawn to order. So, consider a diet attempt as a foray into new eating habits, rather than a constraint on your current ones, and enjoy some exciting new foods.

Pre-planning for difficult situations
Pack yourself healthful food, or at least plan out what you are going to eat for the day at breakfast, rather than just waiting to see what you come across. If you have a plan for food consumption for the day, you are less likely to skip meals, or make poor choices out of hunger, stress, or temptation in the moment.

Ask or observe respected role models

Interview friends or family who have maintained a healthful weight to see how they did it. They may be able to link you into local programs or networks that can help or give you specific tips on how to manage weight given the realities of your local environment. Moreover, the practical tips and modeling of effective behaviors will make it easier for you to learn and adopt new behaviors. The experience of successful people who share your local environment can be extremely helpful.

Researchers have studied people who were successful at losing weight and keeping it off for a long time. While some of the basic findings are not surprising, such as that these people tend to eat relatively low-calorie diets and exercise more than normal (McGuire et al., 1998), other findings may be less obvious (Kruger et al., 2006). Compared to unsuccessful dieters, those successful at weight loss and maintenance are less likely to use over-the-counter diet products. They are more likely to prepare their own food, not eat out frequently, plan meals, and report cooking and baking for fun. They are more likely to regularly monitor their behavior and success by tracking calorie and fat consumption, measuring the amount of food they eat and weighing themselves daily. They are more likely to lift weights, and therefore build energy-demanding muscle mass. Being more involved with your food tends to help rather than hinder weight loss attempts. Model your weight loss plans after those that were successful and you will increase your chance of success.

Play!

Perhaps the most important aspect of developing a weight loss or maintenance plan is making it fun! Your new behaviors must become self-reinforcing if you are going to keep them up. Find active things you like to do and do them more. Learn to play with food, cook, experiment, and try new things. Indulge yourself in healthful treats on a regular basis. Spend more time with happy people with healthful habits, and do not let yourself be pulled down by others' criticism or excuses for stale, old, unhealthful routines. Give yourself permission to take care of yourself and rest. Regardless of public perceptions, effective people do not deprive themselves of sleep, fun and stress-relief, or they would cease to be effective quickly. Get up, try new things, and engage in life actively and with passion, and behavior change will become easier and even habitual itself. Get out and play!

Exercise: Is your Prefrontal Cortex Pulling its Weight in your Weight Loss Efforts?

Various regions of your prefrontal cortex are necessary for enacting strategies to improve eating or other health behaviors. Practicing these strategies may not only help with weight maintenance, but also may strengthen these areas of the prefrontal cortex and develop new skills with benefits across multiple domains. Moreover, being sure to engage all these regions of your prefrontal cortex in your efforts to improve weight management may make your attempts less sensitive to lapses when one type of strategy fails. Below we provide a checklist of common weight control strategies that engage each key region of the prefrontal cortex. Go through the checklist and mark each strategy or element that is true for you. When you are done, sum up the number of elements that you marked for each brain region. Compare these numbers. Are there regions of the prefrontal cortex that you are using less than others? If so, consider adopting some of the strategies within that domain. When it comes to extra pounds and your prefrontal cortex, you have to use it to lose it.

Dorsolateral Prefrontal Cortex (DLP, Daily Life Planning): Planning and Flexibility To Pursue Goals

___1. I have specific, measurable, long-term health goals.

___2. I am monitoring my weight and other health goals on a regular basis.

___3. I am able to flexibly revise the plans I have to include new healthful choices.

___4. I have developed a schedule to incorporate sufficient physical activity to achieve or maintain a healthy weight.

___5. I have identified physical activities that I can do on a daily basis.

___6. I have a flexible way of switching from one physical activity to another if one form is not available.

___7. I have informed myself of the health risks associated with weight gain.

___8. I have developed a way to track my progress on a regular basis.

___9. I have developed a way to reinstate healthy eating after relapses.

___10. I am able to regulate what I eat on weekends or in social settings.

Total for Dorsolateral Prefrontal Cortex _____

Anterior Cingulate Gyrus (ACG, Action Control Guide): Motivational Commitment

___1. I am committed to initiating behaviors that lead to long-term goals.

___2. I am committed to maintaining behaviors that lead to long-term goals.

___3. I am able to stay with my program even when it is hard to resist eating.

___4. I stay motivated when I experience a lapse or relapse.

___5. I stay motivated after I have been successful in reaching a goal.

___6. I stay motivated even if I go on an occasional binge.

___7. I have remained motivated to remain on program for at least a year.

___8. I believe it is worth the effort in the future to stick with my plan.

___9. Overall, I remain motivated, in spite of negative moods or apathy.

___10. I am willing to stick with my plan indefinitely.

Total for Anterior Cingulate Gyrus _____

Ventromedial Prefrontal Cortex (VMP, Valued Momentary Pleasures): Emotion-Driven Eating

___1. I am able to sense if I am making a poor eating choice.

___2. I am usually able to resist nutritionally poor, comfort foods.

___3. I am able to distinguish between being full versus emotionally fulfilled by food.

___4. I listen to my gut level emotions to avoid making bad eating choices.

___5. I am usually able to resist impulse buying when shopping.

___6. I do not tend to overeat when I am sad.

___7. I do not tend to overeat when I am angry.

___8. I do not tend to overeat when I am lonely.

___9. I do not tend to overeat when I am celebrating a success.

___10. I do not tend to overeat when I am tired.

Total for Ventromedial Prefrontal Cortex _____

Orbitofrontal plus Ventromedial Cortices (OFC, One's Friends and Confidants): Social Eating

___1. I can taste something really good without having to eat more.

___2. I can sense when not to take even the first bite of something very enticing.

___3. I accept that others can eat things that I cannot.

___4. I am able to identify how eating too much could harm myself and thereby also be a source of distress to others close to me.

___5. I can resist overeating on Thanksgiving and other such occasions.

___6. I have developed an effective way to communicate my eating preferences to those close to me.

___7. I can resist eating unwholesome food served by others.

___8. I have been able to recruit others to help me stick with my program.

___9. I usually make good nutritional choices while eating socially.

___10. I can communicate my needs in a way that leads to meaningful dietary change.

Total for Orbitofrontal plus Ventromedial Cortices _____

Chapter 7: Changing Habits in your Health Care System: Addressing the 5 Challenges to Improve Patient Outcomes, Support Staff Wellness, and Reduce Cost

Example Introduction

Just as each of our habit behaviors influences our health, the practice habits of health care staff have an immense effect on the health outcomes of their patients. Health services and quality improvement research is rife with examples of substantive improvements in patient outcomes with only simple changes to health care workflows, provider education, reminders and decision support, practice organization, etc. Patient health is not only determined by what treatments a health care system offers and/or the expertise of their clinicians. Patient health outcomes are also highly influenced by the structures and processes developed to support health care providers in reaching patients when they need intervention and in making decisions that support the patients' long-term well-being. Clinicians, just like patients, have health and wellness as their goal and work hard to help as best they can. But also just like patients, clinicians are vulnerable to environments that make health-promoting choices difficult and habits that help in the immediate moment but cause longer-term challenges to health and well-being. Attention to the same 5 challenges can help health care systems optimize provider health care delivery habits in ways that have profound impacts on patient outcomes.

In this chapter, we will discuss ways in which the 5 challenges affect health care practice patterns and review strategies that can improve clinicians' practice habits. By reshaping health care systems in ways that acknowledge and embrace the humanity of those that work within them, we can improve patient health outcomes, clinical efficiency, and health care provider wellness and satisfaction. To make optimal decisions that support long-term patient wellness, health care providers need to practice in environments that (1) don't over-value quick fixes, (2) provide them with opportunities to address stressors, and problem-solve and work together to flexibly address needs, (3) provide realistic, healthful, and supported work expectations, (4) reinforce use of effective, evidence-based services and practice patterns, (5) intentionally support communication across clinics and services, and collaboration within and across teams, and (6) clearly prioritize areas for changes or improvement.

Following, we will consider how each of the 5 challenges contributes to the habits of health care providers, managers, and health care system staff in ways that influence the health outcomes of their patients. We will consider common challenges that alter health care system practices and evidence-based suggestions for methods or designs that can successfully reshape practice and improve patient care.

Using the 5 challenges to change clinical practice and reduce patient mortality related to complex chronic pain and opioid prescribing

Before we dive into each of the 5 challenges, here I share a personal example of how my team worked within the Veterans Health Administration to try to improve patient outcomes related to pain management and opioid prescribing. As background, my team consists of a diverse group of health care implementation specialists and data scientists and are tasked with improving behavioral health care practice across the Veterans Health Administration's 141 health care systems.

Given high rates of overdose, suicide, and other negative outcomes among complex patients on opioid medication, my team explored ways to try to improve clinical practices to improve patient safety. We had been monitoring clinical practice across VHA health care systems and providers for years, assessing consistency of use of recommended risk mitigation strategies and treatments from clinical practice guidelines for opioid therapy, suicide prevention, and substance use disorders treatment. We interviewed and shadowed primary care providers in their day-to-day practice (Trafton et al., 2010). Providers shared that it wasn't resistance to the guideline recommendations that prevented them from implementing them, but rather competing priorities. The recommendations simply took too much time to be done routinely in care without compromising attention and services for patients' other needs. They suggested that if we could help them recognize when these recommendations should take priority over other clinical needs, then they could make sure they fully attended to opioid risk mitigation in the patients who needed it most, without compromising care for other concerns, such as diabetes, hypertension, cancer screening, etc. So, we built a predictive model to estimate risk of suicide and overdose events or death based on prior years of health care data, and incorporated estimates of risk for each patient into a decision support system, which we named the Stratification Tool for Opioid Risk Mitigation (STORM) (Oliva et al., 2017). Providing STORM to clinicians did support increased use of risk mitigation in higher risk patients, but when we reviewed patients the model identified as high risk, there were still obvious problems with care coordination for these complex patients. We decided to undertake design of a health care system intervention to improve risk mitigation for our highest risk patients on opioid therapy.

We considered each of the 5 challenges in design and evaluation of this intervention (Chinman et al., 2019; Minegishi et al., 2019):

(1) Triggers: Providers appeared to be frequently unaware of care that patients were receiving from other providers. Complex patients were often being seen across clinical departments (e.g., primary care, mental health, and specialty pain clinics) and across health care systems with different medical records. Each clinician was separately responding to their specific clinical habit triggers for prescribing treatments, aggressively treating patient symptoms within their specialty concern in isolation. As a result, patients were often receiving multiple treatments that increased risk or reduced effectiveness in combination (e.g., co-prescriptions of opioids and sedating medications, or behavioral treatments for addiction plus "as needed" controlled substance prescriptions). Here we sought a solution that encouraged collaborative input towards a single treatment plan that all treating clinicians would help implement, rather than each applying their individual practice habits for their area of expertise.

(2) Opportunity enrichment: Providers reported lacking training in pain management and addiction treatment. They also felt competing pressures from patients seeking pain solutions versus oversight and legal authorities seeking to blame clinicians for unfortunate patient outcomes. Here we sought a solution that would provide peer support for clinicians and expand considered treatment options to include services that individual primary care physicians and specialists were not traditionally trained to deliver. We made it a goal to provide a community of practice to clinicians, so that they had others to help problem-solve challenging cases, as well as peers who could review

practices and back-up clinicians when they felt pressure to stop providing a specific treatment for a patient. Lastly, we sought to provide suggestions for risk mitigation and alternative treatments for each patient, providing guideline-based suggestions for care and risk mitigation to ensure clinicians were aware and reminded of options.

(3) Empathic Stress: Providers felt under pressure to address the immediate distress of their patients. Seeing their patient in pain, they felt obligated to give them something to help now! Providers found it difficult to separate themselves from the patient's emotions while the patient was in front of them, making it difficult to design a treatment plan that would be most likely to help the patient long-term. Here, we sought a solution that provided clinicians time to consider patient treatment needs without the stress of having the patient in pain in the room.

(4) Reinforcing new habits: Following clinical practice guidelines for opioid prescribing required clinicians to learn and consistently implement new and often time-consuming practices to reduce risk. We sought to reinforce completion of these new practices through a variety of means. We automatically updated a checklist of recommended risk mitigation interventions, visually checking off interventions as each was provided to the patient in clinical practice. We also created summary tools that provided normative feedback, by providing side-by-side comparison of rates of completion of recommended interventions by a specific prescriber, clinical care team, or facility as compared to national averages. These summary tools provided rates of providing interventions within patients clustered by estimated risk of suicide or overdose, helping to assure clinicians that differences observed were related to practice habits rather than clinical complexity or risk in the patients they treat. These summary tools were not only provided to hospital leadership, but also to clinical pharmacists trained and tasked to help educate and coach providers and teams through effective completion of the interventions (Midboe et al., 2018). Lastly, we sought to make new practices easy to do by automating and prompting recommended workflows and simplifying documentation (e.g., using medical record templates and tools).

(5) Executive support: Providers reported that competing priorities, organizational barriers (e.g., to communication and collaboration between services, time-consuming lab or documentation processes) limited their ability to follow clinical practice guidelines for opioid safety. To increase leadership support and attention and provide dedicated time for clinicians to focus on opioid safety for the health care system's most complex patients, we developed and released health care system policies that required development of an interdisciplinary team to review patient cases at highest risk, along with regularly updated performance measures to track whether the policy was implemented and leading to desired practice changes. Progress was discussed in senior leadership meetings to emphasize the importance of these efforts. By using predictive models to prioritize patients for attention, we sought to help clinicians navigate competing priorities, helping to ensure attention in cases where it was most likely to impact long-term patient outcomes.

The designed intervention:
An interdisciplinary team consisting of at least pain, behavioral health, and rehabilitation specialists conducted a review of each patient case identified as "very high" risk based on the STORM predictive model. The team made recommendations for a consolidated

treatment plan, which was added to the patient record and shared with the patient's original treating providers. In some cases, the team scheduled visits with the patient to ensure delivery of risk mitigation interventions or recommend shifts in treatment plans.

Outcomes: To test whether the intervention had benefit, we conducted a staged roll-out of the targeted prevention program, initially referring a restricted population (the top 1% of patients based on estimated risk of overdose or suicide) for review and then expanding the population to the top 5%, with randomly shifted timing for the expansion at different health care facilities (i.e., a stepped wedge design). We found that being targeted for the interdisciplinary review reduced complex patient mortality by 22% in the next four months, demonstrating that the intervention improved treatment effectiveness with minimal investment (Strombotne et al., 2023). Since this evaluation, the case review effort has been expanded to include other high-risk populations with signs of inconsistent or poorly integrated care (e.g., patients with recent non-fatal overdoses) and this new clinical practice has been maintained at all VA health care facilities.

Considering each of the core challenges to new habit formation helped us design an intervention that was effective and practical to implement in health care systems, leading to broad and maintained adoption of this novel clinical practice.

Challenge 1: Identifying over-valued triggers for clinically unhelpful practices
Generally, when non-optimal clinical practices become common, there is some short-term incentive driving the clinical decision. Often, this is simply empathy for the patient. Sharing a patient's distress or pain can be challenging and can over-value clinical responses that provide the patient quick symptomatic relief or help the clinician quickly disengage from the patient. Both responses relieve the clinician of the pain of observing someone in pain. Sometimes that response is completely in line with long-term recovery needs, and the reward experienced by the clinician and patient from the quick relief appropriately trains the clinician to respond more decisively in the same way in the next similar case. For example, resetting a dislocated shoulder both provides relief in the moment, and starts the patient on a road to recovery. Successfully resetting a few dislocated shoulders will make a clinician more confident and effective in treating patients with dislocated shoulders. But other times, the short-term fix can cause long-term problems for recovery, and clinicians and health care systems can wind up creating new health care challenges on top of the original ones.

Some examples of clinical habits that provide quick relief but worsen long-term patient outcomes include:

> Antipsychotic prescribing in nursing homes. Here, patients with dementia and hard to manage behaviors (e.g., aggression, agitation) may get prescribed antipsychotic medications to sedate the patient and minimize risk to staff and patients due to the disruptive behaviors. While this practice reduces risk or frequency of behaviors that are upsetting to patient and provider alike, the sedation and side-effects of the medication may reduce patient quality of life and increase risk of mortality. While the antipsychotics manage the immediate behavior, they worsen longer-term well-being and longevity, which is obviously in conflict with clinical goals. Other

behavioral strategies to address the challenging behaviors can be effective and have positive long-term effects. However, changing clinician practice can be difficult, particularly when providers do not have alternative methods to address behaviors available to them due to lack of availability or training, or when staffing shortages limit clinical support or time needed to use other effective approaches.

Monitoring for drug use when prescribing controlled substances. While clinical practice guidelines strongly recommend screening for drug use before and during treatment with controlled substances, getting clinicians to regularly drug screen when prescribing controlled substances like opioids or benzodiazepines was a challenge. The long-term benefits of drug screening for preventing development of substance use disorders or overdose were not effective motivators to drive clinical practice change. Two main barriers limited use of drug screening. First, many clinics were not set up to collect urine for testing and/or did not have arrangements with on-site labs to collect samples. Second, many clinicians felt ill-prepared to discuss drug use with their patients in the cases where drug testing identified non-prescribed or illicit drug use. Not drug testing relieved the fear of having uncomfortable discussions with patients, and the challenge of urine sampling. Until system changes addressed these barriers (e.g., by setting up urine collection and drug testing protocols, and providing clinician training in how to discuss and address drug use), professional pressure had little effect on targeted drug screening practices for patients receiving controlled substances.

Graduating patients from psychotherapy. Clinical trials of psychotherapy have shown that intensive courses of structured psychotherapy (e.g., 12 weeks of weekly cognitive behavioral therapy) improve patient health outcomes across a variety of disorders and psychotherapy protocols. However, in practice, patients may continue to receive psychotherapy from the same psychologist, often with less intensive contact (e.g., monthly visits) for years. Studies suggest that the incremental benefits of additional psychotherapy decline with increasing numbers of sessions (Stulz et al., 2013). As such, the population value of a psychotherapy visit decreases the longer a provider continues to see the same patient. In short, a provider's decision to continue to see the same patient for years, means that another patient who has yet to receive psychotherapy and would gain more from initial sessions does not receive that care from them. As such, the long-term benefits of psychotherapists on a patient population would be maximized by graduating patients to maintenance care, such as on-going mutual support programs led by peers, after an evidence-based course of treatment. This would open psychotherapy to additional patients. Graduating patients, however, involves addressing patient anxiety about minimizing a therapeutic relationship that has been beneficial and transitioning them into new unfamiliar services. This patient anxiety and need to hand-off the patient creates both less-familiar work and distress for the provider; the required work and relationship distress can both be simply relieved by scheduling the patient for another session. Adding to these natural rewards, many health care systems prioritize and reward provider productivity in terms of quantity of billable sessions completed. Stable long-term patients are more likely to show up for their appointment and less likely to experience crises that might require more time or follow-up than available in a standard scheduled appointment. Scheduling stable patients with proven ability to engage in planned services will increase clinician productivity measures compared to seeing new, unstable patients with psychosocial challenges to engaging in care. The short-term benefits of scheduling another session with the patient in the room can drive clinical habits that minimize the population benefits of therapy services and limit treatment access for new patients.

Other obvious examples of unhelpful clinical incentives stem from the desire to please the patient, which can be intensified by pressure to score highly on patient satisfaction surveys or avoid complaints to the patient advocate. Patients may come to a visit wanting a diagnostic test, medication, or treatment that they have heard about; if that service isn't appropriate to their case, it can be a challenge to tell the patient "no" or explain why that isn't a good idea. For example, patients may perceive a decision to not request imaging as the clinician either not believing their symptoms or being cheap to save the health care system money. It may take considerable effort and time to explain that not ordering imaging is an evidence-based decision to prevent the patient from receiving unnecessary radiation exposure or overly aggressive treatments that are more likely to harm than help. The short-term benefits of pleasing the patient may drive clinicians towards providing costly and non-evidence-based services that are unlikely to provide the patient long-term benefits.

Recognizing situations where short-term incentives are encouraging clinicians to behave in ways that limit patient recovery is the first step to reshaping systems and/or patient-provider interactions to support optimal care. Given the size and complexity of health care, identifying these problems before they become widespread can be difficult.

Performance measurement systems can be helpful for monitoring big picture care practices in relationship to clinical practice guidelines or health care goals. Review of practices with an eye towards lack of alignment with guideline recommendations or inefficiencies can identify areas in where short-term incentives may be discouraging guideline-consistent care. From there, observation of care practice and/or discussion with clinical teams and patients can help to uncover specific incentives or challenges that may be unintentionally driving non-optimal care and help to identify opportunities to shift practice.

Slowing triggered clinical responses
A first step to shift clinicians away from an undesired practice is to limit triggers that initiate the practice. A simple way to address unhelpful triggers toward problem-causing, quick fixes in clinical practice is to insert delays or extra effort into the process for responding to the trigger. This could be as simple as a click-through pop-up window on a computerized medical record that provides a warning and rationale for questioning the clinical decision, or something that slows the decision further, such as an external review/approval process or extra required documentation. Slowing down the response to the trigger both delays the reward, and thus reduces its perceived value, and provides time for executive brain circuits to consider the decision from a longer-term perspective. This delay won't prevent the clinician from using treatments when they are important and

appropriate for a patient but may help clinicians' catch themselves when immediate relief or patient approval might otherwise drive a clinical decision that isn't the best for the patient's long-term wellness or recovery.

The downside of this approach is that if the delay doesn't alter clinician behavior in ways that reduce downstream health care needs (e.g., by redirecting them to an alternative treatment option that may be harder to initiate but improves patient outcomes long-term), it will simply add inefficiency to the process of providing a non-optimal treatment and/or getting non-optimal patient outcomes. Thus, when adding a delay or extra effort to discourage a clinical practice, health care systems should have a clear vision regarding what the clinician should do instead, and ideally redirect the clinician down that path during the delay process.

For example, imagine a health care system wanted clinicians to reduce opioid prescribing for musculoskeletal pain, as clinical evidence suggested minimal benefit and significant risk of harms. They could put in delays to prescribing opioids, for example, requiring the clinician to write a justification for the prescription, conduct urine drug screens and prescription drug monitoring program checks, complete patient education and document informed consent before the prescription could be ordered. These interventions would certainly delay the decision to prescribe and increase clinician effort needed to order the prescription. One would expect that these requirements would increase clinicians' hesitancy to prescribe, and the pre-prescription interventions themselves might reduce patient risk and be beneficial to patients prescribed opioids. So, this could be a beneficial intervention on its own. But if the clinician doesn't have other treatment options to consider, the requirements may not reduce opioid prescribing. It will just take the providers a lot longer to prescribe opioids. If the health care system instead changed the clinical workflow to facilitate use of recommended treatment options, clinicians may gravitate towards using the recommended option, rather than prescribing opioids. For example, when a provider tried to order an opioid, the health care system could provide the clinician with information about available evidence-based treatment options, along with ready-made patient education materials to support shared decision-making with the patient, and a streamlined process to make referrals to recommended options such as physical therapy, cognitive behavioral therapy for pain, and/or recreational therapy (e.g., swimming or yoga classes). In this design, instead of simply delaying a clinician decision, the health care system encourages an alternative behavior.

Clinical interventions to prevent harmful habit behaviors are more effective when the provider is trained to not only be mindful about their triggers and urges but also to conduct a different behavior in response to the trigger. For example, it is more effective to not only train patients attempting to quit smoking to be aware of when they have cravings and pause, but also teach them a new response to the craving, such as chewing gum or taking 15 deep breaths to reduce stress. Likewise, health care system interventions are more effective when they not only generate delays, but also redirect clinicians towards desired clinical practice. As a side benefit, providing an alternative can greatly reduce clinician frustration with the delays and extra work that the approach might otherwise produce.

Identifying and minimizing triggers

In some cases, it is possible to identify specific triggers that elicit predictable, but unhelpful, clinical responses and eliminate them. In these cases, triggers are often unintended consequences of components of clinical workflows, or management or oversight pressures or incentives. Open communication with and between clinical teams is often the best way to identify these triggers; clinicians and local managers often recognize the problematic behaviors quickly and will readily share their frustration or confusion with a safe and interested manager.

A deep dive into two previously discussed examples of problematic clinical triggers can help illustrate methods and benefits of addressing them. One example of a trigger for unhelpful and unintended clinical behaviors is the pain as a 5th vital sign standards that were put in place by The Joint Commission hospital accrediting body in 2001. In an attempt to address the widespread problem of untreatment of chronic pain conditions, these standards recommended assessing for pain severity in standard care, potentially at each health care visit. While this practice did successfully bring attention to the problem of chronic pain in patients, the focus on pain severity oriented clinicians and patients towards goals of quickly lowering pain intensity (Ahluwalia et al., 2018). Moreover, clinicians in most settings did not have the ability to provide interdisciplinary treatments to support chronic pain recovery and realistically only had prescribing options in their toolkit. Thus, in some settings, the pain vital sign assessments developed into clinical triggers for prescribing analgesic medications. This analgesic prescribing was both not effective for promoting chronic pain recovery, but also increased risks from overuse of analgesics. most notably risks of opioid overdose and addiction, but also risks from overuse of anti-inflammatory and psychotropic medications. After recognizing the effect of this assessment on prescribing practices, health care systems and The Joint Commission undertook efforts to minimize the pain severity assessment-triggered analgesic prescribing behavior. They specifically changed the pain assessment focus from pain severity to pain-related function and personalized recovery goals (Baker, 2017). This reframing of the assessment eliminated the trigger to treat immediate pain experience (i.e., prescribe analgesics), and instead prompted discussion of ways to improve long-term wellness and function. This was paired with efforts to create alternative clinical responses for clinicians by expanding pain management options available by referral. Together these are helping to reshape clinical practice away from analgesic over-prescribing and towards recovery-focused treatments for chronic pain conditions.

Attempts to maximize productivity of psychotherapists provide a second example of unintended consequences of well-meaning efforts. With a goal of providing access to psychotherapy for additional patients, many agencies have implemented performance goals rating psychotherapists' performance based on productivity standards, specifically completion of a maximized goal for number of clinical sessions, hours of face-to-face clinical time, or work relative value units. This approach incentivizes psychotherapists spending as much time as possible in face-to-face therapy with patients and minimizing the amount of time spent with each patient. While this approach simplistically seems like it would increase patient access to care by ensuring as much clinician time as possible is available for appointments, in practice it unintentionally creates incentives that reduce access to care to those most likely to benefit from services. For example, productivity standards punish clinicians when a patient doesn't show up for an appointment, as the clinician will not get credit for that missed face-to-face treatment time. This can encourage two practices that are unhelpful for patients and can even reduce patients' access to care. First, punishment for missed appointments encourages clinicians to discharge patients who are struggling with treatment engagement as early as possible, potentially reducing access to treatment for the patients who need help the most (Hatchett and Coaston, 2018). Second, creating incentives to avoid missed appointments rewards keeping stable, recovered patients in on-going treatment, thereby discouraging graduation of patients who are well enough to reliably show up for services and who need minimal support during and between sessions. As such, a focus on psychotherapist productivity unintentionally pressures clinicians to focus attention away from the patients with the greatest challenges and needs, and toward the patients with the least need for treatment. These unintended incentives are counter to therapists' clinical judgment and these pressures can reduce their job satisfaction, potentially to the point of reducing the quality of the services they provide (Franco, 2023). While productivity standards may increase the amount of time providers are in face-to-face visits with patients, they may shift that time away from visits that produce the most benefit for patients, reducing the amount of patient benefit per minute of clinical encounter. Productivity standards for psychotherapists risk increasing the amount of time they spend in the room with a patient while reducing the overall population benefit of the care they provide.

How could performance standards be changed to address this problem? Conceptually, health care systems should shift performance standards away from seeing more patients towards healing more patients. This could be done by changing clinical productivity standards for psychotherapists to, for example, measure rates of patient graduation from therapy after meeting goals for symptom reduction or functional improvement. Such an approach might have the additional benefit of encouraging measurement-based care, where patient treatment progress is assessed over the course of care to guide treatment planning. If assessing patient improvement is too complicated, health care systems could simply assess rates of patient completion of episodes of care (e.g., at least 6 sessions in 10 weeks). This would reward provider efforts to support treatment engagement and adherence in new, unstable patients and eliminate rewards for maintaining patients in treatment once the incremental benefits of more sessions are minimal.

In both examples, small shifts in health care system design have outsized effects on clinical practice, changing who gets care and the type of care they receive. Where health care system design creates incentives for practices that aren't optimal for patient health, systems can unintentionally waste resources or even harm patients. Investigating drivers of problematic clinical behaviors can help to understand the triggers for these practices and suggest solutions that reduce or eliminate those triggers. It can be challenging to find and understand these unintended triggers and incentives for non-optimal clinical practice. Helpfully, clinicians tend to be sensitive to and upset by situations where they feel pressured to behave in a way that isn't aligned with their patients' best interest. Processes that assess areas of clinician dissatisfaction and encourage clinicians to raise concerns can be extremely helpful for pin-pointing areas of practice in which unintentional incentives are causing health care system problems.

Challenge 2: Creating opportunity-rich environments for providers and patients

Just like patients, providers require regular opportunities for immediate reward to strengthen the inhibitory indirect pathways that slow habit responses. Health care delivery can be highly rewarding and provide endless opportunity for problem-solving and fulfilling interactions with patients and peers. However, it is not automatically so. Without a supportive environment, clinicians' jobs can instead feel like a stressful slog, with undue pressure to solve-problems that they don't have solutions for, to disappoint patients who want something they can't provide, and to act calm and positive when experiencing negative emotions or stress. Designing clinical environments such that clinicians have regular opportunity for immediate reward and relief can help them make better decisions for their patients and their own wellness.

Creating a culture rich in social support

Positive social interactions and social support are some of the most rewarding and readily available opportunities in a healthful community or work environment. Creating health care and community environments that nurture positive social interactions and social support can help slow reward and relief-seeking decisions and enable providers and patients alike to focus on long-term health goals. There are many ways of improving health care environments, from hiring and training health care managers and supervisors who model and reward positive, prosocial, team- and mission-focused efforts, to adopting organizational structures and health care delivery models designed to support clinician well-being.

While local hospital and clinic culture and team dynamics and relationships may have the largest impact on provider experience of social support day to day, formal interventions may beneficially impact providers' sense of support and well-being. Qualitatively, clinicians reported finding benefit from peer-to-peer support interventions, including emotional debriefing after traumatic or stressful events, peer coaching, and formal counseling and mentorship opportunities (Crandall et al, 2022). Facilitation of group interactions between clinicians was also appreciated. Beyond qualitative feedback on social support interventions, interventions have not been well-studied. However, a meta-analysis investigated social support interventions for young (age 18-24) health care professionals (Waqas et al., 2020). Included studies examined professionally led cognitive behavioral therapy groups, peer-led support groups, activities to increase awareness of or mobilize social resources, and incentives and material support for provider groups with extra challenges (e.g., front-line workers during the pandemic, or international clinician trainees). Overall, the meta-analysis found that interventions to increase social support effectively reduced symptoms of anxiety, depression, and short-term burnout, without changing perceived stress experienced by the clinicians. The interventions reduced the negative impact of workplace stress without reducing the stressors. Qualitatively, the young clinicians reported that the programs improved their sense of belonging and improved relationships at work. Group discussions were described as particularly helpful and well accepted. Clinicians reported that the interventions increased mentorship and training relationships, improved communication skills, and improved ability to address conflicts. Professional-led groups were more effective than peer-led groups and face-to-face interventions were more effective than those on digital health platforms. The quality of the intervention was found to be more important than the duration for effectiveness. While these early studies suggest that providers generally find these interventions helpful and acceptable, concerns were often raised about provider privacy and confidentiality. Moreover, clinicians emphasized the need to avoid problematic power dynamics, as might be caused by participation of supervisors or senior team members. While including managers and supervisors in interventions to help build social support and coping resources for health care providers and workers may be counterproductive, having managers emphasize the importance of relationship building, support activities, and provide time for supervisee participation is key to success.

Making identifying errors and risks rewarding: Supporting problem-solving at the health care system level

Health care is a complex, high-pressure, high-consequence industry where layer upon layer of organization and process must work effectively to treat a patient optimally and safely. Clinicians and other health care workers are human and inevitably make mistakes. To ensure patient safety, processes must be optimized to develop and maintain systems that minimize errors and minimize harms when errors do occur. This optimization process inherently requires identifying and learning from errors. How mistakes are handled can have a big effect on both the success of safety efforts and provider stress and collaboration (Dekker, 2016; Rodziewicz et al, 2023). A focus on catching and blaming clinicians for mistakes can lead clinicians to hide mistakes and distance themselves from others when they make mistakes. This "hide and avoid" approach might decrease the likelihood that the clinician as an individual will get blamed or punished for an error, but it doesn't reduce the risk of an error. A punitive approach not only tends to keep mistakes hidden, but it also reduces opportunities for collaborative problem-solving and development of system-fixes that prevent errors from being made again.

From an individual clinician perspective, a system focused on identifying rule-breaking and errors limits opportunities to improve clinician well-being; punitive approaches encourage effort towards hiding from oversight, rather than identifying challenges that clinicians can find solutions to address. Each of those identifiable, solvable challenges is a reward opportunity. Shifting focus towards finding and solving health care system challenges that could lead to errors, patient risks, or negative outcomes, increases opportunities for reward for health care staff. This broadened access to reward opportunities should reduce impulsivity among health care staff, creating a less habit-driven, more thoughtful team, able to focus on long-term outcomes.

Numerous agencies have developed "just culture" efforts to encourage an approach that reinforces identification and sharing of errors as part of a patient safety quality improvement program (e.g., Boysen, 2013; Murray et al., 2022; NHS, 2023; Agency for Health Care Research and Quality, 2019; U.S. Department of Veterans Affairs, 2023). "Just culture" quality improvement programs seek to reshape systems, training, processes, environment, and culture to make errors less likely and less harmful. "Just culture" emphasizes responsibility to bring attention to and address risk for errors, with a focus on problem-solving rather than blame. Clinicians are held accountable for decision-making and intent, rather than errors or outcomes that may have been due to systemic problems or vulnerabilities. Moreover, "just culture" acknowledges and addresses the reality that being involved in a clinical error that causes harm can be traumatic for a clinician (Wu, 2000), and explicitly includes efforts to console and counsel providers in cases where mistakes stem from system vulnerabilities (Boysen et al., 2013; van Baarle et al., 2022). Encouraging open communication and expression of emotion may support implementation of "just culture" safety efforts. Fostering participation in problem-solving efforts across all health care system staff and building trust between health care leadership and staff can also support implementation (van Baarle et al., 2022, Murray et al., 2022). Hierarchical, authoritarian leadership structures may impede efforts.

"Just culture" or learning health care systems provide space for innovation and sharing of diverse perspectives from those involved in health care. Rule-focused approaches can tend to be top-down and emphasize the perspective of those in leadership positions. Solution-focused quality improvement initiatives recognize that vulnerabilities may stem from any part of the health care system. A challenge in the human resources department might delay hiring and leave a clinical team short-staffed, causing process gaps. A contracting problem might cause a shortage of needed supplies. Non-optimal scheduling practices might make it impossible to get patients seen by the most appropriate clinicians at the right frequency. Errors and unintended outcomes may stem from challenges that originated far from the patient-provider interaction that may have immediately preceded the negative outcome. Encouraging communication and problem-solving efforts across the entire health care system is foundational to effective problem-solving, expanding the breadth of problem-solving (and thus reward opportunities) and the scope of possible solutions.

A reward-rich health care system is one where problem-solving opportunities are plentiful and teams can make their working environment and patient outcomes better with every solution they offer and apply. While changing health care system culture is not something that can be done overnight, roadmaps and implementation guides have been developed to support efforts towards a "just", "learning" health care system culture. We recommend some of the following as starting points to guide local health care culture towards this goal:

> Agency for Health Care Research and Quality's Communication AND Optimal Resolution (CANDOR) Toolkit: https://www.ahrq.gov/patient-safety/settings/hospital/candor/modules.html

> United Kingdom's National Health System Patient Safety learning hub: https://www.patientsafetylearning.org/the-hub

> And their Blueprint for Action: https://ddme-psl.s3.eu-west-1.amazonaws.com/content/A-Blueprint-for-Action-240619.pdf

> VA's "just culture" focused approach to patient safety: https://www.patientsafety.va.gov/about/approach.asp

VA's Just Culture decision making tool:
https://www.patientsafety.va.gov/docs/Just-Culture-Decision-Support-Tool-2022.pdf

Encouraging Long-term Recovery Focus in Clinical Practice:
Generally, health care has been offered as a service for help-seeking patients. When a person has a problem, they seek out health care and are scheduled with a provider who designs and enacts a treatment plan to address the issue for which the patient is seeking help. In this model, patients are almost always in some sort of distress when they interact with their clinicians. A health issue is bothering them enough to drive them to ask for professional help. The health issue may be urgent or non-urgent, but in this model, there is always an acute need that is the focus of both patient and provider attention. As such, both patient and provider are oriented towards quick fixes to an immediate stressor. But, as we have discussed frequently in this book, quick fixes aren't always the best for long-term outcomes, and they may ignore important health habits needed to meet life goals and/or prevent negative health outcomes. To attend to longer-term health, a different model of health care interaction is needed; one in which patients and providers interact outside of encounters made to address patient distress. Providers need to be able to talk with patients at times when both patient and provider can think clearly about long-term health goals and strategies to meet them. Health care systems need to reach out to patients proactively when they aren't help-seeking for an immediate problem in hopes of understanding long-term goals and values and optimizing health behaviors to meet them.

Multiple strategies to encourage health care attention beyond acute care needs have been developed. Each of these seeks to create health care interactions where providers can better understand a patient's goals, values, motivations, life stressors, and barriers to health and focus on developing realistic plans to prevent negative outcomes and improve health over the long-term. This altered focus reduces pressure to attend to immediate needs and stressors, reducing the drive for immediate relief or reward-seeking by both patient and provider, and enabling more conscious, deliberate, multidimensional treatment planning. From a neurobiology perspective, it shifts decision-making from habit/reward-learning circuit focused-processes to executive/prefrontal cortex focused-processes.

Primary care practices generally encourage well-person visits where preventative interventions, such as disease screening, health behaviors, and vaccination may be the focus of the visit. Whole health and population management approaches can augment typical primary care strategies to further provide time and focus on long-term goals and needs.

Whole health
Personalized whole health approaches to treatment planning emphasize engaging with the patient to understand their personal mission, motivations, and purpose behind treatment-seeking as well as their health and wellness goals. Here, clinicians are encouraged to help the patient assess the context around health problems, towards better understanding what outcomes are important for a patient. While lab values and clinical assessments may

provide helpful information to providers regarding health status in a patient, they rarely provide motivating goals from a patient perspective. Consider a patient with diabetes. While improving blood glucose levels may be a reasonable goal from a clinician's perspective, that goal is not only exceedingly abstract for a patient, but also comes with the threat of needles and unpleasant labs for assessment. Suggesting the patient change life habits to get lower scores on a lab may feel intrusive and meaningless to a patient. But the patient's poor blood glucose management, and the unhealthful diet and inactivity that may underlie it, may have effects on mood, energy, ability to participate in activities, appearance, and downstream health risks or consequences. Minimizing these negative effects may be highly motivating for the patient. Identifying outcomes that matter to the patient can support goal-setting and monitoring that provides meaning and motivation for health behavior change for the patient. A patient may be willing and able to make health behavior changes to, for example, be able to play with their grandkids, that they wouldn't consider if framed as an effort to lower scores on a lab.

Encouraging patients to think through their personal goals can help providers develop treatment plans that prioritize improvements that matter to the patient. Achievements towards these personal goals can help motivate the next steps in wellness behaviors. Developing understanding of personal health goals, and framing and monitoring effectiveness of treatment plans based those goals can improve patient success in making positive changes in health behavior and in adhering to medical treatments. Tools to help foster discussion and treatment planning around personal health goals have been developed and piloted, to the satisfaction of patients and providers alike. For example, the Veterans Health Administration's Personal Health Inventory (available at: https://www.va.gov/WHOLEHEALTH/docs/PHI-long-May22-fillable-508.pdf) was found to be well accepted and helpful in samples of providers and patients in clinical care (Howe et al., 2017; Barnhill et al., 2022). By reshaping health care interactions to focus on goals and achievements that are meaningful to the patient, the health care system increases clinician opportunities for reward via gratitude from patients, awareness of the personally meaningful benefits of the clinician's work, and positive interpersonal interactions.

A main challenge to implementing personalized goal-setting approaches is creating clinician time to have discussions with patients. In studying reasons for low adoption of the VHA's Personal Health Inventory, providers expressed concern that time constraints would limit their regular use of the tool (Howe et al., 2017). Assessment and treatment planning around personalized health goals does not necessarily reduce the need for medical assessment and monitoring of health conditions. Considering the diabetes example above, a physician would still likely monitor HbA1c labs and optimize medications while treating a patient with diabetes who is taking medications, making diet changes, and walking daily towards a personal goal of having energy to play with their grandkids. Understanding a patient's personalized health goals does not necessarily practically reduce the tasks the physician must complete within a patient health care visit, even if it does improve outcomes. Recognizing that physicians are both expensive and in short-supply in most health care systems, it is likely not practical to expect physicians to elicit and map patient personalized health goals as part of their individual visits. Instead, a health care system may need to build broader health care teams to support this personalized goal-setting approach with, for example, health coaches or peer support specialists available to have structured discussions with patients and share summaries with the rest of the health care team (e.g., Denneson et al., 2023).

Population health and care management

Population health approaches serve to shift the role of a provider from treating problems that a local patient pool has successfully sought and scheduled treatment to address (i.e., optimizing services within scheduled appointments), to optimizing wellness for an assigned population of patients. Having an assigned patient population shifts responsibility for recognizing when health care interventions are needed from the patient alone to the patient and their providers. In a population health model, providers have incentives to attend to the health care needs of assigned patients whether they are actively seeking services for immediate concerns. Electronic medical record systems can support providers in population management, enabling them to look across their assigned patient population for signs of, for example, underutilization of services, poor treatment adherence, worsening health markers, or missed opportunities for prevention. For example, electronic population management systems can flag patients who don't refill their prescribed medications on time, who aren't up to date on needed labs, vaccinations, or screenings, who have missed or not scheduled expected appointments, or whose labs or screenings show negative trends. This can enable providers to reach out to patients to reengage them in services or problem-solve barriers limiting effective treatment adherence. This proactive approach to optimizing health across an assigned population is a common component of care management programs, and there are examples across many conditions demonstrating benefits, particularly in reducing emergency visits and admissions and increasing recommended engagement in preventive care.

As an example within the Veterans Health Administration's 141 health care systems, my team implemented a population management system to track patients with psychiatric admissions, supporting discharge planning that included not only the inpatient providers, but also the patient's local primary care and outpatient mental health teams. The data system shared key information across the inpatient and outpatient teams and tracked post-discharge engagement with the patient's outpatient mental health providers, enabling early recognition of problems with follow-up care. Implementation of the data system nationally, increased rates of successful post-discharge mental health care engagement by 5.7%, equivalent to roughly 600 additional patients per month successfully transitioned to outpatient mental health care (Schmidt et al., 2022). We have since shown that this successful engagement in outpatient mental health is associated with lower mortality over the next year. By anticipating challenges during this high-risk health care transition and using population health approaches to proactively connect patients in care, we were able to reduce adverse outcomes in this vulnerable and high-cost patient population.

Studies of similar approaches to improve both preventive care and chronic disease care have emphasized the importance of not only having informatics tools to support population management approaches, but also dedicated care management staff to review data and address signs of under-treatment. For example, a pediatric clinic successfully implemented a population management approach to increase receipt of all 13 recommended preventive care interventions for a population of underserved children under 2 years of age by nearly 20% (Khoury et al., 2022). Over time, clinical outcomes tracked the availability of an assigned care coordinator for the program, improving only during periods that the case coordinator was attending to supporting preventive services. Likewise, Ashburner and colleagues trained 18 primary care practices in use of an informatics system to support population management of diabetes, cardiovascular disease, and hypertension (Ashburner et al., 2017). Eight of the 18 practices were also assigned a half-time dedicated population health coordinator to provide health coaching, motivational interviewing and chronic disease management support based on the population health informatics tool. They supported scheduling and overdue lab completion, conducted chart reviews, and huddled with clinicians to encourage proactive intervention where treatment was not optimal. Patients in primary care practices assigned the population health coordinators showed greater improvements in targeted chronic markers (i.e., low-density lipoprotein cholesterol, glycated hemoglobin (A1C) and blood pressure) but not non-targeted measures (i.e., cancer screening), after implementation of the program. Creating health care practices where care teams are encouraged, informed, and provided time and support to anticipate and engage with patients outside of scheduled care visits can prevent and manage disease and improve outcomes of care.

Long-term health, wellness, and recovery requires creating a life that is meaningful and enjoyable for the individual. Creating opportunities for patient interaction outside of acute treatment needs (e.g., well visits, population health approaches, targeted prevention programs) inherently shifts clinical decision making away from a focus on providing immediate relief towards a focus on long-term health goals. Restructuring health care systems to provide time for clinical interactions that are not driven by immediate patient needs may create new opportunities for clinical interventions that support long-term patient health, wellness, and quality of life.

Ensuring a full toolbox is available to clinicians

Maslow's hammer, the adage that states "If the only tool you have is a hammer, it is tempting to treat everything as if it were a nail", is a common challenge in health care delivery. When health care providers work relatively independently (e.g., in a private practice model with referrals to each specialist), the treatment plan recommended for a patient may be shaped more by the specialties of the providers seen than what is evidence-based practice for a health condition. Each provider seen may tend to view the patient as a candidate for their instrument, assessing whether the patient might benefit from the service they specialize in, rather than considering what might be best for the patient if all options were considered. Not only can this lead to non-optimal or even dangerous care for patients, but it can often be upsetting or frustrating to providers. For example, a medical doctor might know that physical therapy may be a better option than medication or surgery for a patient, but if the doctor does not know how to get the patient into physical therapy or physical therapy is functionally not accessible to a patient, the doctor may feel compelled to offer the medication or surgery that they are able to provide. As a real-life example from my work, during the peak of opioid prescribing, we found that the lower the availability of mental health and physical therapy providers at a health care system, the higher the rate of opioid prescribing was for the patient population. Our interpretation was that when a provider couldn't get their patients seen by a mental health provider or physical therapist in a timely manner, they were more likely to prescribe the patient an opioid medication. In all likelihood, the provider knew that the opioid medication was not a first-line treatment option, but when other options were not accessible, the readily accessible option of an analgesic prescription was offered. While clinical practice guidelines assume that all treatment options are available to all patients, in the real world, treatment plans are shaped by local availability of options.

From that perspective, health care quality depends on clinicians having knowledge, access, and easy pathways for collaborations with providers with other specialties. Ensuring that systems of care are rich in a variety of care modalities, provider types and specialties, and treatment options, and include highly available experts for consultation and referral, will provide clinicians with opportunities to optimize each patient's care plan, rather than simply choose whether to hit each patient with their personal clinical hammer.

While it may be difficult for a health care system to alter the local health care landscape, there are actions any health care system can take to increase awareness of treatment options, and collaboration between providers with different specialties and training.

Examples include:

> Team-based care: As described in more detail in Challenge 4, having an interdisciplinary team of providers work together to design and implement treatment plans can help each team member consider options more broadly to include at least interventions in the whole team's rather than just the individual provider's toolkit.

> Formal collaborative agreements between clinical departments, health care systems or provider networks, community programs, and agencies: Developing collaborative agreements between health care delivery organizations that should be working together to address common patient needs can help increase awareness of treatments available elsewhere and clarify processes for successful referrals and collaborations.
>
> Crucially, the success of collaborative partnerships depends on clinicians being trained and comfortable with the process for collaboration; it is not enough for the resource to be available. The clinician must know when and how to use it. I've seen numerous cases where a health care system went to considerable effort to build up new clinical resources to address known needs for a treatment in the local patient population. But, once in place, the new clinical resource received no referrals or consultations, until intentional clinical training on the new resource and referral process, plus relationship building between referring and treatment teams (e.g., by social introductions), occurred.
>
> Collaborative agreements require intention and effort to develop, and even when clinical teams desire partnerships, they may not know how to approach developing one. While the details of an effective partnership will differ depending on the partners involved and their shared goals, all partnerships benefit by working out, specifying, and documenting the intentions, processes, and boundaries around

the collaboration. Generally, partners should develop a Memorandum of Agreement (MOA), a written document that describes the intended collaboration and expectations of each participating group. There is no required structure for an MOA, however, MOAs should contain standard components to cover common elements of a partnership. The Substance Abuse and Mental Health Services Admininistration (SAMHSA)'s Strategic Prevention Technical Assistance Center provides a brief description of what to put in an MOA as well as a standard template at: https://www.samhsa.gov/sites/default/files/resourcefiles/sptac-creating-memorandum-agreement.pdf

Directories of and protocols to access telehealth services: Particularly since the COVID-19 pandemic forced rapid innovation around delivery of services via telehealth, many health care interventions can be delivered via clinical video telehealth or telephone. This is particularly true of behavioral health interventions, which are less likely to require lab testing, physical exams, and procedures that require physical interactions between the patient and health care staff. Creating directories and clarifying referral and payment processes for health care services that may not be available locally can help expand the treatment options that are functionally available for the provider to consider. Creating warm hand-off procedures so that a provider can initiate behavioral health care immediately when a need is identified in a health care visit can be particularly beneficial. For example, a trial of methods for warm hand-off of patients to a behavioral health provider over telehealth during a primary care visit increased patient likelihood of accepting a treatment referral and engaging in on-going mental health treatment (Fountaine et al., 2023). Developing streamlined systems for identifying services available via telehealth and connecting patients to them can greatly increase options for providers and patients alike.

Directories of and referral protocols to community services: Creating directories and warm hand-off practices to community services can also expand opportunities available to clinicians when working with patients. One well-studied example of the benefits of clinical protocols to engage patients in community services focused on clinical collaborations with local mutual help groups, such as Alcoholics Anonymous, to support recovery from addiction. While mutual help participation has been shown to be highly effective for improving alcohol use disorder outcomes (Kelly et al., 2020) and predictive of better drug use outcomes (Humphreys et al. 2020), health care systems rarely develop protocols to collaborate with local mutual help groups to engage patients who might benefit from participation. In a randomized trial, Timko and Benedetti (2007) compared the effectiveness of providing patients starting an outpatient treatment episode for substance use disorder with either a schedule of local 12-step mutual help meetings or an intensive referral consisting of counselor-mediated introduction to a 12-step volunteer and a review of 12-step journals that recorded meeting attendance during clinical care. The intensive referral process not only increased mutual help attendance, but also improved patient abstinence rates by 10% at one year after the intervention. Empowering clinicians by supporting clinical referral behaviors that help patients engage successfully in often free community services expands clinicians' toolkits, and thus opportunities to succeed in their environment, with little cost to the health care system.

Develop local guidebooks of available self-management services for patient and provider education: A wide variety of patient self-management interventions and approaches have been developed and shown to improve behavioral health symptoms and outcomes when patients use them. As selected examples, computerized and bibliotherapy versions of cognitive behavioral therapies are available and have been shown to be effective in meta-analysis for treatment of depression, anxiety, panic disorders, and insomnia (Andrews et al., 2018; Efron and Wootton, 2021; Simon et al., 2023). Participation in regular exercise or physical activity has been shown to have significant effectiveness for, as examples, treatment of mood disorders and improving cognitive function and sleep quality in older adults (e.g., Schuch et al., 2016; Stubbs et al., 2017; Gallardo-Gómez et al., 2022; Morres et al., 2019; Hasan et al., 2019). Numerous mobile applications, as well as private clubs and community organizations are available to enable, provide support for, and encourage safe exercise options. Mutual help group participation has been shown to be the most effective option for alcohol use disorder recovery (Kelly et al., 2020) and may be beneficial for a variety of behavioral health concerns. Even minimal attention and support from health care providers can improve engagement with and outcomes of these self-management options. For example, a systematic review of self-management interventions for obsessive compulsive disorders found these interventions had large effects when health care providers supported engagement with minimal contacts, moderate effects when engagement was mostly self-driven, and small effects when the patient self-management intervention was completely independent from the health care system (Pearcy et al., 2016). Developing an organized guidebook to orient patients and providers to locally available and effective self-management options may increase patient use of these options, particularly if providers recommend, monitor, and reinforce patient engagement in these self-management practices. Having a core set of recommended options that the clinician knows well may be particularly beneficial, as this allows the provider to answer patient questions, set expectations, and discuss and troubleshoot patient challenges or concerns with use of self-management options.

In all the examples above, the goal is to expand each clinician's toolkit, by providing them with new collaborative skills or habits that enable them to respond to common patient needs more flexibly and effectively. With an expanded array of effective options to consider and apply, the provider increases opportunities in their environment to meet their primary clinical goal, improving wellness of their patient. This should make their job more rewarding and reduce impulsive habit-driven clinical decisions. Rather than getting out their hammer and, for example, prescribing another psychotropic on top of the last one that didn't work or evaluating a patient for a surgery with low likelihood of benefit, this broadened landscape of treatment opportunities allows the provider and patient to step-back and consider other approaches and tools.

Challenge 3: Reducing stress

Like patients, clinicians under stress will be prone to making health care decisions that prioritize immediate relief and/or reward over longer-term goals. Clinician stress can be a problem for therapeutic relationships, as exaggerated relief-seeking can make it difficult for providers to tolerate empathic distress with their patients. When they are stressed, providers may not be as able to listen and relate to a patient's pain, anxiety, distress, and problems without reacting to end the shared distress. A provider might end their empathic pain simply by cutting the visit short or discouraging the patient from sharing or emoting around things the provider is too stressed to hear. Or a provider may pick a quick solution to end the visit, for example, writing a prescription and sending the patient on their way, rather than having to hear additional content that might be distressing but clarify more effective ways of addressing the patient's problem. Alternatively, a provider may experience burn-out and depersonalization, where they simply cannot connect and empathize.

Clinician stress can have negative effects on both the clinicians themselves and their patients. Clinician burnout describes a state where a clinician experiences emotional exhaustion, a reduced sense of accomplishment and depersonalization as a result of chronic stress related to excessive work demands and inadequate resources (West et al., 2018) Rates of burnout in physicians and other clinicians have been reported to be high (e.g., ~50%) and increasing (Shanafelt et al., 2015; Linzer et al., 2022). Health care systems suffer when clinicians struggle with burnout; Burnout can reduce provider productivity, increase likelihood of staff turnover, increase risk of medical errors, and lower patient satisfaction, each at substantial cost to the health care system (West et al., 2018). Clinicians with burnout are at elevated risk of developing mental health conditions, including substance use, depression, and suicidality. Studies of patient and provider perceived health care quality suggest that patients and providers both report lower quality of care when physicians are experiencing greater burnout, even when objective measures of care quality do not identify an effect (Rathert et al., 2018). Where studied to date, measures of clinician burnout were sometimes, but not consistently associated with care quality, effectiveness, and clinical error rate; diagnostic criteria for mood disorders rather than burnout measures better identified when clinicians were experiencing functional challenges likely to cause clinically meaningful differences in care quality (Mangory et al., 2021). Whether clinical decision-making deteriorates at the time the clinician recognizes burnout, or when the stress becomes harmful enough to cause a mood disorder in the clinician, chronic, uncontrollable stress can encourage impulsive habit-driven health care decisions.

Health care systems and other organizations often attempt to address clinician stress and burnout by offering wellness programs to staff. These programs may offer intuitively helpful resources for improving health during the workday or after work hours at no/low cost to staff. Examples of offered resources include on-site fitness classes, mindfulness training, or self-management support such as fitness or diet trackers. Studies suggest that mindfulness training programs may reduce clinician burnout, and resilience and stress reduction training may decrease clinician depression and stress (Naehrig et al., 2021; Kunzler et al., 2020; Shiri et al., 2023). However, these may not address the underlying drivers of clinician stress and burnout. Without other workplace intervention, these well-meaning programs may even increase stress on staff, adding in reminders of one more thing that they aren't able to do properly, and/or increasing anxiety about their own non-optimal health behaviors (Chard, 2018).

Employee wellness programs assume that staff health and lifestyle behaviors are the main cause of worker stress. In health care settings, that may not be a correct assumption. For example, a survey of a diverse and representative population of 10,325 health care workers in France in May 2021 found ~30% of health care workers reported symptoms consistent with depression, with similar rates across all health care professions (Fond et al., 2022). Even when burnout was not considered, workplace factors had stronger associations with depression than personal health risk behaviors (e.g., overweight, sleep duration, hazardous drinking, activity level). Workplace factors with the highest association with depression included burnout, sustained bullying in the workplace, and lack of decision-making latitude. Lack of emotional support from colleagues, job fragmentation and unpredictability, and job complexity/intensity were also significantly associated with depression. Similarly, a survey of over 20,000 advanced practice clinicians during the COVID-19 pandemic found that chaotic work environments, poor teamwork, and lower control over one's work were highly associated with burnout (Linzer et al., 2022). In the 2022 General Social Survey Quality of Worklife Module, health care workers that reported trusting management, having supervisor help, and having enough time to complete work had lower likelihood of burnout (Nigam et al., 2023). Together these suggest that workplace challenges are main causes of clinician distress, burnout, and mental health conditions, and encourage interventions focused on improving workplace conditions, climate, and function.

To effectively reduce clinician stress, health care systems must examine the environments in which clinicians work day-to-day and seek to understand and mitigate common stressors. Talking to or soliciting feedback from health care system teams, including non-clinical staff, is generally the best starting place for addressing local clinical stressors. Health care system staff are generally good at identifying situations or concerns that repeatedly frustrate or scare them, if provided the opportunity to share in a safe and trusted venue. These discussions can help identify and prioritize local staff concerns, which can then be explored and addressed through shared redesign and quality improvement efforts. Notably, including affected staff in the redesign process can itself enhance a sense of control over common health care stressors. This increased sense of control may reduce stress, even in cases where the challenge cannot be eliminated (e.g., having to interact with distressed patients).

Examples of common modifiable health care designs that put stress on clinicians:
> Long shift lengths: Long clinical shifts can lead to lack of sleep that can impair clinician health and increase risk of clinical errors. For example, rates of procedural complications were significantly higher in the last 4 hours of 12-hour emergency medicine residents shifts than in the first 8 (Gatz et al., 2021). Ensuring clinicians get adequate rest is non-controversially considered important for their wellness and patient safety. However, a one-size-fits-all solution to that common goal is unlikely given the diversity and complexities of medical settings and practices. Studies of

reducing shift lengths have generally found shortening shift lengths to reduce rates of medical errors, motor vehicle crashes, and percutaneous injuries among clinicians, but studies have been poor quality and unable to identify a standard optimal shift duration (Reed et al., 2010). In some settings, trade-offs between reducing shift-length and maintaining continuity of care, and/or ensuring access to training opportunities may make longer shifts preferrable for clinicians. Simple policy restrictions on resident duty hours were associated with less emotional exhaustion and dissatisfaction with well-being among residents but were not found to consistently improve patient outcomes (Sephien et al., 2023, Bolster and Rourke, 2015). Ensuring clinician input into shift planning and design within clinics may help balance the competing challenges of ensuring adequate clinician rest and addressing the complexity of clinician hand-offs.

Unrealistically short-appointment booking: Booking clinicians too tightly can cause them to be chronically late to patient appointments and to prioritize completing a clinical visit quickly rather than with the most effective clinical intervention. This time pressure can interfere with patient and provider satisfaction and limit a clinician's connection with their patients (Dugdale et al., 1999). The stress from time pressure on clinicians can shift decision making towards quick solutions to patient distress, such as medication prescribing (e.g., Grol et al., 1985). For example, a study of the opioid prescribing behaviors of 5603 primary care physicians found that the more behind schedule the clinician was at the time of the patient visit, the more likely they were to prescribe the patient an opioid analgesic. A patient seen when the clinician was more than 60 minutes behind schedule was 17% more likely to receive an opioid prescription than when the clinician was less than 10 minutes late (Neprash and Barnett, 2019). The later a clinician felt and the more behind they were on appointments, the more likely they were to prescribe an opioid analgesic, a quick to implement but relatively high-risk treatment to address pain. Even simple organizational stressors such as time pressure on visits can significantly alter treatment decisions with potential long-term consequences for patient outcomes.

Inadequate security: Clinicians must work with distressed patients and can sometimes become the targets of violence. This reality puts health care workers at high risk of experiencing violence in the workplace. The U.S. Occupational Safety and Health Administration (OSHA) reported that 70-74% of the roughly 25,000 workplace assaults that were reported each year between 2011 and 2013 occurred in health care or social service settings. For example, a study of 917 psychotherapists in Europe found that more than half (51.3%) reported experiencing patient attacks or threats of violence in their careers (Daniels and Anadria, 2019), and a study of 140 clinicians in an Emergency Department found that all reported being verbally abused, with 87% of nurses and 37% of providers also reporting experiencing physical violence (Boles et al., 2022). Lack of violence prevention programs, or inadequate security support and response can leave clinicians vulnerable, defensive, and stressed in their interactions with patients.

OSHA has developed guidelines for building comprehensive workplace violence prevention programs in health care settings (Occupational Safety and Health Administration, 2015; Occupational Safety and Health Administration, 2016). There is not a "one-size fits all" approach that will most effectively reduce violence in all health care settings. Strategies need to be tailored to the clinical setting, patient population, environment, and other local characteristics to address the risks of the specific health care clinic. But, OSHA lays out a common approach to help all health care settings develop and optimize strategies to minimize violence. Foundational to the recommendations are a need for universal participation and transparency. Health care management must emphasize the importance of violence prevention, commit to efforts publicly (e.g., through written plans, posted signs, committees to support organized efforts), and participate actively in on-going efforts to improve. Health care workers must be engaged in violence prevention efforts and feel comfortable, supported, and safe in consistently reporting incidents. Health care systems must have systems in place to track incidents of violence and non-judgmentally review and respond to ensure health care worker safety and prevent future incidents. These response and evaluation systems should focus on continuous improvement, seeking to learn from events or reported risks and to adapt to prevent future occurrences. The violence prevention program should include initial and on-going efforts to assess risks within each clinical setting and implement strategies to address them. Health care workers and ideally also patients should be centrally involved in identifying risks as well as solutions. In addition to walk-throughs and inspections of settings for common environmental risks (e.g., lack of escape routes, barriers to visual observation, understaffing, light furniture that could be used as a weapon), violence prevention efforts should assess the concerns, experiences, and recommendations of health care workers, administrators, and patients within a setting, using methods such as focus groups, surveys, anonymous suggestion systems, or team meetings.

Hazard prevention programs should include both "engineering controls", consisting of changes to a workplace to minimize hazards, and "administrative and work practice controls", consisting of protocols to help prevent or minimize harm in dangerous situations. Engineering controls might include installing panic buttons, adding mirrors to improve visibility, or adding features to make waiting or treatment areas less stressful and more calming. Work practice controls might include having clear protocols for incident response and trained security personnel available to implement them, developing dress codes that reduce opportunities to harm staff (e.g., avoiding necklaces, providing ID badges without last names), or ensuring staff transporting or visiting patients off-site have check-in procedures and reliable means of communication). Lastly, all staff should receive safety and health training, including on violence prevention protocols in their setting, ways to recognize warning sign or risk factors for assault, methods to deescalate anger and aggression, self-defense, and methods of reporting risks and incidents. These guidelines provide both a call to action and a blueprint for health care systems to reduce threats and/or harm to staff.

Rotation of clinical staff: Effective teamwork is crucial for efficiency, safety, and effectiveness of clinical teams. Having turnover in team membership can add challenges to communication, process, and trust. Some organizational practices inherently create inconsistency in team composition. For example, rotating trainees or clinicians across numerous units or having a pool of clerks or nurses who rotate coverage across many clinics may inherently increase the variation in clinical team members from day to day. While this may make it easier to ensure each clinic is fully staffed each day (e.g., by adding flexibility to address absences or spreading less desirable assignments across qualified staff) and/or provide trainees or staff broader exposure to facilitate learning, the inconsistency in team membership may have negative consequences. For example, a large academic medical center decided to investigate the impact of maintaining greater team consistency by varying how they assigned medical residents during their 16-week inpatient medicine rotation (Iyasere et al., 2022). In one arm of their designed randomized trial, residents stayed on a single medical nursing floor (i.e., with a single nursing team) for the full 16 weeks. In the second arm, they split their 16 weeks across 4 general medicine floors with 4 assigned nursing teams per usual practice. Despite similar performance of the general medicine units before the trial, the unit where residents stayed the full 16 weeks reported better team function after, including better ratings of leadership and management, support for and communication with team members, ability to negotiate with patients, and positive interactions between team members. Moreover, the unit with the consistent residents outperformed the other units in medical simulations. While this small trial is not necessarily generalizable, it does highlight the frequently ignored benefits of team consistency and familiarity for provider wellness, team function, and clinical safety and effectiveness.

Lack of team or health care system support: Having a tight-knit, supportive team that communicates and works well together is key to minimizing stress on providers. For example, a mixed method study in an urban teaching hospital emphasized the importance of having trusted, consistent, interdisciplinary teammates who communicate together effectively for preventing burn-out, and highlighted isolation, particularly among physicians, as key risk for burnout (Lu et al., 2023). Emphasizing that the crucial elements of team support involve qualitative rather than quantitative availability of team support, a study examined whether availability of mental health providers for warm hand-off in primary care using a Primary Care Mental Health Integration model reduced burnout in primary care providers. While use of and communication with the integrated mental health staff did not reduce primary care physician burnout, better communication, and satisfaction with team function within the primary care team was associated with lower primary care physician burnout, demonstrating the importance of strong interpersonal connections between the team members who work most closely together (Leung et al., 2020).

One method to improve team function is to use a formal Crew Resource Management (CRM) team training approach, borrowed from aviation team training practice. CRM uses structured information-sharing methods, demonstration-based methods, and simulation or role-playing methods to train teams to work together effectively. Because this is a time consuming and expensive approach, it is typically only used in high-risk clinical settings. Reviews have found CRM approaches to have large effects on clinician knowledge and behaviors and small effects on attitudes, although effects on patient outcomes are still unclear (O'dea et al., 2014; Buljac-Samardzic et al., 2021). Expanding and targeting use of CRM team trainings to improve communication and teamwork within lower functioning teams might reasonably be expected to lower provider stress.

Interestingly, a study examined a gaming approach to fostering improved team communication and function in medical simulations. They examined differences in team communication strategies between novice (i.e., medical student) versus experienced teams. They found that experienced teams were more likely to prompt for additional information and input from other team members, acknowledge task requests, explicitly distribute and clarify workload and tasks among team members, encourage open communication, prompt for reevaluation, and provide better justification for decisions (van Peppen et al., 2022). Outside of formal team trainings, encouraging practice of concretely helpful communication behaviors such as these might improve communication and minimize clinician burnout and stress. More generally, soliciting input, debriefing and problem-solving around team communication and support may have benefits for reducing clinician stress and improving patient safety.

Lack of availability of needed services by referral or in the community: For many behavioral health disorders, the most effective and recommended services require specialized training (e.g., in specific evidence-based psychotherapy protocols) and/or intensive courses of treatment (e.g., daily or weekly sessions for a 3–4-month period). Primary care or general mental health clinicians typically do not have the specific training, and/or space in their schedules to deliver these types of services to patients, and instead will rely on referral to intensive specialty mental health programs. Such programs may be in scant supply and/or offered too far away from a patient's home to make attendance logistically feasible. When providers are unable to get their patients into recommended intensive treatments, they are left to improvise within the limits of their personal knowledge, available treatments, and scheduling capacity. This may lead, for example, to an over-reliance on psychotropic prescribing for behavioral health conditions, as providers use the only tools available to them within a framework of infrequent (e.g., monthly, or quarterly) encounters with patients. Carrying a caseload of patients in need of unavailable higher levels of care can be stressful and demoralizing for providers. For example, in the Veterans Health Administration, therapists who experienced greater institutional support for evidence-based psychotherapy (e.g., greater ability to schedule episodes and transition patients down to a lower level of care after treatment completion) were significantly less likely to experience burnout and had increased job satisfaction even after controlling for therapist workload (Sripada et al., 2023). Seeing patients when you cannot get them the treatments you think would be best for them is emotionally challenging and frustrating for providers.

Efforts to ensure that guideline-recommended care for common behavioral health conditions is readily available can reduce provider stress and improve patient outcomes.

Interventions to reduce stress in clinical care

As we learned in chapter 3, the defining difference between an exciting healthy challenge and a traumatic harmful stressor is often only real or perceived control over the situation. A sense of control over a potential stressor can prevent the cascade of stress circuit effects on cognition, emotion, and physiology that lead to short-term-focused decisions and increase risk of long-term health conditions. As the above examples illustrate, there are many potential contributors to workplace stress, and there is unlikely to be a single optimal solution or intervention that minimizes stress in all health care settings. But ensuring that health care workers contribute to the design of health care systems, provide regular and on-going feedback about challenges that they don't have ready solutions for, and have supportive peer and leadership structures to collaborate and cope around difficult situations can help workers experience and build a sense of control over challenges in their workplace. From within that supportive and collaborative structure, teams may consider numerous options for addressing the uncontrollable challenges in their local work setting.

We have or will discuss many health care interventions and structures that may help address common challenges. For example, in challenge 2, we described quality improvement and safety practices that focus on fixing systems rather than laying blame. These may reduce fear of retribution for accidents and encourage problem-solving around trouble spots in care. We also describe population and care management approaches that can help get patients needed services proactively. Intervening upstream can reduce risk of crises and emergencies in patients with chronic conditions, reducing stress in patients and clinicians alike. In challenge 3, we highlight that mindfulness interventions can have moderate effects on clinician well-being and that violence prevention is crucial to address in health care settings, making up two important components of systems to reduce negative consequences of clinician stress. In challenge 2 and 4, we describe health care delivery practices such as team-based care, group practice models, consultation services, and service agreements that can support collaborative, interdisciplinary care, and provide opportunities for health care workers to seamlessly support one another through otherwise difficult or uncomfortable patient cases and interactions. Working in systems that inherently encourage peer support in health care treatment planning and delivery may reduce isolation and frustration that can contribute to chronic stress. With time and attention to identifying stress-points in health care settings and creative use of less commonly implemented health care designs and interventions, health care leaders and workers can create working environments that minimize health care worker stress, burnout and depression and improve the safety and effectiveness of care.

Challenge 4: Creating and Reinforcing New Habits

Clinical evidence and health care practice is constantly evolving, requiring clinicians to learn new clinical practices, restructure their workflow, change their communication methods, etc. Learning new habits requires not only having the knowledge and skills to do a new behavior, but also ensuring that the new habit is triggered at the right time and reinforced such that it is repeated at the next appropriate time. Continuing medical education focuses on knowledge and skills building, leaving health care systems to create supports and rewards to encourage use of the new clinical behaviors where they are helpful. Some common strategies can help health care systems make it easier for clinicians to do the right thing and get reinforced for doing so.

Making it easier to do the right thing: Setting up workflows to favor evidence-based practice:
Decision Support
One of the most challenging things about clinical care delivery is the breadth of patient needs, complexity of decision-making, and time pressure of service delivery. The overwhelming number of competing demands understandably clutter providers working memory with tasks and problems, leading to cognitive overload. Providers can't possibly remember every detail about every patient, nor do they have time to do comprehensive reviews of patient records and clinical practice guidelines to guide each treatment decision. To help ease provider's cognitive overload, health care systems can help develop decision support to trigger and walk clinicians through guideline-recommended care protocols tailored for patient's needs. These may be low-tech or high-tech, but their success depends on their being embedded smoothly and carefully into clinician workflows, such that they facilitate rather than disrupt clinician-patient encounters.

Examples of decision support features that have been shown to successfully encourage consistent use of guideline recommended clinical practices include (Sutton et al., 2020):

Clinical reminders: These are typically either pop-up alerts or pre-visit summaries of care interventions that are overdue or appropriate given a patient's health history or demographics. For example, these are frequently used to encourage screening interventions, ensure that follow-up labs and assessments are conducted, support prescription renewals, etc.

Alerts: These are frequently used to manage potentially dangerous medication interactions or allergies, but may also be used to warn about urgently overdue labs or assessments, etc.

Checklists and documentation templates: Checklists and documentation templates are frequently used to support clinicians through complex procedures or bundles of clinical interventions that may be needed for patients with common conditions. These checklists help to ensure that key steps in a clinical process are not missed or overlooked and can support care coordination to enable team-based care delivery. Documentation templates serve a similar function in cueing clinicians to complete and document all needed actions in a care intervention or protocol, though typically with an added focus on facilitating complete and proper record-keeping and coding.

Complex decision support: Complex decision support systems may help tailor patient care based on applying details of a specific patient case (e.g., as extracted from an electronic medical record or entered by a clinician) to a guideline-based algorithm to generate care recommendations for clinician consideration. Complex decision support systems may also help to make patient-relevant clinical knowledge or resources handy, for example, by identifying and providing links to patient education materials, key references for a recommendation, or local resource lists that may be helpful for a particular patient.

Prioritization systems (e.g., risk assessment systems, predictive models): Predictive models or risk assessment tools can help clinicians better recognize relative risk across patients and prioritize additional risk mitigation interventions or more frequent follow-up for those at elevated risk.

There is considerable evidence that these decision-support structures can successfully reshape clinical practice. For example, meta-analysis across 42 studies of the impact of clinical reminders on clinician behavior found moderate sized effects on the practices clinicians were reminded to do (Holt et al., 2012). A meta-analysis of pharmacy alerts found some less consistent results, with 53% of 23 studies showing positive effects, 34% showing no effects and 6% showing negative effects; positive effects were observed in 5 of 6 studies of drug-condition alerts, and 2 of 6 studies of drug-drug interactions (Page et al. 2017). A review of 70 studies of decision support systems found that when decision support systems were automatic and computer-based, included recommendations, and were embedded in clinical workflows at the time and location of decision-making, they significantly improved clinical practice over 90% of the time (Kawamoto et al., 2005). Decision support systems can be so effective in triggering clinician practice habits that their biggest challenge has become their success. Alerts and reminders can successfully orient clinicians to a question that needs to be asked or a task that needs to be done, but employed too liberally, the alerts themselves become overwhelming and distracting (Ng et al., 2023). Alert fatigue can lead to the alerts being ignored or even dismissed unread, even as they disrupt the clinic visit. Unless the workflow provides reasonable time to address all the alerts, recommendations, and checklists, decision-support can lead to tasks being rushed so much that they become ineffective. As an example, I have seen clinics where excessive pressure on behavioral health screening in primary care led to useless implementation, with well-validated screening tools being boiled down into a rushed query of "You don't have problems with drinking, domestic violence, depression, or anxiety, do you?". This abbreviated and leading approach to screening led to unbelievably low rates of documented positive behavioral health screens among their patient population. As such, it is important to review decision support from a holistic perspective within actual clinical workflows. If the decision support creates rather than relieves clutter and distraction within clinicians' workflow, then it may worsen rather than improve clinical care.

In contrast to decision support systems designed to trigger and facilitate recommended clinical behaviors, decision support can reduce non-optimal practices by adding in barriers or delays to implementing those unfavored behaviors. Barriers may be as simple as a medical record pop-up window that provides a caution message and/or asks for a justification for the choice to be documented. Hiding unfavored options under layers within medical records can also be an effective discouragement (Burton et al., 2021).In some cases, hospitals may require additional levels of approval through a supervisory or administrative chain of command. Making the clinically unfavored decision more difficult, time-consuming, or uncomfortable for a clinician to choose can significantly reshape clinical behaviors.

Providing peer support and monitoring

Normative feedback is a highly effective approach for reshaping health behaviors. While it has been studied most as a method for reshaping unhealthful behaviors in teens and young adults, it has been used with substantial success for shaping clinician behavior as part of multiple quality improvement strategies.

VA's Academic Detailing Service combines targeted clinician education with data tools that enable comparison of a clinician's practice habits with other clinicians nationwide. Clinical pharmacists meet with providers and share information about how their practices differ from guidelines or norms among other clinicians. They then provide them with one-on-one training and clinician and patient education materials with practice information on how to change behaviors. Knowing that your practice is different than other clinicians and that a peer is monitoring what you and others are doing can motivate changes toward clinical recommendations, particularly when paired with demonstrations of how to do the recommended practice within the clinician's specific clinic setting. This normative feedback approach has generated large, rapid changes in targeted provider behaviors. For example, an Academic Detailing campaign focused on reducing sedative-hypnotic prescribing to older adults reduced rates of new starts of sedative-hypnotic prescriptions in older adults by over 50% in providers who received a training session. Practice changes were maintained for at least 18 months (Ragan et al., 2021). A study of an Academic Detailing campaign to encourage use of guideline-recommended pharmacotherapy for alcohol use disorders found an 68% increase in use of these treatments at facilities that implemented the Academic Detailing campaign as compared to facilities that did not (Harris et al., 2016). As with patients who would benefit from behavior change, providing normative feedback to clinicians regarding target behaviors (e.g., your practice habits in comparison to peers) along with an offer of assistance to support a shift to recommended, more normative habits can be an effective intervention, producing significant long-lasting shifts in behavior with brief interventions.

Many models for programs that provide training and supported practice of new clinical behaviors have been developed. In addition to the Academic Detailing model described above, another well-studied and effective model that has successfully encouraged new clinical behaviors in extended networks of clinicians is the Extension for Community Healthcare Outcomes (ECHO) model (Arora et al., 2014). ECHO uses on-going group teleconsultation with specialists and case-based learning to support generalist providers such as primary care physicians to adopt and utilize health care practices typically only provided by specialists. Originally designed to increase access to care for hepatitis in rural regions with no local access to specialists (Arora et al., 2011), this model has been adopted and used widely to spread specialist clinical knowledge and practices across health care specialties and systems (e.g., recent examples in behavioral health include cognitive behavioral therapy for psychosis (Kopelovich et al., 2023), disaster mental health response (Hambrick et al., 2023), and pediatric depression treatment (Cinko et al., 2023). Minus the broader programming provided in the ECHO model, teleconsultation programs generally can be helpful for supporting clinicians attempting new clinical practices or applying clinical practices to a complex or challenging patient cases, in that these programs also make specialists available on demand to educate and coach providers through patient cases. A key challenge with standard teleconsultation programs is that they generally rely on the generalist clinician to recognize when they need help; without support to identify cases where consultation is warranted, providers may not know to seek out consultation when they and their patients might benefit, and these teleconsultation programs may be underused.

Performance Measurement systems also provide monitoring, typically with standardized metrics based on health care administrative data or chart review. Health care systems may use these as oversight tools to drive quality improvement or Ongoing Professional Practice Evaluations. In these cases, these performance measures are often used to compare practice across providers, clinics, or health care systems, and identify potential problems for solving. Alternatively, performance metrics can be used to create Contingency Management programs for clinicians, with incentives, usually in the form of recognition, positive reviews, or performance-based bonuses tied to completion of the desired health care practice. Just as with patient treatment, providing direct incentives for completing desired or new clinical practices is likely to be most impactful when the clinical behavior is uncomfortable and not inherently rewarding. For example, performance-based bonuses are reasonable to consider in cases where the most effective treatments for patients are time-consuming, stressful, or unpleasant, poorly reimbursed, or otherwise punishing or not rewarding from the provider perspective. Also like with patients, providing feedback on practice behaviors in as close to real-time as possible will increase the effectiveness of the incentives and better reinforce the clinical behavior. For example, providing feedback in regularly updated patient tracking dashboards that update as clinicians do or do not implement the target practice will likely shift clinical practice more than providing metrics on past year performance at the time of annual performance reviews.

Creating Systems that Support Providers in Care Delivery

Delivering recommended health care interventions frequently requires clinicians to do behaviors that aren't particularly rewarding for them in the moment. Interventions may require providers to do uncomfortable or frequently punished behaviors, such as bringing up uncomfortable topics (e.g., regarding substance use, suicidality, anger, weight issues, sexual behaviors, etc.), recommending behavior changes that the patient may be defensive about, stopping or stepping down treatments that aren't benefiting the patient, or asking the patient to undergo unpleasant tests. Even when interventions may have significant health benefits for the patient, the provider may not experience these clinically gold-standard behaviors as interpersonally rewarding in the moment. Being human, providers may struggle to adopt health-promoting interventions that are personally uncomfortable or distressing to deliver or are likely to elicit negative reactions from patients. Understanding this challenge, health care systems must consider ways to help make gold-standard practices rewarding from the clinician perspective, as well as the patient perspective.

As we discussed earlier, decision support systems can help with this problem to some extent. For example, providing reminders and templates that walk clinicians through uncomfortable interventions can make them less uncomfortable, and providing "credit" for completing the task (e.g., via visual checkboxes on decision support or higher scores on performance measures) can create an immediate reward for carrying out the gold-standard intervention.

Other organizational strategies can also be helpful. Team-based care can provide social reinforcement for implementing uncomfortable interventions. Providers on the team can reinforce and encourage recommended practices for each other, support, problem-solve and provide back-up to implement challenging practices and provide accountability to discourage their teammates from avoiding uncomfortable practices with challenging patients or during stressful periods. Team-members may also provide immediate "second opinions" in cases where new health care recommendations are unfamiliar or second-guessed by patients, potentially even supporting each other in visits where challenging conversations are anticipated. Having team-members available may help providers implement new practices, particularly when clinicians are expected to do interpersonally uncomfortable, anxiety-provoking, or frequently punished behaviors (e.g., bringing up uncomfortable topics, making high pressure clinical decisions on complex cases).

Providing an example of the potential benefits of team-based care delivery, the Veterans Health Administration (VHA) piloted a reorganization of general mental health service programs, shifting from a model where patients were typically assigned to individual clinicians for specific services (e.g., to a psychologist for therapy and a psychiatrist for medication management) to a team-based model. This modeled used principles from the Collaborative Chronic Care Model (CCM) and was called the 'Behavioral Health Interdisciplinary Program' (BHIP) by VHA (American Psychiatric Association, 2023). In the team-based model, an interdisciplinary team of providers were assigned a population of patients for whom they were responsible for general mental health service delivery and care coordination with specialty mental health services (e.g., residential care, intensive outpatient substance use treatment, etc.). The team developed and managed treatment plans together and met in daily huddles to discuss cases and coordinate services. The reorganization enabled providers to support each other around challenging practices and patient cases and brought multiple perspectives to problem-solving. Additionally, the population-based assignment enabled development of decision-support focused on tracking patient receipt of guideline-based interventions and adherence to care plans (e.g., refilling medications on time, not missing appointments, timely receipt of needed labs and assessments), providing clinicians with on-going feedback on their success in delivering services as intended. Even in early implementation, "staff specifically highlighted the potential for the BHIP model to improve staff working relationships and enhance communication, collaboration, morale, and veteran treatment consistency" (Barry et al., 2016).

I observed the benefits of interdisciplinary team-delivered care when implementing demonstration trials integrating services for chronic pain into public primary care clinics for persons with HIV (Trafton et al., 2012). These clinics treated complex patients who frequently had not only HIV and chronic pain, but also substance use and/or mental health disorders, and psychosocial challenges. This pilot program brought together an addiction psychiatrist, a psychologist with expertise in cognitive behavioral and acceptance therapies for chronic pain, and a social worker focused on facilitating community engagement, particularly with rehabilitative exercise and social activities. Each of the clinicians had deep experience and expertise in working with complex patients with addiction and pain. They were explicitly focused on goals of getting patients actively engaged in practices (e.g., reframing, relaxation strategies, exercise, addressing catastrophizing, anxiety, and depression) that both reduce pain and facilitate recovery, and minimize reliance on potentially addictive medications and disengagement from work, social, and other responsibilities in response to pain. While straight-forward in theory, working with patients with chronic pain and frequently co-morbid addiction was difficult in practice. Over years of experiencing pain, patients may develop pain behaviors, including emotive responses (e.g., grimacing, catastrophizing) and help-seeking responses that are extremely effective in eliciting observer empathy and impulses to immediately rescue the patient. These pain behaviors can drive clinicians to prescribe medications, such as opioids or benzodiazepines, that might provide quick relief but worsen behavioral responses, or reinforce patient beliefs and habits that maintain disability (e.g., non-return to work or rest in response to pain).

Despite their expertise and explicit awareness of this challenge, the three clinicians would still struggle to not respond to patient cues and drift from recommendations that required the patient to struggle through new responses. Aware of this very human, and deeply empathic tendency, the team would pre-huddle on challenging patient cases to set goals for the visit, and sometimes even see a patient in pairs. Together the clinicians could split focus, with one engaging fully with the patient, and the other monitoring the interaction, and redirecting their teammate if they became too entangled emotionally with the patient to encourage recovery-focused plans. Providing care actively as a team enabled the providers to carry out guideline-recommended treatment plans without needing to disengage from their patients emotionally, maintaining compassion, but not unhelpful clinical responses to empathically experienced pain.

The CCM and team-based reorganization showed benefits for patients and the health care system as well. Patients experienced a reduction in inpatient hospitalizations and a 24% reduction in all-cause mortality (Bauer et al., 2019, Ruderman et al., 2023). Implementation of the BHIP model was found to be cost saving to the health care system through reduction in inpatient mental health care costs (Miller et al., 2020). Specifically, outpatient implementation was estimated to cost $40 more per patient in general mental health services but was associated with an overall reduction in patient costs of $78 per patient. From a team perspective, the average team invested $27,985 to implement the model, but saved $47,500 in patient health care costs during the next year.

As discussed prior, team-based care also brings interdisciplinary perspective and care options to treatment planning for patients, expanding opportunities for clinical success in the local health care environment. When patients are seen by an individual provider, the provider will naturally gravitate towards recommending those treatments that they have expertise and ability to deliver. A team brings a broader array of expertise and more clinical options to address patient challenges.

Delivering care to patients in groups

Like team-based care models, group-based practice offers benefits for supporting new habits in both clinicians and patients. Delivering health care to groups of patients is a well-established practice for some types of psychotherapy (e.g., cognitive behavioral therapy). Not only does group practice allow a provider to see more patients in less time, but the modality itself may be particularly beneficial for patients. Group format can have numerous benefits (Kirsh et al., 2017). Having multiple patients with similar health challenges together offers opportunities for many types of beneficial interactions. Patients may better understand how to apply skills by observing others try to use them. They may benefit from examples of changes or supports that were helpful for others in the group. They may gain self-efficacy by interacting with people like them that are further along in recovery from their health condition. They may get new ideas by problem-solving their challenges with experienced others. They may gain social support and feel less isolated by meeting others struggling with similar problems. They may learn of helpful community resources or create supports together (e.g., a walking group, a book club).

Nevertheless, even in the case of therapy, group-based care is under-utilized. While models for group-based shared medical appointments have been developed, they are very rarely used. Those that have implemented them often rave about the benefits, as interactions with patients frequently solve some of the motivational challenges that can otherwise plague provider attempts to address medical conditions with strong behavioral components.

For example, a colleague found herself the lone addiction psychiatrist at her medical center after a few local retirements. This left her with far more patients with opioid use disorder than she could reasonably see with an individual practice model, and innovating out of necessity, she set up a shared medical appointment model for patients with opioid use disorder in collaboration with a nurse and a psychologist. Patients would be seen in groups where sessions would include both medical assessment (e.g., by the nurse and psychiatrist, with individual break-aways as needed) and psychotherapy and mutual support. Her experience with this shared appointment model was so positive, she contacted me in hopes of sharing her model with others. In particular, she was deeply impressed with how the shared appointments addressed the challenge of getting new patients to engage in treatment. Whereas in an individual appointment model she often spent a lot of time convincing patients to try effective treatments, and then stick with them during the early challenging days of behavior change, in the shared medical appointment model she found she just had to get them to agree to come sit in a group appointment. There, the patients further along in treatment would share their success, address questions and concerns from the perspective of someone who made a similar choice recently and encourage the new or ambivalent patients into treatments that work. When the new patients came back, the other patients would help motivate continuation and problem-solve barriers. The provider was there to provide medically accurate information, address misperceptions, and ensure appropriate treatment planning and monitoring, but experienced patients were able to address the complex motivational and logistical challenges that prevent early patient care engagement in ways that a non-peer simply couldn't. Moreover, the experienced patients benefited from helping the new patients. By voicing what was working for them, they brought attention to their own effective strategies, reinforcing their own new behaviors, increasing their own self-efficacy and sense of self-worth, and creating a group of peers to monitor and support them in the case when they veered from the path that was working for them. In short, the shared medical appointment model allowed the psychiatrist to focus on optimizing medications and addressing co-morbid medical needs, while the group format allowed the patients themselves to address many of the common challenges to behavior change, minimizing fears about making changes, increasing confidence around safety and ability to change, and providing support and reinforcement during attempts to initiate new habits. Demonstrating that my colleague's experience was not unique, Sokol and colleagues provide a very helpful series of case studies of group visit models for treatment of opioid use disorder which help to demonstrate the diverse ways in which this modality of care can be used to successfully deliver services (Sokol et al., 2020).

Shared medical appointment models have been developed and used for weight loss, prediabetes and diabetes, glaucoma, cancer follow-up care, congestive heart failure, asthma, women's health, long-COVID, and other chronic conditions (Walker et al., 2022; Papadakis et al., 2021; Edelman et al., 2015; Tam et al., 2022; Marshall et al., 2022; Shibuya et al., 2020; Wall-Hass et al., 2012; Carlsson et al., 2021; Gerontakos et al., 2023; Lin et al., 2022). Studies of shared medical appointments suggest that they often improved patient satisfaction, perception that care was meeting their needs, and trust of their providers (Wadsworth et al., 2019; Kirsh et al., 2017). Patients and providers expressed that they provided more time for discussion and relationship building, and improved communication. Patients expressed improved sense of community and reduced isolation, an increased sense of empowerment in managing their health, as well as experiencing care as more accessible and timely. Reviews to date have found that studies of shared medical appointments are too weak and diverse to determine if they improve health outcomes, but in small studies where outcomes have been measured, they tend to find equivalent or better clinical outcomes with the shared appointment model, suggesting that significant negative health outcomes of the approach have not been encountered.

Group visits may have additional benefits from the perspective of reducing problematic provider pressures that may trigger unfavored clinical habits:
1) Having other providers in the room may make it easier for providers to say no to patients when they ask for treatments that aren't appropriate. For example, providers may find it easier to discourage patient enthusiasm for non-evidence-based treatments a patient may have seen in a commercial, found on the internet, or heard about through social media. They may also be better positioned to help patients understand treatments that are popular because they are addictive (e.g., cannabis, benzodiazepines) or promoted deceptively or repeatedly on addictive or manipulative media. Having

multiple providers in a visit helps establish clinical consensus and expertise with a ready second opinion immediately available.

2) The format may make the provider feel less rushed and provide more time to understand patient symptoms, functional challenges, and the context, causes and consequences of their illnesses. This may reduce time pressure and stress on the clinician that might otherwise favor a hasty prescription or referral.

3) Providing treatment in a group setting may reduce provider safety concerns (e.g., as compared with being alone in a room with a patient). Notably, safety concerns have anecdotally encouraged some mental health providers towards preferring increasingly virtual practice models, which a subset of patients may dislike.

4) As described in the example above, this may provide checks on providers empathic connections with patients, which can drive unnecessary diagnostic testing, symptom- rather than recovery-focused care decisions, etc. When providers get pulled into patient fears and distress, they may suggest over-aggressive health care interventions, even when safer (or no) medical intervention is recommended (e.g., back surgery and MRIs for back pain, etc.). Having multiple providers in the room helps them provide checks on each other's emotional involvement and/or exhaustion.

5) When clinicians are trying to change practice habits, having another clinician in the room can help reinforce new protocol, process, and communication strategies, speeding and hardening adoption.

6) Allowing patients to observe the clinician interact with other patients may help to build respect and trust for the clinician, reducing patient anxiety and thus provider discomfort (Kirsh et al., 2017).

Use of group modalities creates opportunities to support and reward both clinicians' and patients' health and health care behaviors that might otherwise be challenging to adopt. Group dynamics create opportunities for efficiencies, problem-solving, and reinforcement that can increase self-efficacy for providers and patients alike.

Just as with patients, adopting and habituating a new clinical behavior requires more than just knowledge of what one should do. Clinicians' require training on how to logistically implement the new behavior in their specific work place. They require environments that make it feasible and easy to do the new behavior. Most importantly, they require reinforcement for completing the new behavior. In some cases, patient gratitude or improvement may provide immediate reinforcement. But in many cases, patient benefit will be on a delay, and the health care system may need to engineer reinforcers, such as streamlined or less stressful work practice, monitors that acknowledge work well-done, peer recognition of new expertise, or even concrete incentives such as bonuses for newly implemented skills. Health care managers and systems must work to create reinforcement systems where needed to help clinical teams optimize and continuously strive to adopt best practices in health care.

Challenge 5: Creating an executive system that supports problem-solving to optimize health benefits for health care enrollees

A health care system needs an active, engaged, and long-term-goal-focused executive system to strategize, organize, facilitate, and reinforce desired changes in clinical practice.

Just as in individuals, a long-term-health-focused executive system is crucial to the well-being of the system and the individuals who work within it or rely upon it. Health care executives and managers create the infrastructure and environments essential for the first 4 challenges. Supporting challenge 1, health care executives and managers can help develop and troubleshoot clinical processes to ensure that guideline-recommended practices are easy to do, and systems are in place to help clinicians through pressures to provide quick relief or solutions at the expense of creating later problems or risks. Having robust quality improvement and/or organizational design and engineering teams evaluating health care practices and working with clinical teams to address challenge points is crucial to optimizing care and avoiding short-term solutions that worsen health care outcomes.

Supporting challenge 2, health care executives and managers set up health care networks, create collaborative agreements, set up systems for communication between health care services and providers, create organizational structures, and set policies and cultures that shape the landscape of opportunities available to clinicians. Health care executives engineer the environments in which clinicians work, determining what options and solutions are available to clinicians seeking to solve a patient's health challenges. By creating robust structures that enable clinicians to communicate and collaborate within interdisciplinary teams, with specialists, and with community programs and supports, health care executives create opportunities for providers to recommend optimal, evidence-based services from across the spectrum of clinical medicine, rather than rely on the treatments within their personal expertise. By integrating clinical teams in logistical and administrative decision-making, health care executives help ensure that health care decisions and outcomes are not limited by non-optimal prioritization of supplies, infrastructure, scheduling, cleaning, and other supports that are crucial to the successful delivery of health care.

Likewise, health care systems need to consistently and non-judgmentally identify errors and safety issues and support efforts to reduce the likelihood of recurrence. Health care executives must build up both a culture that supports reporting of problems as well as efforts to develop and implement solutions. This requires management to prioritize both learning and safety, rewarding staff for proactively bringing up challenges and concerns and/or suggesting improvements to practices or systems. Avoiding blame and judgment for existing non-optimal practices and emphasizing a focus on patient safety and wellness is crucial for finding problems and reducing defensiveness around efforts to change. By fostering a culture in which problems are non-judgmentally aired and shared toward developing and implementing systems solutions to address them, health care executives turn challenges and errors into opportunities for improvement.

As with patients, clinicians in low opportunity environments will tend toward habit-driven actions that provide immediate reward or relief, rather than long-term solutions. By creating an opportunity-rich environment for clinicians, health care executives encourage clinicians to attend to the long-term health and wellness of their patients, rather than focusing attention on quick fixes to cover symptoms or complete a visit.

Supporting challenge 3, executives and managers have influence over policies, culture and work environments that can either induce or minimize stress in providers and patients. We discussed numerous common examples of stressors in clinical environments, and ways in which these might be addressed to improve clinician well-being and therefore decision-making. Soliciting feedback and engaging with providers and patients is central to all efforts to reduce workplace stress. Problems and challenges stop being stressors when the person experiencing them gains a sense of control over the problem. When a solution or escape is readily available, persisting in a difficult experience is not necessarily stressful. Creating cultures where workplace and life stressors are shared and solutioned collectively can help providers, clinics and health care systems responsively adapt to shifting and evolving stressors faced in delivering care. While not every challenge is avoidable, ensuring the workplace is explicitly focused on recognizing and supporting problem-solving around challenges in itself increases provider control over stress.

Supporting challenge 4, managers set the culture and practice environment in which clinical habits are learned and reinforced. Health care executives can develop measurement systems that help clinicians and administrators monitor health care system or clinician behaviors. These monitors allow executives to provide recognition and rewards for behaviors that they want to encourage and help recognize behaviors, processes, or structures that are causing problems, so that the executives can support and target problem-solving. The measures themselves can help support clinicians in personal efforts to learn new skills or improve practice behaviors, by providing transparent and time-trended measures of their and their peers' performance. The measures can reinforce their own behaviors by making improvements visible and help them find models or mentors by highlighting peers who have mastered the practice behavior. Health care executives lead crucial efforts to prioritize attention on the clinical practice or health care system behaviors that are most important to learn or improve, setting quality improvement agendas and monitors that support them. To ensure success on prioritized learning efforts, health care executives critically support development of blueprints to break down targeted behaviors into component pieces and provide support for addressing challenges and learning required at each step. By structuring learning efforts and bringing attention to relative and incremental performance, health care executives can support continuous improvement and mastery of new practices within their health care systems.

Supporting challenge 5, managers must have systems in place to enable informed decision-making. Just like our frontal cortices, health care executives must consider long-term and cross-system effects of health care practices and design. Our frontal cortex assesses information from all over our brain to review and predict long-term effects, potential punishments or adverse consequences, misalignments with goals or mission, and even inefficiencies of the behaviors recommended or completed by our reward learning systems. The cortex can stall choices or practice behaviors when there are concerns that they may have undesirable longer-term effects and can shift decisions towards a new behavior when habitual practices are deemed non-optimal. Similarly, health care executives must review information from across the health care system to ensure that decisions made in one part of the system do not conflict or cause problems for other parts of the system. They must assess the long-term outcomes of health care practices to ensure that practices aren't short-sighted and/or cause later negative consequences. When non-optimal practices are identified, they must support innovation and learning to develop new practices that address or avoid identified problems and lead to better outcomes.

Ensuring clinical practices optimize patients long-term health

Understanding long-term patient outcomes is crucial for guiding health care executive decisions towards effective health care delivery processes. While this sounds straight-forward superficially, in practice, it is difficult to link specific health care system and provider behaviors and practice patterns to long-term outcomes. Because health care treatments are offered to patients based on their need for the treatment, receipt of a treatment is tightly linked to the clinical indication for the treatment. If you simply look at the outcomes of patients who get a treatment, the outcomes will reflect both the effect of having the disease for which the treatment is prescribed, as well as the effect of the treatment. As such, patients who receive treatments are generally sicker and have worse outcomes than those who don't. Looking at associations between getting a type of care and having negative outcomes can be extremely misleading. For example, patients that receive a second-line chemotherapy treatment might have higher rates of dying of cancer than those that don't, as only those with cancer that didn't respond to first-line treatment are likely to get that second-line treatment. Needing a second-line chemotherapy is an indication that one's cancer is aggressive or treatment resistant. The effectiveness of the treatment can be hidden by the negative effects of needing the treatment. Gold standard methods for avoiding this problem and determining the effects of a practice behavior require conducting a well-controlled randomized clinical trial. However, randomized clinical trials are expensive and take years to conduct, and in some cases may not be ethical to implement. Moreover, findings of the trial may or may not generalize to patient populations or practice settings different than the one in which the trial was conducted. Given these limitations, more timely and agile methods that can be used in regular practice environments are needed to provide feedback on the long-term risks and benefits of health care practices.

Randomized, and/or staged implementation of new health care practices can provide methods for separating the effects of a disease from the effects of receiving a new treatment in regular health care practice. For example, it is often not feasible for health care systems to train and support all health care providers in learning and implementing a new health care practice at the same time. If the health care system intentionally stages learning and implementation across providers, teams, or clinics over time, then they can use the time-matched non-implemented groups as a control during the implementation period. If the health care system randomizes the order of clinician or clinic participation in implementation activities, then they could create a randomized trial that can provide information about the effect of implementing the new intervention.

In the many cases where adoption of new practices is not so controlled, quasi-experimental designs can also provide information to evaluate the longer-term effects of health care practices. These methods vary in approach and in limitations, but they often can be strengthened with intentional and collaborative design of the evaluation with the clinical care programs being evaluated. This might be as simple as better capturing decision-making around an intervention or practice (e.g., if a patient was considered appropriate for a treatment but preferred a different option), agreeing to standard assessment protocols (e.g., consistently using a specific lab to monitor treatment progress), or consistently documenting reasons for stopping a treatment (e.g., because the patient got better, or because the treatment didn't work). Engaging health care teams in both decisions about what practices are important to evaluate and how to best answer key questions can lead to more interpretable answers and thus better executive decision-making. Integrating intentional program evaluation into clinical operations can provide health care managers and executives with meaningful information about the risks and benefits of health care practices as delivered in their health care system to their patient population. Partnerships between experts in evaluation design and analysis and clinical teams are crucial in these efforts. With the findings from these evaluations, health care clinicians, managers, and executives can make informed choices about what practices to continue versus change.

Managing health care finances

Health care executives additionally have the difficult job of managing the financial health of a health care system, ensuring the system brings in enough resources and distributes them to support and enable effective care practices. The complex and variable landscape of health care finance systems, combined with the complexity of health care practice makes this an enormously difficult task. Payment systems can be a significant barrier to adoption of health care practices that have been shown to improve patient outcomes, even when those practices are cost-effective. Fee for Service (FFS) health care models pay providers for medical procedures rendered. These models incentivize efficient delivery of well-reimbursed procedures, regardless of their impact on patient health outcomes. Health care executives managing under these incentives are pushed to prioritize becoming attractive, efficient, high-volume providers of services for which the cost to deliver a procedure is significantly below current reimbursement rates. Meta-analysis of studies comparing FFS payment models to others suggest, for example, that FFS programs may tend to treat higher income patients and might provide more unnecessary care (Jia et al., 2021), and such models are believed to discourage prevention and care coordination (Reindersma et al. 2022).

Conversely, capitated payment models, where health care systems get a periodic lump sum payment for each patient enrolled, have greater incentives to focus on prevention and avoid unnecessary care and expensive inpatient or emergency services. However, capitated payment models may restrict access to effective but costly services and avoid enrollment of high-risk or high-cost patients (Reindersma et al., 2022). Numerous other payment models exist and are being innovated upon rapidly, each providing somewhat different incentives for optimizing components of services and risks for gaps, inefficiencies, and ineffectiveness of health care. Shifting payment landscapes can cause confusion and frustration among executives and discourage investments with longer-term benefits (e.g., prevention programs). Being aware of financial constraints and incentives within your health care system when trying to implement a practice change can help address concerns and support practice designs that are financially supported and sustainable.

Despite the potential influence on executive priorities that payment systems can provide, studies have found that shifts in payment systems have inconsistent and often nonsignificant effects on clinical practice (Jia et al., 2021; Park et al., 2018). Upliftingly, qualitative studies suggest that clinicians are primarily motivated by their ability to help people and will rapidly adopt practice changes that they see improving patients' well-being, and balk at practice changes that they see taking time and energy without clear benefits to patients. A qualitative study of clinician and executive response to alternate payment models (APMs) concluded "physicians were broadly supportive of APMs that enabled their practices to make noticeable improvements in patient care. In such cases, physicians reported intrinsic satisfaction with clinical improvements, sometimes even when these improvements did not result in financial bonuses. However, when APMs' principal impact on physicians was to create new documentation and reporting burdens—or there was no perceptible improvement in patient care—physicians generally reported disengagement and skepticism that anything had improved, even when they received bonuses" (Friedberg et al., 2020). The alignment between provider motivation and satisfaction and patient benefit suggests that health care executives may achieve greater long-term gain by focusing on aligning financial incentives to support clinical goals than aligning health care systems and practices to optimize financial gain under existing incentives. While ensuring enough immediate revenue to cover costs is important, advocating for changes in payment systems, contracts and financial processes and incentives that limit providers from effectively treating patients or focusing on care may be essential for maintaining provider and patient engagement and satisfaction with the health care system. Payment systems must be informed by provider and patient experience in care delivery, as ability to help patients and focus on that mission is as or more valuable than direct compensation to most providers.

This joy-inspiring reminder that clinicians are overwhelmingly driven and motivated to help patients helps to highlight the role of the health care executive from this mission-focused perspective. The health care executive should support clinicians towards most effectively and efficiently improving the wellness of patients. That means making it easy to provide highly effective treatments, for example, by creating and resourcing opportunities and systems that encourage best care. It means streamlining processes so that clinicians have time to help as many patients as possible with optimal interventions. It means creating participatory cultures and processes so that clinicians can trouble-shoot challenges, communicate effectively and openly, collaborate seemlessly, and support and care for themselves, each other, and their patients through often difficult situations and complex interventions. It means setting priorities, developing learning environments, and transparently evaluating progress, so that the health care system and everyone in it can continue to improve and address new health care challenges. It means taking time to acknowledge, reflect upon and express gratitude for the amazing work done every day by everyone in our health care systems towards helping people live their best lives.

And with that, I thank you, the reader, for taking the time to delve into strategies to help patients, peers, and yourself habituate behaviors, thoughts, and feelings that lead towards health and meaning throughout the fun and challenge that is life.

Appendices

Appendix 1: An Introduction to Basic Brain Circuits Involved in the Five Challenges

Meet the cast: A brief introduction to the neuroanatomical players in the book
In discussing the brain processes involved in changing health behavior, we have mentioned the brain regions involved. Connecting the jobs and functions involved in the processes with a few of the key brain regions that control them can help us decipher neurobiological research studies, and the effects of disorders and treatments that change these brain regions.

In understanding how the brain makes decisions and how to shape them, it is primarily important to understand the functional processes involved in the decisions. Neuroscientists and psychologists have done a lot of work to determine how decisions are made and the processes occur. They have also tried to determine which brain regions are involved in carrying out these processes. The difficulty here is that our brains use very distributed networks to complete most functions. It is rare that there is a single localized brain area responsible for any important function. Circuits are spread out and redundant. Additionally, our brains never waste real estate. Any given region of the brain or cluster of neurons is almost always used for multiple purposes. Brain regions will be involved in multiple processes. Therefore, it is not possible to create a one-to-one map of neural form to function. For the brain regions discussed in this book, trying to explain all the functions and processes in which they are involved would be a monumental task and a giant tangent from our goal of understanding how to modify health behaviors. Instead, we have broken the basic functions of circuits discussed in this book into key components or roles and will briefly describe key parts of the brain that contribute to these functions and how they interact with each other.

Role 1: Your Agent – Someone to find and alert you to opportunities to improve your well-being.

Your brain has a highly automated system that scans your environment while considering your skills. Its function is to alert you to opportunities that you could avail yourself of to improve your well-being. The extended *amygdala* and *ventral tegmental area (VTA)* are key brain regions involved in this function. These regions primarily look for opportunities to make your life better in the here and now. This may be an opportunity to get something nice, an opportunity to solve a problem that is bugging you, or an opportunity to gain relief from a threat. These regions evaluate such opportunities based on all the information they can gather from their extensive networks. They give special attention to your prior experiences with the opportunity. For example, if a particular person has been particularly attentive and helpful to you in the past (perhaps they comforted you when you were lost and anxious in a new city, guided you to a nice meal, and then taught you how to navigate the subway system), then a chance to interact with that person again would be identified as a highly valuable opportunity. The extended amygdala and VTA generate reports on how much you stand to gain from taking an opportunity and send these reports to the nucleus accumbens in the form of dopamine neuron firing. A copy of this report is also sent to the prefrontal cortex to be used for long-term decision-making (Hampton et al., 2007). The prefrontal cortex has some ability to modify the report based on additional information it has about competing goals, special contexts, or other more nuanced concerns. The extended amygdala also generates emotional reactions to these opportunities and creates logs or memories of your experience with prior opportunities, but these jobs will be less of a focus of this book.

The extended amygdala and VTA seek opportunities that may be beneficial for you and brings them to your attention. They tend to look in places where they have found opportunities before and tend to determine the value based on their previous experiences with similar opportunities in the past.

Role 2: Your Short-Term Financial Advisor– Someone to guide you regarding how to spend your effort (e.g., work or money) to help you in the here and now.

Your brain also has a system to help direct your energy, work, or resources to maximize immediate benefits to your well-being. This system makes recommendations about how much money or work to spend on trying to obtain each opportunity that your Agent identifies. Your *nucleus accumbens* (located in your ventral striatum) is a key brain region involved in this function. The nucleus accumbens weighs your Agent's estimates of the potential value of an opportunity and considers your need for rapid gain versus long-term stability. The nucleus accumbens gets constant information about opportunities for immediate gratification from your Agent, and uses this information to calculate how much work you should be willing to do to (i.e., how much you would be willing to pay) to take advantage of that opportunity. Should you be making investments now? Is this opportunity worth putting your work or money into? Do you really need to be working to improve your state right now?

Unfortunately, your nucleus accumbens only considers a very short time horizon (e.g., seconds to hours) in making its recommendation. It is kind of an extreme version of those financial advisors who might try to convince you that buying a house with a variable rate mortgage that you will only reasonably be able to afford for the next two years is a good idea. The immediate benefits are considered strongly, but a separate system considers the long-term consequences. Your nucleus accumbens will help you consider your need for housing and the immediate costs and benefits of taking out that mortgage (e.g., the how nice the house is, the cost this month). Other systems, such as circuits involving the prefrontal cortex, consider the longer-term impact of the decision and these have veto power over this circuit centered on the nucleus accumbens.

Your Short-Term Financial Advisor listens to: 1) the extended amygdala to find out about opportunities (Role 1), 2) the medial prefrontal cortex to find out about our overall financial outlook: Can I keep the opportunities coming? Do I feel in control of my environment? Do I have the ability to find resources when I need them? (Role 7), 3) the prefrontal cortex to make sure that there are not any rules against going after that immediate reward (Role 6), and 4) the dorsal raphe nucleus to find out about our current needs: Are all our body parts well fed and happy? Are we being threatened by outside invaders? Are there any environmental crises? (Role 4). It then talks to circuits that know how to carry out the work (see Role 3) and tells them how much and what to do.

Role 3: Your Well-Trained Laborer or Professional Athlete – Someone to carry out the complex, highly trained work or behaviors necessary to obtain the identified benefits.

Your brain has highly developed systems to guide your brain and body through the complex movements and reactions needed to successfully perform work toward a goal. The *striatum, caudate* and *basal ganglia* are key brain regions involved in this function. This system learns motor patterns following intensive practice. It can carry out complex behaviors without requiring focused attention. Like a professional athlete, it can do very difficult behaviors because it has practiced them extensively. However, it is not highly involved in making choices about when to do these behaviors. It needs a coach to tell it what behavior to do and how much energy to put into the behavior at any given time. In these situations, the nucleus accumbens provides the coaching advice. The nucleus accumbens may tell it to "do play C this time", "go hard on this one", "or use that new move that we practiced", and these brain regions will do their best to carry out these instructions.

Role 4: Your Watchdog or Sensational Journalist – Someone to alert you to the threats around and within you and sound warnings.

Having an alarm system to alert you about danger is crucial for survival. Thus, the brain systems that provide this function evolved early and have been conserved. Your brain has a highly developed alarm system that warns you about threats and triggers emergency responses. The *dorsal raphe nucleus,* located deep in the brain, is the key region of this system.

The dorsal raphe nucleus gets constant information about possible threats of all sorts and transmits warnings all over the brain. It pays attention to potential problems with our internal state as well as potential threats from our environment or others. It then publicizes information about any detected threats by sending an alert to systems all over the brain. For example, it checks whether our cells are healthy. If not, it might issue headlines such as "Muscle Cells Hungry in the Arm" or "Freezing Temperatures in the Fingers". It checks whether we are being threatened by outside invaders. If so, it might issue headlines such as "Mosquito Stings Mid-back, Immune Fighters Initiate Swelling", "Boss Gives Us the Evil Eye After Comment in Meeting" or "Bad Bacteria Invade Stomach Riding on Chicken Sandwich". It checks whether we are endangered by environmental crises. If so, it might issue headlines such as "Extremely High Levels of Caffeine Found in Water Supply" or "Loud Noises Disrupt Sleep". It sends out alerts about any and all potentially dangerous situations that it observes and encourages the rest of the brain to initiate stress responses to deal with the threat immediately. It plays the important role of alerting us to possible dangers, although sometimes its suggestions may be alarmist and extreme.

This watchdog sends information to your agent (Role 1) and your short-term financial advisor (Role 2) suggesting that they amplify estimates of the benefits of and put more work or resources into opportunities for escape or immediate gratification. Thus, your watchdog encourages your brain to focus on the short-term when it thinks you are threatened or stressed. The watchdog also sends information to the executive system (Roles 5-7) to assess the threat and plan a response, helping focus attention on the threat so that the brain can use its problem-solving skills to ensure your safety and well-being.

Role 5: Your Management Executives – Someone to set priorities and determine where to focus effort.

At any given time, your brain is receiving information about many possibilities and concerns in your internal and external environment that you may want to pursue. Obviously, the brain cannot address them all at once. For example, you cannot behave to address a need for sleep, an opportunity for a meal, an upset child, and a chance to improve your housing all at the same time. Your brain needs management executives to set priorities and focus effort to efficiently and effectively address your needs and avail yourself of opportunities. This relatively complicated function is performed by highly integrated cortical circuits.

The *dorsolateral prefrontal cortex* and the *anterior cingulate cortex* appear to work together to help determine where to focus effort. They monitor goals, punishments, failures, and rewards and decide which tasks to prioritize at any given moment. They may inhibit tasks given low priority and enhance attention and effort on tasks given high priority. We include them together because it is not clear exactly what each area is doing (Mansouri et al., 2009); they seem to act as partners on many tasks. Together, they manage the many tasks being conducted by the brain at any time, making sure that everything gets done safely, efficiently and in a timely manner.

Role 6: Your Strategist – Someone to let you know when it is time to change strategy and forge a new course.

Most of the time, the best response to a problem is to do what worked well in the past. Thus, our brains have a tendency to recycle responses when we encounter similar situations. This leads to the general behavioral truism that "past behavior is the best predictor of future behavior". However, sometime situations change and it is necessary to alter strategies and devise new responses to optimize our behavior and maximize the benefits we obtain. Our brains have thus developed a strategist to identify when new responses are needed and shake us out of our behavioral ruts.

Your *orbitofrontal cortex* tells you when it is time to make a change. It lets you know when you need to try something different than your stale old routine. The orbitofrontal cortex tells the rest of the brain things like "I know that worked the other time, but conditions have changed" or "Last time we tried that it failed miserably. We need to try a new strategy." Its job is to help us notice when the outcomes of our behavior are not positive in our current situation, even when that same behavior may have benefited us in another situation. It notices when contingencies change and makes sure that we change our behavior in response.

Role 7: Your Executive Press Secretary – Someone to quell panic and restore calm when potentially concerning situations are under control.

While it is important to have a highly sensitive alarm system or vigilant watchdog, it is equally important to have a smart, rational, calm overseer to assess whether identified threats really pose an immediate danger before initiating emergency responses. Clearly, it would be wasteful and potentially harmful to call in the National Guard every time the watchdog barks. Thus, our brain needs a clear focus to assess the situation and distinguish between threats on which we already have a handle and threats that are immediate, potentially harmful, and without an existing solution. Our brain needs an Executive Press Secretary to filter through the headlines, guide decisions about how to respond, and issue statements to calm the rest of the brain when emergency responses are not necessary.

A portion of the *ventromedial prefrontal cortex* is key for performing this function. The ventromedial prefrontal cortex keeps a close eye on identified potential threats, assesses the actual threat based on our past experience, and issues announcements when the situation is under control. It lets the rest of our brain know when we do not need to worry about potential threats because we know from experience that we can handle them. The ventromedial prefrontal cortex calms the rest of the brain when threats are discovered, stopping the brain from panicking and triggering all sorts of protective defense systems (i.e., our stress response). Like most defense systems, our stress response system conducts immediate actions that may rapidly resolve the threat, but are highly costly and often cause additional long-term problems. The ventromedial prefrontal cortex pays attention to the sensational media warnings, checks with advisors when necessary, and issues statements instructing the rest of the brain to "stand-down" and avoid over-responding to the threat. In other words, the ventromedial prefrontal cortex tells us when "the situation is under control".

Limbic versus executive roles

Roles 1-3 are primary functions of the brain's limbic reward circuit. Here, basically, your agent identifies opportunities and estimates the benefits of each. He sends that information to your short-term financial advisor and to your executive system so that they can determine how much and what sort of effort one should expend towards each opportunity. Your short-term financial advisor manages your well-trained laborer who performs the behaviors as planned. Role 4 is a component of the automatic maintenance systems that are housed in the midbrain and brainstem, the lower part of your brain that connects with the spinal cord. Your watchdog sounds the alarm to both your limbic reward circuit and your executive system when possible threats are detected. Roles 5-7 are components of the executive system led by parts of the prefrontal, frontal and limbic cortices. Here, your management executive prioritizes attention and behavior using information from your agent, as well as about your long-term goals, longer-term consequences, and detailed context. Your strategist monitors outcomes of your choices and changes course when things aren't working. Your executive press secretary assesses and puts out potential fires, to help avoid unnecessary panic and maintain the calm necessary for optimal management and strategic decisions.

In understanding some of the characteristics and limitations of our neural actors, it can be useful to consider our limbic reward circuit versus our executive functions as a whole.

Characteristics of the limbic reward circuit
Your limbic reward circuit is involved in important functions including the formation of new habits. In addition, it plays a crucial role in forming associations between cues and rewarding events. The limbic reward circuit plays a key role not only in addictions to cocaine and amphetamines, opiates, nicotine, marijuana, and alcohol, but also addiction-like symptoms associated with eating disorders and obesity. Further, healthy addictions, including stimulating physical activity (e.g., moderately intense exercise), mental activity (e.g., listening to music) and social activity (e.g., getting approval or affection from a friend), as well as combinations of these (e.g., sexuality), also engage the limbic reward circuit.

Your limbic reward circuit is a series of brain structures that work together to help guide you through your day-to-day world. Its main job is to automatically select well-learned behaviors to optimize short-term improvements in your overall condition. It chooses between your habits to find the one most likely to make your life better in the next few minutes. To illustrate, your limbic reward circuit may currently be weighing the options of continuing to read, taking a nap, taking a bathroom break, preparing yourself a snack, or checking your phone for messages.

The reward system monitors our internal and external environment for opportunities to improve our well-being and ward off threats. It directs our well-trained behaviors to respond to these opportunities to provide immediate reward or relief without distracting ourselves from our other goals or focuses. For example, this is the system that helps us successfully eat a whole box of popcorn without missing a bit of the movie we are watching. We do not need to consciously attend to the popcorn, contemplate whether to eat each piece, or think about putting the popcorn in our mouth and chewing. Our reward system can notice the popcorn and decide to trigger eating behaviors depending on our need to relieve hunger or enjoy a salty treat, while we focus on the action in the movie.

Your limbic reward circuit is highly efficient and does not require conscious effort to make its decisions. In some ways, it might be considered your behavioral autopilot system. For example, it can direct you to eat a whole bag of chips while you watch TV, smoke a cigarette while you talk with a friend, comfort your child while you cook dinner, drive to work while you plan your day, or jog while you enjoy music. It plays back standard behavioral habits that have worked well in situations you have experienced before. For example, if pouting got you sympathy and care when you felt tired previously, your limbic reward circuit will encourage you to pout the next time you are tired. Furthermore, your limbic reward circuit will guide your behavioral choices unless it is overridden by the conscious control of your executive system.

Your limbic reward circuit's choices are limited to things that you have already learned and mastered. It cannot generate new behaviors or help make different choices than the ones you previously learned in similar situations. Your limbic reward circuit is also shortsighted. It cannot consider the long-term consequences of its choices, but rather picks what will work best to alleviate or improve your current immediate situation. However, this does not imply that the limbic reward circuit's decisions are haphazard, simple, or rash. They are very carefully chosen based upon a broad consideration of known elements in your current environment, your lifelong experience in your world, and the behaviors you know how to do. This circuit receives a complicated mix of information collected from all over the brain. It uses this diverse information to guide its decisions. It also uses an elegant learning process both to learn when different behaviors are beneficial and also to constantly update your knowledge of opportunities in your world.

Your limbic reward circuit uses a consistent and relatively simple logic to make decisions about whether to carry out habits to gain relief from an unpleasant situation or gain benefit from an opportunity. When rewards or relief are achieved, the system will favor repeating that behavior again in the future. However, it does not involve multi-step planning or consideration of the effects downstream. The limbic reward circuit relies on the executive system both to plan for the future and to veto its plans when they may have undesirable longer-term consequences.

Characteristics of the executive system
The executive system is composed of prefrontal and frontal cortical circuits. The prefrontal cortex is a collection of brain structures found on the surface of the brain just behind your forehead as well as deep cortical structures that are in the prefrontal region. This part of the brain is evolutionarily new; humans have an abnormally large prefrontal cortex compared to most other animals. We are consciously aware of mental processing that occurs in our prefrontal cortex, and we are generally able to describe the logic used during prefrontal-cortex-driven decisions. The prefrontal cortex includes a number of more specific sub-regions, such as the orbitofrontal cortex (OFC), the dorsolateral prefrontal cortex (dlPFC), the anterior cingulate cortex (ACC), and the ventromedial prefrontal cortex (vmPFC). The functions of these sub-regions are key to the processes described in this book. These cortical regions, their functions, and the circuits with which they communicate are described in more detail in Appendix 3.

The prefrontal cortex considers our values, beliefs, long-term goals, unique situational factors, expectations, social context, and other more complex concepts in making decisions about how to behave. It can both turn on and hold back our habitual behaviors, as well as choose to try a new behavior that has not yet been mastered. While the prefrontal cortex does not always make choices that are good for us in the long-term, it at least has the ability to consider long-term effects in its decision-making process. Moreover, we are generally conscious of the decisions our prefrontal cortex is making. This awareness can be helpful when we are trying to find ways to change our behavior patterns.

The balance and interplay between the influence of our limbic reward circuit and our executive prefrontal cortex will help determine whether our choices tend to be impulsive versus deliberate. Our training and experience will determine whether the habits driven by our reward system are healthful or not. Our beliefs, goals and social networks will determine whether our prefrontal cortex biases us toward healthful or unhealthful behaviors, and immediate rewards versus long-term goals. Training new habits and changing our beliefs, goals and social networks can help us alter our health behaviors.

The prefrontal cortex works to prioritize goals and focus our attention and effort on our current priorities. It assesses the success of our decisions and develops and redirects strategy when things are not going well. The prefrontal cortex oversees and overrides our behavioral autopilot when necessary. It watches other people interact with the world and learns from their experiences, even when these experiences are relayed second-hand. The prefrontal cortex uses sophisticated logic and complicated analysis of data collected from a wide variety of sources to make decisions. This helps the prefrontal cortex make balanced decisions in complicated circumstances, but also makes the prefrontal cortex relatively slow. All that analysis takes a long time. While the prefrontal cortex can make executive decisions even when life gets confusing it cannot do so quickly, leaving your behavior under the control of your autopilot in the meantime. If your autopilot is badly programmed, these lags can be a problem.

How our brain actors work together to make health-related decisions
In our model, decisions about how to behave are controlled by two main brain circuits, the limbic reward system and the executive system. The limbic reward system can make decisions quickly, efficiently, and without conscious effort; however, it can only consider the short-term effects of choices. The executive system can make decisions after considering many options and the short- and long-term consequences of the behavior; however, since this process is more flexible and complex, it generally takes longer to make a decision. Both systems are crucially important for guiding health behaviors.

Effects of psychiatric disorders and treatments on these key brain structures
Some clinicians find it easier to understand and remember brain anatomy and circuits in terms of the effects they have when they dysfunction. Thus, now that we have explained how these brain structures and processes interact during normal function, we provide a description of these key brain regions as they have been found to contribute to psychiatric or behavioral disorders and their treatment. As we noted before, almost all brain regions are involved in multiple functions so there is a caveat to this section: the problems resulting from damage of these key brain regions are substantially greater than loss of the key functions we focus on in our model and this book.

Limbic and motor systems
Striatum: The striatum includes several large structures located behind the frontal lobes and deep to the cortex. Clients with damage to the striatum (e.g., Huntington's disease) exhibit many different forms of frontal-lobe pathologies, or symptoms seen in patients with damage to the frontal lobe, in part because the connections between striatum and the frontal lobe have been impaired. Further, these clients exhibit automatic, habitual movements known as chorea. The chorea may be suppressed for a while by intentional effort, but without ongoing suppression by the striatum circuits, these habitual movements will return. Damage to the striatum releases all sorts of trained-in habitual movement patterns. Generally, because all these behaviors are released simultaneously, this appears as undirected movements rather than specific habit behaviors.

Basal ganglia: Once habits are trained and stored in the basal ganglia, these habits can be performed without conscious awareness or the need for conscious memory centers. If we have undamaged basal ganglia, we will not forget how to ride a bicycle or to brush our teeth even if we lose conscious memories. Clients with damage to the hippocampus or other parts of the brain that form conscious new memories, develop severe deficits of short-term memory. They are not able to consciously remember things that they have learned or experienced. But they can still learn procedures and acquire habits as long as the basal ganglia are intact. But habit learning by the basal ganglia requires programming, specifically through practice of the behavior in conjunction with activation of the reward system.

Clinical improvement in clients with obsessive-compulsive disorder has been associated with a reduction of activity in parts of the basal ganglia. Specifically, clients with obsessive-compulsive disorder treated with either cognitive behavioral therapy or selective serotonin reuptake inhibitors (SSRIs) showed a significant decrease in activity in the right caudate (Linden, 2006; Benazon, et al., 2003). The basal ganglia, in particular the caudate, receive outputs from the three regions of the frontal lobes described below. These key frontal lobe centers may be able to modify activity in the basal ganglia and thus influence habits through these connections.

Amygdala: The amygdala comprises two almond-shaped structures located deep in the brain, each on one side of the head. People with damage to their amygdala lose the ability to assess the importance or salience of emotional cues. Several clients with selective bilateral damage to the amygdala have been studied and their behavior described (Adolphs et al., 2007). For example, SM was found to have a normal range of emotion, but was extremely dispassionate, particularly when describing traumatic experiences, and lacked a normal sense of distrust or danger (Tranel et al., 2006). She could not really tell when music was scary, sad, or calming, even though she was able to perceive the music and identify when music was happy (Gosselin et al., 2007). Clients with amygdala damage did not display an aversion to loss in gambling tasks (De Martino et al., 2010). They are generally able to recognize and respond to emotion cues, but these cues do not induce the same fear, anxiety, caution, and avoidance as individuals with intact amygdala.

Clinical improvements in clients with anxiety and mood disorders have been associated with changes in activity in the amygdala. In studies for PTSD, phobias and major depression, individuals that responded to cognitive behavioral therapy showed a reduction of activity in the amygdala (Bryant, et al., 2008; Schienle et al., 2007; Siegle et al., 2006).

Executive systems
Orbitofrontal cortex: This region is located behind the top of the bony orbits of your eye sockets. Damage to this region impairs social intelligence and reward assessment. People with damage to this region exhibit disinhibition; in other words, they demonstrate a lack of social judgment, tactlessness, limited insight, and other aspects of impoverished social intelligence. People with this damage also neglect personal care (Cummings & Mega, 2003).

What underlies the impairment of social intelligence? One possibility is that since the orbitofrontal cortex is necessary to change strategy in new situations, people with damage to this region cannot help but carry out their standard responses even in situations where such behavior is inappropriate.

The orbitofrontal cortex is in an active conversation with reward centers of the brain. Whereas the reward centers quickly compute the short-term benefits of an action, biased toward immediate gratification, the orbitofrontal cortex is able to delay habitual responses and collaborate with other executive system regions to come up with a more nuanced response. Again, it can block a trained habit to try a new behavior. Clients with obsessive-compulsive disorder (OCD) get stuck repeating certain behaviors. When these clients are treated with cognitive behavioral therapy, they have a better response to therapy when there is increased activity in the left orbitofrontal cortex (Porto et al, 2009). Similarly, in clients phobically afraid of spiders, those who gained long-term benefits from cognitive behavioral therapy (i.e., reversing their habitual emotional response to spider cues) also showed greater activation of the orbitofrontal cortex (Schienle et al., 2009).

Dorsolateral frontal cortex: This region is located in the area of the frontal lobes behind the forehead and above the orbital area. Damage to this region impairs executive functions, leading to difficulty coming up with a new action plan in response to changing events, difficulty in making plans, poor abstraction, and impaired ability to generate strategies for problem-solving.

From these findings, it can be inferred that this part of the brain helps a person make health-related decisions about what behaviors to change and how to change them, after receiving input from the orbitofrontal cortex suggesting that a new strategy is needed. The ability to identify and respond to problems (e.g., following an obstacle to or cessation of a healthy behavior) requires effective use of the dorsolateral frontal cortex. Doing the same maladaptive behavior over and over again is an example of perseveration. Being creative, flexible and developing a backup plan requires a healthful dorsolateral frontal cortex. These actions can help maintain and reinstate behaviors following relapse.

Modification of activity in the dorsolateral prefrontal cortex has been associated with treatment-related improvement in a number of mental health disorders. These changes have been seen in the dorsolateral prefrontal cortex of clients who received antidepressant therapy (Fales et al., 2009). Although cognitive behavioral therapy is not consistently effective in treating clients with schizophrenia, improvement in these clients was associated with greater activity in the dorsolateral prefrontal cortex (Kumari et al., 2009). In major depression, there are indications that people who respond to cognitive behavioral therapy have activation of the dorsolateral frontal cortex as well as selected structures in the limbic system, such as the hippocampus (Seminowicz et al., 2004). However, it is not easy to map which regions of the frontal cortex are most likely to be responsible for the benefits of cognitive behavioral therapy, since other structures are involved including the orbitofrontal cortex and anterior cingulate gyrus (Kennedy et al., 2007).

Anterior cingulate gyrus: This region is located close to the middle of the frontal lobe of each hemisphere. People with damage to this area exhibit impaired motivation including reduced interest, poor initiation of behaviors, reduced activity, and reduced concern. People with damage to this region have difficulty prioritizing an action to motivate its completion. In the extreme case, a client with damage to each side of the anterior cingulate gyrus may develop a condition known as akinetic mutism, in which the person will speak only when spoken to and will not get up out of bed, even to go to the bathroom. They show no initiative whatsoever. The opposite occurs in people with intractable obsessive-compulsive disorder (OCD), for whom there is excessive motivation to repeat a specific set of events. Interestingly, one rather drastic treatment for OCD is the surgical destruction of part of the anterior cingulate gyrus.

People with mood disorders often have difficulty motivating or prioritizing behaviors. People with major depression who had the lowest activity in their anterior cingulate gyrus showed the greatest clinical improvement following cognitive behavioral therapy (Siegle et al., 2006). Also, lower activity in the anterior cingulate gyrus in response to fear cues predicted better clinical response to cognitive behavioral therapy for posttraumatic stress disorder (PTSD) (Bryant et al., 2008). Presumably, people with PTSD who had decreased response to fearful stimuli were better able to dampen anxious responses with the help of treatment.

Appendix 2: How the Brain Changes Itself: A Brief Introduction to Neuroplasticity

To understand how your brain learns and changes it is helpful to understand some basics about how the brain communicates and how it changes with experience. We briefly describe how neurons talk to one another and create useful connections to get things done.

Languages of the brain

Brain regions talk to one another using chemical signals transmitted by the neurons. These chemical signals have two main functions: 1) neurotransmitters send information through existing circuits to deliver information and produce responses, and 2) neuromodulators change existing circuits. Our overly efficient brains often use the same chemicals as both neurotransmitters and neuromodulators, which can make it difficult to explain brain function in simple terms. However, as a rule, the brain uses relatively simple or easy-to-produce chemicals primarily as neurotransmitters, and relatively complex or more difficult-to-produce chemicals primarily as neuromodulators. For convenience, we will classify these chemicals with regards to these primary roles.

Neurotransmitters

Some of these chemical signals are simple commands where one neuron tells another how to respond immediately. Examples of neurotransmitters are glutamate and GABA. These chemicals are simple amino acids, which are basic in structure and easy to supply. Neurotransmitters primarily send information through existing circuits, which allows them to rapidly drive responses.

Neuromodulators

Other chemical signals change the relationship between neurons or brain regions, or change the personality of the neurons involved. These are called neuromodulators. They might make neurons more or less receptive or more or less reactive to another neuron or set of neurons. Examples of neuromodulators are dopamine, serotonin, and peptides (i.e., strings of amino acids such as enkephalin or oxytocin).

Most neurons contain multiple neurotransmitters and neuromodulators and they may release them together or separately. Often a neuron will release only neurotransmitters when it is transmitting a weak or low frequency signal, but then release both neurotransmitters and neuromodulators when transmitting a stronger or higher frequency signal. This allows the neurons to pass on messages using existing networks when standard information is being passed along (e.g., using neurotransmitters only) and modify the networks themselves when new information or associations are identified within our environment or ourselves. For example, because you already know how to read, your brain will primarily use neurotransmitters and existing networks to identify and decode the words on this page. When you encounter a new word of which you do not know the meaning, your brain will need to alter its connections to encode the word within its networks. To learn this new term, your neurons will release both neurotransmitters and neuromodulators; the neuromodulators will change how your neurons talk to one another so that the next time you see this word you will remember what it means.

Excitability and plasticity

Excitability describes how easy it is to get a neuron to pass on a signal. If a neuron fires and sends a neurotransmitter message to a connected neuron, how likely is it that the second neuron will fire and send a neurotransmitter message to its connections? In a way, excitability can be thought of as a measure of the extent to which a neuron gossips. If it is told something, does it pass the message along? How reliably? Increasing excitability of a neuron means that information is more likely to get passed on through a circuit, the same way you know telling something to your most gossiping neighbor ensures that everyone in your neighborhood will soon know the news. Increasing excitability of neurons makes it more likely that whatever thought, behavior, or calculation that those neurons are trying to trigger will occur. The greater the excitability, the more consistent the desired outcome.

Increasing the excitability of a neuron refers to making the neuron more likely to continue to pass on a signal. Decreasing the excitability of a neuron refers to making the neuron less likely to respond to a signal. Neuromodulators help us shape circuits to better filter information and change what we respond to over time. Plasticity refers to your ability to change the excitability of your neurons. A brain that can modify the excitability of neurons quickly and efficiently in response to change is considered very plastic. A very plastic brain learns quickly.

Getting your brain to work optimally requires training your neuronal networks so that important messages are successfully delivered and unimportant ones are dropped. For example, we hope that when someone finds a fire in a building that message is successfully passed on to everyone else in the building, the fire department, and the police. However, when someone sends an e-mail scam, we hope that the message is deleted and not passed to others. In the brain, learning involves building up neuron excitability so that messages that have some importance to you are delivered to all relevant parts of the brain and body while those that are not important are ignored. We must learn which pieces of the information available to us deserve our attention and only send these along through our networks.

Enhancing connections: Changing the efficiency of neuronal communication

Neurons do not directly touch each other but connect to each other at the gaps between them called synapses. These synapses are specialized structures where two neurons communicate. The first neuron has an axon terminal from which neurotransmitters and neuromodulators are released and the second neuron has a post-synaptic density (i.e., a special cell structure to which signaling machinery can be attached) that holds receptors and signaling systems to respond to the transmitted signals. You can think of this being analogous to the mouth of one person and the ear of another. The axon terminal, like the mouth, transmits a signal to be detected by another neuron, and the post-synaptic density, like the ear, collects the signal and processes it to be interpreted by the second neuron. Most neurons, like our heads, have both "mouths" and "ears" and can both send and receive messages. However, a single neuron typically has thousands of "mouths" and communicates to thousands of "ears" located on neighboring neurons, with multiple languages (neurotransmitters and neuromodulators) and volume (excitability) that are modified on an ongoing basis.

The efficiency or strength of a connection refers to how well or how reliably the synapse can send signals from one neuron to another. To continue our analogy, a strong connection would be one where the second neuron consistently "hears" the message being sent correctly. A weak connection would be one where the second neuron does not notice things that the first neuron "said" or "hears" them incompletely. A connection can be strengthened either by making the first neuron "louder", or improving the second neuron's ability to "listen". Neurons have many strategies for improving connections. For example, the first neuron can release more neurotransmitters (i.e., yell louder), it can reshape itself to send a more focused signal (i.e., use a megaphone), or reposition itself to better reach the post-synaptic density (i.e., turn toward its target). The second neuron can make more receptors (i.e., amplify the sound, as with a microphone) or move the receptors around to better collect the message (i.e., turn toward the speaker). Neurons strengthen their connections when connections are used frequently, thereby developing networks of neurons that communicate efficiently to complete a function.

Appendix 3: A Conceptualization of Five Loops that Modify Habits

We are what we repeatedly do.
Excellence, then, is not an act, but a habit.
- Aristotle

Introduction

Throughout this book, we have presented information on the neurobiological underpinnings of habit learning from a functional, process perspective. This functional perspective is helpful for understanding what information the brain considers, how it combines and processes information, and how it learns and regulates habit behaviors. However, a focus on process may not paint a clear picture of the structure that underlies the functions. You may understand what the brain does, but not understand how it is organized. Here, we seek to remedy this gap. Now that you understand how the brain develops and modifies habits, we will share a view of the neuroanatomy that does this work.

This Appendix is for those who seek a deeper, more nuanced understanding of how the intertwined structures and circuits of the prefrontal cortex and basal ganglia can instigate or modify habits. By providing a visualization of some of the integrated brain circuits or loops that enact processes underlying habit learning and expression, I (W.G.) hope this section will provide a greater understanding of the cortico-subcortical loops involved in the formation and retrieval of habits.

The prefrontal cortex, constituting a third of cerebral cortex, is critically involved in the formation of new habits. Most of the activity within the prefrontal cortex is implicit, that is, removed from our consciousness. For example, when you meet someone for the first time, your prefrontal cortex rapidly and almost automatically makes cognitive and moral judgments, rating your new contact on likeability, social and sexual attraction, or repulsion (Forbes & Graffman, 2010). By contrast, explicit, conscious activity of the prefrontal cortex is attention dependent, and includes our ability to redirect focus and to plan; in essence, to invent our future.

The formation of new habits and the transformation of old habits rely in large part on five key areas of the prefrontal cortex and their connections to the basal ganglia. The five prefrontal regions I will discuss are in constant communication, so it is difficult to say that any component of habit learning or expression relies on only one of the regions. Nevertheless, understanding common paths of information flow highlights how very different structures in the brain work together to process and use types of information.

Garrett Alexander (Alexander et al., 1986), a neurologist, is credited with the discovery of functionally distinct circuits or loops linking the cerebral cortex to the basal ganglia. Subsequent research has revealed how habits involving the prefrontal cortex are organized in the human brain, and their relation to key disorders, human abilities, and impairments. This information has helped to provide a fundamental understanding of how we can use our brains more effectively to acquire adaptive habits.

The five prefrontal areas each have loops as described below:

1. *The ventromedial prefrontal cortex circuit (lower loop):* The ventromedial prefrontal cortex, situated at the midline and at the lowest level of the prefrontal cortex is involved in reward-based behavior and social conduct.

2. *The subgenual anterior cingulate cortex (middle loop):* The anterior cingulate gyrus, located near the middle of the frontal region, is critically involved in enabling us to focus attention, address conflicting information about how to respond (i.e., conflict monitoring), and regulate affect. For example, the anterior cingulate's conflict monitoring abilities allow us to ignore distractions when involved in a task. This loop is involved in the expression of obsessions and compulsions.

3. *The lateral orbitofrontal loop:* The orbitofrontal cortex participates in acquiring and then modifying rules and strategies based on current context and contingencies, probabilistic learning (i.e., learning to make choices that consider the likelihood of an outcome based on past experience), and prospective memory (i.e., the ability to remember to do something in the future). This loop helps us adapt and behave flexibly in a diverse and changing environment.

4. *The dorsolateral prefrontal cortex circuit (upper loop):* The dorsolateral prefrontal cortex, located on the sides of the frontal region, engages in executive planning, organizing, and creating. This circuit regulates habits by supporting storage and retrieval of task-relevant information and providing spatial working memory (i.e., the short-term ability to remember where things are in your environment, for example, where you just left your keys). This loop is involved in placebo effects.

5. *The premotor loop:* Situated above the dorsolateral cortex, the premotor loop is critically involved in enacting movements associated with acquired habits. The premotor loop maps out an immediate plan to move your body to execute the habit behavior.

The basal ganglia: Core systems conserved from our reptilian origins

If you were a lizard, you would possess an ancient version of the caudate nucleus, a brain region that looks rather like a fetus, with a large head, and a curled-up body and tail (see central grey structure in Figure 1). At the tip of the tail is the amygdala. There is a boulder-shaped structure that sits next to the caudate nucleus, called the putamen. Together, the caudate and putamen are referred to as basal ganglia, a name comprised of the term "basal", meaning it occupies the lower half of the interior or basement of the brain, and the term "ganglia" referring to clusters of nerve cells (see clusters of dots in the caudate in Figure 1). The basal ganglia provide lizards and humans with the ability to store and retrieve habits. In mammals, these brain regions have been augmented by the development of the four-layer limbic cortex and the six-layer neocortex (e.g., see dark grey shaded prefrontal cortex regions at the front of the brain in Figure 1). Primates have developed additional abilities to plan and control habits with refinements of prefrontal cortex circuits. Yet, even the most advanced components of the prefrontal cortex still have direct connections with the basal ganglia (see arrows depicting projections from cortical regions to ganglia in the caudate in Figure 1). A visualization of how cortical loops intertwine with the basal ganglia is displayed in Figure 1.

Figure 1: The Basal Ganglia Communicates with Prefrontal Cortex. Illustrated by Nelson Hee.

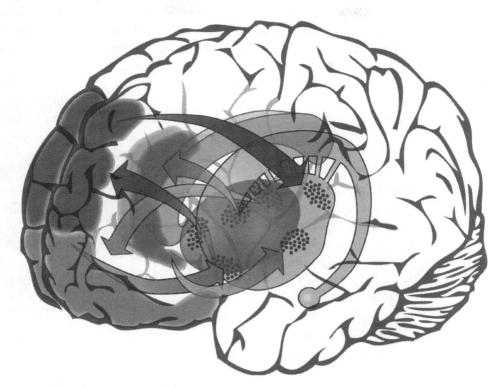

These ancient loops residing in the human brain can be thought of as highways that form and return from their point of origin. These loops are not entirely independent. There are off ramps for one loop to connect with a neighboring loop. The highways between stops consist of white matter tracts.

To be more precise and less comprehensible, the circular tracts have three lanes with information orbiting the loops at different speeds. The lane that is the fastest (i.e., the hyperdirect path) is required for stop-go functioning in some of the loops. Damage to the hyperdirect path can disrupt movement in Parkinson's disease. The middle lane (i.e., the direct path) operates at a slower conduction speed due to stops along the way. The slow lane is called the indirect path. The direct path is excitatory, and the indirect path is inhibitory. This creates a push-pull effect that enables the prefrontal cortical fields to help direct information traffic through these loops.

To be even more precise and less understandable, imagine that there are five elliptical tracts arranged in three dimensions from top to bottom in each hemisphere of the brain. Each tract includes three lanes with different orbital speeds. Each tract resides in different cortical fields and subserves different abilities. Together they comprise 10 tracts in all, with unequal abilities in each hemisphere, and interactivity between tracts. Activity within these tracks occurs constantly, providing the autopilot system that enables us to carry out a wide range of habits.

The structure of the loops intertwining the prefrontal regions with the basal ganglia provide important clues to understanding habit learning, particularly how the prefrontal regions can program new habits within the basal ganglia and how maladaptive habits can be restrained and retrained. The study of these loops has assumed an increasingly important role in characterizing neuropsychiatric disorders, their anatomy, and successful treatments (Taber et al., 2010; Haber, 2016).

I now describe features of the five cortico-subcortical loops, their anatomy, functional characteristics, and how they are involved in the formation of healthful and pathological habits.

1. THE VENTROMEDIAL PREFRONTAL CORTEX CIRCUIT: LOWER LOOP

The lower loop, situated behind the eye sockets, forms the floor of the prefrontal cortex and is critically involved in habit-related functions. Here, I focus on the role of the lower loop in the regulation of social conduct, however, its interactive dialogue with the amygdala and nucleus accumbens underlies its role in substance use disorders and other manifestations of uncontrolled appetites.

Figure 2: The Ventromedial Prefrontal Cortex Circuit. Illustrated by Olivia Ray.

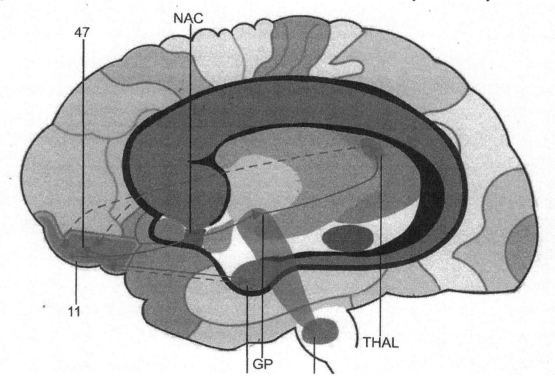

Figure 2 illustrates the Ventromedial Prefrontal Cortex circuit. The circuit's cortical components are shown at the front of the brain. The ventromedial prefrontal cortex is comprised of regions labeled here as Brodmann's areas (BA) 11 and 47, using a numbering scheme developed in the early 1900s by the German anatomist Korbinian Brodmann. The loop includes a one-way connection to the nucleus accumbens (NAC). The NAC operates at the interface between motivation and action formation, supporting decisions regarding when to conduct a learned habit to obtain benefit. The loop continues from the NAC traveling to the globus pallidus (GP), a deep brain region whose name means "pale globe" in Latin. The GP is involved in all five habit loops, yet its exact function and how it processes information is not fully understood. The GP provides a passage for connections that include dopaminergic neuron projections that originate mainly in the substantia nigra (SN). Although the dopaminergic projections are very complicated, for the purpose of this illustration, they appear as a simple cone. From the GP, the loop continues to the thalamus (THAL), the Greek word for chamber. The thalamus is a common stop in all of the 10 habit loops and transmits the information back to the cortical fields of origin, in this case, the ventromedial prefrontal cortex.

Conditions related to ventromedial prefrontal cortical damage

Social disinhibition: Orbitofrontal lesions generally produce dramatic changes in social behavior, characterized by disinhibition (Cummings & Mega, 2003), impaired empathy, blunted moral judgment and risky decision-making (Fuster, 2008). Patients exhibit poor social judgment, make tactless and inappropriate remarks, commit antisocial acts, enjoy inane humor, and engage in inappropriate sexual or social behaviors.

Acquired Sociopathy: Patients with damage to both sides of area 11 develop a condition that has been termed acquired sociopathy. They exhibit impaired reasoning, lack of empathy, deficient impulse control, a lack of regret, and a lack of sensitivity to peer pressure (Fellows & Farah, 2007; Bault, et al., 2019). When the amygdala is also damaged, resulting gaps in fear, anxiety, and other emotional responses may further unleash impulsive behaviors (Damasio, et al., 1990; Damasio, 1994; Bechara et al., 2000). When the amygdala is damaged or disconnected, the perception of emotions being experienced by others is also impaired.

Psychopathy: In fMRI studies of psychopaths, Kent Kiehl reported immature activity within a ring of tissue including the ventromedial prefrontal cortex and its connections with the amygdala and the most anterior aspect of the temporal lobe, the temporal pole (Kiehl, 2006; Kiehl et al., 2018). In a predominantly inherited disorder that produces a form of frontal temporal dementia, patients may exhibit disinhibition, risk-taking, and dishonesty. People with sociopathic and psychopathic tendencies due to ventromedial prefrontal cortex dysfunction can make others uncomfortable, as the resulting lack of social awareness and empathy can be alarming. Yet, remarkably, patients who suffer the loss of the ventromedial prefrontal cortex usually do not show impairment on standardized tests of intelligence.

Hyperphagia: Excessive eating follows certain forms of damage to the ventral and orbitofrontal cortex. The right side of the ventromedial prefrontal cortex is preferentially activated by smells and tastes and in collaboration with the limbic reward circuits, the ventral prefrontal cortex contributes to estimates of the expected value of food and other rewards (Kringelbach, 2010).

Data from imaging studies

Food reward appraisal

In healthy individuals imaged via fMRI, the ventromedial cortical region shows elevated activity when the person is given a small amount of chocolate. If additional chocolate is provided, it begins to lose its reward value. At the point of satiety, the ventromedial cortex no longer shows increased activity (Muller-Vahl et al., 2009).

Substance use disorders

Abnormal activity in the orbitofrontal region can be detected in drug-dependent patients experiencing craving and binging. Reductions of the gray matter in the ventromedial and orbitofrontal cortex have been documented in persons who experienced cocaine use disorder but are now abstinent (Goldstein et al., 2006).

Together, these findings suggest the ventromedial prefrontal cortex loop plays a key role in estimating, modifying, and making choices related to reward value. Dysfunction in this loop tends to lead to risky and impulsive decision-making and an insensitivity to resulting negative consequences that normally regulate reward-related decisions. Without effective functioning of this loop, people may develop habits that lead to long-term problems and social disapproval.

2. THE SUBGENUAL ANTERIOR CINGULATE CORTEX CIRCUIT: THE MIDDLE LOOP

Figure 3 illustrates the subgenual anterior cingulate cortex circuit. The cingulate cortex is depicted as a band near the front of the brain and extends from the parietal lobe forward to the frontal lobe as a long rainbow-shaped structure. Here, we focus on the anterior cingulate cortex, mainly Brodmann's areas 25 and 32, regions implicated in attention and mood-regulation processes. The loop originates in BA 25 and 32, and travels through the head of the caudate nucleus (CAU), to the nucleus accumbens (NAC) and thereafter to the globus pallidus (GP). The path traverses the putamen, a part of the brain conserved from reptiles that concerns movement-related habits. After interacting with dopamine-containing neurons from the substantia nigra (SN), the path enters the thalamus and returns to BA 25 and 32.

Figure 3: The Subgenual Anterior Cingulate Cortex Circuit. Illustrated by Olivia Ray.

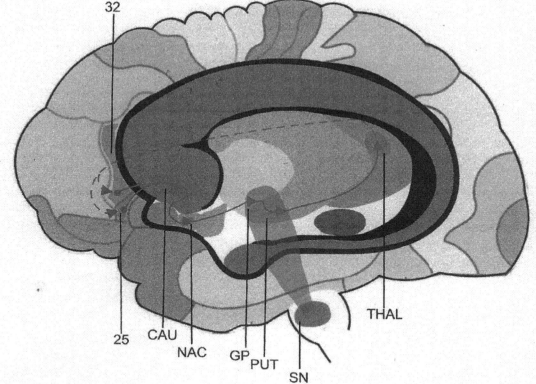

Effects of naturally occurring lesions to structures in the middle loop

Apathy: Patients with damage to the anterior cingulate may exhibit a reduction of motivation and goal-directed activities and loss of concern. Such patients show reduced curiosity, loss of interest in usual social, professional, and recreational activities and a lack of interest in learning and new experiences. Their normal response to errors is blunted, as is the response to an unexpected reward.

Hypokinesia and akinesia: Naturally occurring lesions that include bilateral involvement of the anterior cingulate can produce a profound loss of concern and may also be accompanied by reduction of movement (i.e., akinesia). An extreme manifestation, akinetic mutism, produces apathy, immobility, and lack of speech in affected patients. Patients will eat only if fed, urinate or defecate if taken to the toilet, and speak or move occasionally when prompted, but otherwise there is a profound inhibition of self-directed behavior.

Findings from imaging studies

Obsessive-compulsive disorders (OCD)

People with OCD tend to have heightened activity in the anterior cingulate and its subcortical projections. Meta-analyses of brain volume changes in OCD indicate a significant reduction in brain volume in anterior cingulate and orbitofrontal cortices. The abnormalities have been interpreted as a disruption of the frontal neostriatal circuit (Rotge et al., 2009).

OCD spectrum disorders

Abnormalities of activity in the middle loop have also been reported in people with OCD spectrum disorders (Saxena, 2008). In these conditions, disproportionate attention is often directed toward somatic concerns; for example, dysmorphic disorder (preoccupation with an imagined defect in appearance), hypochondriasis (preoccupation with somatic symptoms), compulsive hair pulling, and compulsive skin picking.

Tourette syndrome

Tourette syndrome is characterized by multiple motor or vocal tics and stereotypies and complex repetitive and unwanted behavioral patterns. Imaging studies of patients with Tourette syndrome identified abnormal activity in the anterior cingulate and its subcortical projections (Muller-Vahl et al., 2009). This abnormal activity is thought to result from activation of dopamine circuits. The elevated dopamine is thought to result in symptoms of hyperkinesia. Cocaine, which enhances dopamine signaling by blocking dopamine transporters, can also induce tics. Reduced cingulate cortical thickness has been reported in people with Tourette syndrome (Worbe et al., 2010).

Effects of anterior cingulotomy for obsessive-compulsive disorders (OCD)

The most common symptoms of OCD include recurrent thoughts of contamination, doubt, aggression or sex, and recurrent compulsions to wash, check, hoard, count or engage in other rituals. These symptoms can usually be treated with psychological and pharmacological therapies. However, a small group of patients, who are resistant to these treatments and suffering from disabling OCD, have been shown to benefit from the surgical destruction or disconnection of the anterior cingulate (see Cummings & Mega, 2003). In this rare, severe, treatment-resistant subgroup, surgically-induced apathy may effectively counter the obsessions and compulsions produced by this disorder.

Together, these findings suggest that the subgenual anterior cingulate cortex loop is involved in modifying habit choices and behaviors based on perceived threats or anticipated punishments. In the absence of these controls, people lose motivation to act or worry and do not modify behavior or learn new habits to avoid potential threats. With excessive activity in these circuits, people may develop habitual responses to threats that may not exist or are objectively exaggerated, for example, reacting to perceived threats from germs, physical symptoms, public appearance, or social interactions that are unlikely to come to pass.

3. THE LATERAL ORBITOFRONTAL CORTEX CIRCUIT

The lateral orbitofrontal cortex (OFC) represents the largest Brodmann area in the human brain. The lateral orbitofrontal loop, illustrated in Figure 4, sits above the lower loop. The loop connects OFC to the caudate (CAU), continues to the globus pallidus (GP), and then the thalamus (THAL) before returning to the OFC, predominantly BA 10.

Figure 4: The Lateral Orbitofrontal Cortex Circuit. Illustrated by Olivia Ray.

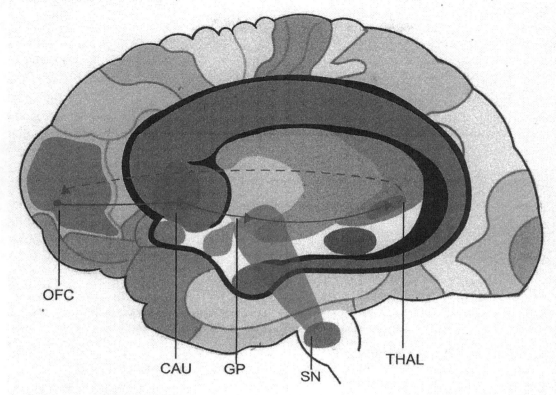

Effects of Naturally Occurring Lesions

Reversal Learning: Damage to the anterior and lateral aspect of the orbitofrontal cortex produces a severe impairment in the ability to switch strategies in response to wins or losses in a probabilistic task (Hornak et al., 2004). While healthy individuals altered strategies in response to experience to optimize gains, patients with bilateral orbitofrontal cortex damage adapted poorly.

Probabilistic Learning: Damage to the OFC is associated with difficulty in learning new associations between cues and outcomes after previous associations between cues and rewards have been learned. In other words, when reward contingencies in an environment change, persons with damage to OFC have difficulty adapting to the new contingencies. Demonstrating that damage to OFC prevents persons from learning based on probabilistic outcomes (i.e., by considering average estimated benefits across a large number of trials), small lesions of the right lateral orbitofrontal impaired performance in a task selecting between "advantageous" and "disadvantageous" decks of cards (Tsuchida et al., 2010).

Prospective Memory: Patients with focal lesions of the frontal-most region of orbitofrontal cortex had greater difficulty in tasks that required them to remember to do a task at a particular time while simultaneously continuing another task (e.g., press a button every 30 seconds while answering questions about which presented word was shorter) (Volle et al., 2011). These deficits in time-based prospective memory suggest difficulties in remembering intended actions and cue-reward associations across time, particularly in the face of competing or changing contingencies. A healthy OFC appears crucial for multitasking.

Reality Filtering and habit extinction: Patients with damage to orbitofrontal cortex regions have been observed to have difficulty determining the relevance of their habit memories to their current reality. For example, a former psychiatrist hospitalized with OFC damage from an aneurysm repeatedly tried to leave her room to "go see patients." She was triggered by hospital cues to initiate her well-trained physician behaviors but unable to recognize that in this moment she was the patient. Isolating this deficit, Schneider (2018) found that while healthy individuals could easily differentiate which pictures were shown in a current set of images over repeat trials, patients with OFC damage had difficulty recognizing whether an image was from the current versus a prior trial. Based on findings over tests, Schneider suggests that patients with OFC damage are not able to extinguish learned cue-reward associations or habits based on new input or expectations, and therefore extend prior and now irrelevant task instructions into current efforts.

Findings from Neuroimaging

Prospective Memory: Imaging studies of tasks that require a participant to remember to respond to a cue at a delay (i.e., tasks requiring prospective memory) find that these tasks alter activity in BA10. In such a task, varying the difficulty of memory task shifted activity from medial to lateral divisions of the OFC. Based on activity patterns, Burgess et al., (2003) hypothesized that lateral OFC maintained the memory of the action to be performed.

Risk Appraisal: In the Iowa Gambling Task, participants are challenged to win money over many trials by choosing from alternative card decks: one considered "safe" which provides relatively consistent small rewards and one that is considered "risky" that provides infrequent large rewards and frequent losses. Favoring choice of the "safe" deck will accumulate money, while favoring the "risky" deck will lead to net loss. In healthy individuals, the lateral orbitofrontal cortex shows increased activity when individuals choose the "risky" versus the "safe" deck. Individuals who previously attempted suicide won less money on the Iowa Gambling task and showed less activity in lateral OFC with their more frequent "risky" choices (Jollant et al., 2010).

Together, these findings suggest that the lateral orbitofrontal habit loop is necessary for inductive processes, in other words, for making generalizations across experiences. The lateral orbitofrontal habit loop is needed to learn and remember actions and effects over time and experience. Perhaps most crucially, the orbitofrontal habit loop is involved in recognizing when contingencies change, enabling us to recognize when a habit was beneficial in the past but is not currently. The orbitofrontal habit loop supports change in behavioral choices to adjust to changing contingencies over long- and short-time frames. You can thank your OFC for enabling you to make short-term shifts in intended actions (e.g., shifting from reading continuing educational materials to going to meet with a patient on schedule), as well as for longer-term shifts in intended action (e.g., ignoring childhood habits of spending all your money on candy and purchasing healthful groceries).

4. DORSOLATERAL PREFRONTAL CORTEX CIRCUIT: THE UPPER LOOP

The upper loop, or dorsolateral prefrontal cortex circuit, begins in the dorsolateral prefrontal cortex (DLPFC), the upper component of the frontal lobes (see Figure 5). DLPFC includes Brodmann's Areas 9 and 46. The loop passes through the caudate (CAU) and divides into a branch that enters the globus pallidus (GP) and a branch that passes through dopaminergic fibers of the substantia nigra (SN). Both branches then converge on the thalamus (THAL) and then project back to the DLPFC.

Figure 5: The Dorsolateral Prefrontal Cortex Circuit. Illustrated by Olivia Ray.

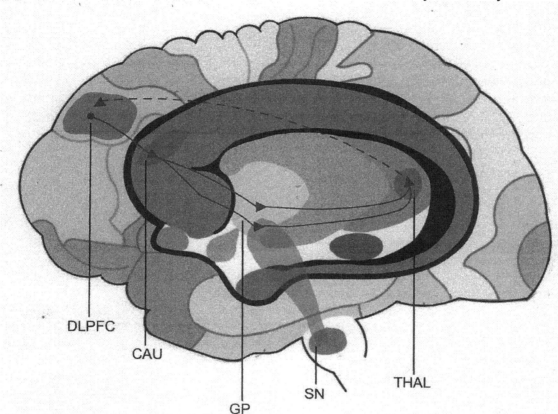

Effects of natural lesions:

Reduction of Distraction: Performance on multiple tasks has been found to be impaired by damage to the upper loop, including tasks involving working memory, delayed recall, and focus when confronted with white noise or the presence of visual distractors during a task (Feredos et al., 2011). These impairments all involve an increase in distractibility when faced with sensory cues or competing internal cognitive processing.

Working Memory: Working memory retains information needed to complete in-process tasks for immediate use, and impairment can manifest in different ways. For example, with failure of working memory one might forget what they were going to do or be unable to calculate solutions to problems in their head. Organization of working memory is widely distributed, consisting of numerous complex processing components to function fully. Dorsolateral prefrontal cortex has been implicated in some of these working memory components, particularly those involving processing of information and action planning using working memories. For example, patients with lesions to the superior frontal gyrus, particularly in BA8, have difficulty with standard working memory tasks, as demonstrated by performance problems on all versions of the n-back test (du Boisgueheneuc et al., 2006). Patients with more focal lesions to dorsolateral prefrontal cortex in one hemisphere did not show performance deficits in basic working memory tasks such as n-back that involve primarily maintenance or monitoring of information in working memory, but did experience performance problems in tasks that required processing of information in working memory, such as doing math or translating words into problems to be solved using information being remembered (Barbey et al., 2013).

Impaired retrieval and fluid intelligence: Long-term memory retrieval can be impaired in patients with damage to the dorsolateral prefrontal cortex. Verbal memory retrieval, such as the ability to think of the names of objects in a given category, is more impaired when the hemisphere specialized for language, usually the left, is damaged. Non-verbal memory retrieval is more sensitive to right hemisphere damage. Patients with dorsolateral prefrontal damage do not generate as many ideas in tests of creativity and exhibit excessive concreteness in their approach to problem-solving.

Transcortical Motor Aphasia: Damage to the DLPFC is associated with a variety of problems with generating and recalling words. For example, patients with brain lesions that included parts of the DLPFC showed deficits in ability to recall words specific to a context in which they were learned (Chapados & Petrides, 2013). Likewise, a reduction of spontaneous speech in the absence of any difficulty articulating words is a core feature of transcortical motor aphasia and is observed in patients with damage to the DLPFC. Word retrieval is a complex process that involves multiple circuits. But consistent with the connections described in the Dorsolateral Prefrontal Cortex loop, damage to the head of the caudate nucleus that results in disconnection of the caudate from the DLPFC also produces word-finding deficits. Breaking the loop at the DLPFC or downstream can result in similar symptoms.

Findings from imaging studies

Approach-Avoidance Conflict: Human behavioral decisions require balancing the potential for reward from approaching an opportunity with potential avoidance of negative outcomes from the same behavior. For example, the decision of whether to eat an ice cream sundae requires balancing the promise of pleasure and comfort to be experienced from eating a tasty treat with the desire to avoid the health and social consequences of high-blood sugar and fat accumulation. Problematic biases in choices towards excessive approach or excessive avoidance underlie many psychiatric disorders from addiction to anxiety disorders. The dorsolateral prefrontal cortex is centrally involved in decisions involving approach-avoidance conflicts. For example, when transcranial magnetic stimulation was used to disrupt activity in the right dorsolateral prefrontal cortex (r-DLPFC), subjects showed reduced sensitivity to the size of the reward available in an approach avoidance decision (Rolle et al., 2022). Conversely, imaging identified increased activity in r-DLPFC with greater reward availability and choices to approach, demonstrating the importance of r-DLPFC in regulating the balance of conflicting motivation to approach versus avoid in the complex choices that we face in daily life.

Together, these findings emphasize the importance of the DLPFC loop in the complex decision-making necessary to plan, focus on, and make balanced decisions around habit-based behaviors. DLPFC supports combining information to understand contingencies and context, weighing of positives and negatives of a decision, and identifying relevant and ignoring irrelevant information. The DLPFC enables decision-making where evaluating pros and cons of a behavior require nuance, consideration, and analysis.

5. THE PREMOTOR CORTEX CIRCUIT

The premotor circuit illustrated in Figure 6 sends projections mainly from the premotor cortex and supplementary motor area (BA 6), as well as the from the primary motor cortex (BA 4) and primary sensory cortex BA1. The information is transmitted to the putamen (PUT), and thereafter to the globus pallidus (GP) and then the thalamus (THAL). From the thalamus, the path continues back to BA 1, 4, and 6, the cortical fields of origin.

Figure 6: The Premotor Cortex Circuit. Illustrated by Olivia Ray.

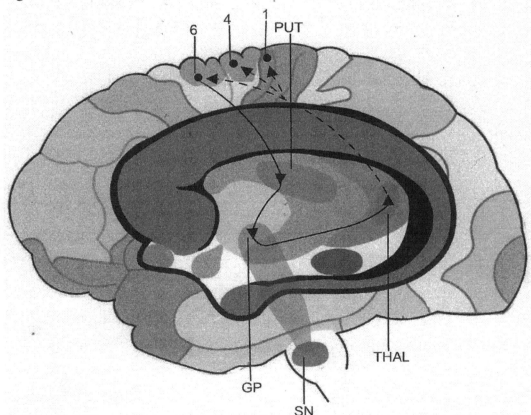

Effects of Naturally Occurring Lesions to the Premotor Cortex

Learning motor sequences: The premotor cortex circuit is important for planning and learning movement patterns required in a behavioral habit. For example, premotor lesions of BA 6 were followed by difficulty acquiring habits involving finger movement sequences on the same side as the lesion (Catalan et al., 1998). The premotor cortex is needed to execute and practice sequential movement patterns towards achieving the automaticity associated with habit behaviors. If practice does not make perfect, it typically makes us better. But without a highly functional premotor circuit, a person has no hope of becoming a concert pianist.

Sense of body ownership: Generally, the feeling that our body components are part of us and other objects are not is so strong that we take it for granted. But in the case of certain brain or bodily injury or carefully crafted illusions, one can demonstrate that this sense of our physical self is only an actively constructed perception. In the rubber-hand illusion, where one's hand is carefully hidden and replaced by a visible fake rubber hand, one can trick healthy individuals into experiencing that the rubber hand is their own. This illusion enabled study of which parts of the brain are necessary to produce a sense of body ownership (Zeller et al., 2011). Lesions to tracts projecting to the premotor cortex were found to be associated with failure of the rubber-hand illusion. Conversely, the premotor cortex was activated during the rubber hand illusion. Together these suggest that the premotor circuit is central to our perception of our body as an integrated and connected whole.

Findings from study of Parkinson's Disease

Situated below the thalamus, the subthalamic nucleus receives inputs directly from premotor cortex and other cortical fields that run through the subthalamic nucleus. The subthalamic nucleus is a key recipient of information from the hyperdirect path of the premotor habit loop (not shown in the illustration). The subthalamic nucleus receives a fast output from these premotor cortical areas. This output provides information interpreted as "stop signals" from the hyperdirect pathway (Temiz et al., 2020). These faulty "stop signals" contribute to the symptoms of bradykinesia (e.g., difficulty planning and initiating movement) and tremor.

Augmenting dopamine-signaling with medications can help counteract the faulty signaling and reduce symptoms. By surgically inserting a device with stimulating electrodes to the subthalamic nucleus, patients with Parkinson's disease who no longer benefit from dopamine-enhancing medications can increase dopamine activity through round-the-clock stimulation of the dopamine neurons. However, a side effect of the procedure is that the other habit loops that pass through the subthalamic nucleus from BA 6, 9, 25 and 32, and possibly BA 10 may also be stimulated. The result is a set of neuropsychological impairments characteristic of defects arising from damage to the upper loop and the middle loop.

Together, these findings implicate the premotor circuit in our ability to perceive our bodies, and plan, sequence and execute movements. While the other loops help determine what behaviors we intend to conduct, the premotor circuit helps determine how to move our bodies to execute the plan.

Employing the five loops in regulating over-eating

Learning, executing, and modifying habit behaviors involve a complex interplay of the five loops. To illustrate, consider an effort to learn to avoid over-eating and eat more healthfully. A successful plan to develop healthy eating habits is likely to require combining the skills sets of all five loops, including developing sustainable systems of social support, environmental contingencies, food replacement strategies, awareness of visceral and emotional states surrounding food, systems of reminders and motivators to maintain or reinstate focus, organizational mastery of goals, contingency planning, staying focused, using fluid intelligence to conceive of alternatives to habitual eating practices, and acting in accord with these principles.

The ventromedial prefrontal cortex loop might help to moderate excessive eating, drinking, smoking, or using other drugs that stimulate the cortical and subcortical dopamine reward circuits. The subgenual anterior cingulate cortex might provide motivation to avoid unhealthy addiction behaviors. The orbitofrontal loop might help you replace your prior understanding of what is good to eat with a new set of rules, trading a learned attraction to junk food for a love of fresh produce. The dorsolateral prefrontal circuit might help you remain focused on your goals and avoid distractions. It might help you focus on the benefits of avoiding rather than eating junk food. Likewise, the ability to devise and execute plans to modify future eating-related behaviors is consistent with the capabilities of the dorsolateral prefrontal cortex circuit. Practicing healthful behaviors, such as chewing slowly and fully, drinking water with meals, avoiding the chip aisle at the grocery store, and not returning to the kitchen for second helpings, requires and engages the premotor cortex.

Some strategies make use of all the habit loops. We provide some ideas and suggestions below:
Habit substitution
Just as "it takes a thief to catch a thief", you may find that "it takes a habit to alter a habit." If you wish to change a habit, it may be helpful to acquire a competing habit. For example, if you wanted to avoid interrupting others when discussing matters that provoke intense emotions, you could train yourself to take a deep breath before speaking. The habit of taking a deep breath can counter and inhibit the habit of making impulsive remarks. By delaying a response, you have time to engage the wisdom of your prefrontal regions to frame a response in ways that are more likely to lead to conflict resolution.

Create Cues to Prompt your Long-Term Goals and Remind You of your Values
Be true to what you value, cherish and believe in by developing a habitual method to remind you of your long-term goals. If you live an authentic life and seek to optimize your health and wellness and the health and wellness of others, you may want to write down your long-term objectives. Dare to dream. It is your life and the opportunities to fulfill it occur only in one lifetime. You can engage the upper loop to invent your future and revise your dreams as needed. View your long-term objectives on a daily basis as a work of art, as the embodiment of your potential. By displaying your goals in verbal or pictorial form, you can habitually remind yourself of your intended path and its destinations.

Review your successes and setbacks
Careful attention to the circumstances that led to a problem can provide key insights that prevent repeat occurrences. It is itself a worthy habit to pay attention to what you did correctly and acknowledge your triumphs in habit formation. Adapt what works, but do not perseverate when a strategy continuously fails. An accurate account also avoids an exaggerated view of setbacks. In sum, documenting the circumstances that led to a lapse,

for example, in healthy eating, social discourse or physical activity, can reduce errors of inclusion, exclusion, or intent that limit success.

Proactive thinking one day at a time
Making intensive lifestyle changes requires maintaining multiple coexisting habits. If you construct a to-do list that is revised on a daily basis, it enables you to engage all three prefrontal regions, including the capacity to plan, sustain motivation, and seek healthful rewards.

Making the Most of the Habit System when Cortical Function Fails: Maximizing Skills of the Reptilian Brain to Counter Effects of Dementia

Advances in the brain and behavioral sciences have led to a critical distinction between memories that arise from conscious, autobiographic recollection and memories that are habit-based. Whereas conscious memories have been termed "episodic", "explicit" or "autobiographic," habit-related memories have been termed "procedural." Following damage to the regions of the brain necessary to form new conscious memories (i.e., the hippocampus and adjacent medial temporal lobe structures), a patient can still learn procedures, such as repeated patterns of skilled movements (e.g., like an assembly line), yet will not remember learning them. Amnesic individuals can also learn key activities of daily living. Procedural memory may also enable people to find their way from one place to another. The hippocampus normally helps with this task by creating a mental map. This mental map allows one to navigate based on visualization of where things are in an environment. But when the hippocampus mental map fails, one can instead memorize a set of directions consisting of a sequence of left and right turns. The sparing of habit-based memories enables people with Alzheimer's disease with profound impairment of short-term memory to practice well-rehearsed rituals; for example, they might be able to continue to practice religious rituals and sing familiar songs (Vance et al., 2009).

Stuart Zola, a leading expert in the study of how short-term memory works and breaks down, is credited with major contributions to understanding the function of the hippocampus, an essential structure for forming conscious short-term memories. One of the hallmarks of Alzheimer's disease and late-onset dementing disorders is pathology affecting the medial temporal lobe, specifically impaired short-term memory and the resulting failure to form new conscious long-term memories. Providing opportunity amidst this challenge, patients with Alzheimer's and late-dementing conditions *can* learn new habits even though they may not realize they have acquired them.

Dr. Zola conceived of a training program to teach patients developing Alzheimer's Disease habits that can significantly reduce the burden of caregivers. The training program was turned into a training tool by MapHabit, utilizing a vastly simplified smart phone that provides an automatic reminder system to trigger learned habits in amnesic patients. The phone is programmed to enable patients to automatically review activities of the day, and cue habits that support activities of daily living. The training program has won several awards for excellence in the treatment of Alzheimer's Disease and in essence makes use of the enduring and dementia-resistant circuits conserved from our reptilian origins (Kelleher et al., 2021; Parker, et al, 2022).

Key Points

- The key structures of the brain that mediate habits emerged in reptiles and survive in the human brain because they serve crucial functions.
- What differentiates the reptilian brain from the human brain is that our species possesses an advanced set of cortical inputs to train, modify, and tailor use of habits.
- Habits are organized in the prefrontal cortex as parallel, partially interacting loops and these comprise at least five circuits in each hemisphere.
- Habits are essential for being able to navigate the complexities of daily living. Were it not for habits, cognition would be overwhelmed.
- Loops that modify habits can shape their use and expression in many ways, including by responding to social context, regulating mood, considering conflicting motivations, and planning creative implementation of habit behaviors, as well as by using induction, deduction, addition, and subtraction to process information and inform decisions.
- All five loops engage in forming, changing, and regulating the expression of habits.
- The non-cortical components of the habit loops that have been conserved from common reptilian ancestors can help the human brain compensate for the loss of short-term memory in the aging brain and in neurodegenerative disorders.

Afterword: Habits and Our Habitat

Dinosaurs lived for more than a hundred million years driven by habit circuits that lacked the additional learning capabilities, planning abilities, and habit modification skills that the evolutionarily more recent prefrontal cortex enables. One would assume that these additional capabilities would make us more evolutionarily resilient than our reptile ancestors and the lizards that survive them. For example, we can understand and foresee the risks posed by Earth colliding with asteroids or other causes of dramatic climate and habitat change. The human brain can also imagine and develop feasible and actionable plans to address foreseen risks. We have the capacity to engineer solutions to address global threats and modify our individual behaviors towards averting catastrophes, such as the comet that caused the extinction of the dinosaurs. For example, scientists in the U.S. National Aeronautics and Space Agency (NASA) Planetary Defense Coordination Office are working to develop strategies to reduce the risk of harm from a celestial object impacting the earth.

However, our habit circuits assess choices from our individual perspectives, and sometimes our individual perspectives are not optimal for the survival of the human species. For example, we have created energy sources and convenient plastic products that make our daily lives easier, but unsustainably pollute our world. Likewise, we have developed weapons to defend our civilization that have the potential to destroy habitats globally. Some of our invented solutions have created side-effects that constitute real existential threats to humanity. We need experts who not only understand where conflicts between near-term individual benefit and population risk exist, but also understand how to guide individuals toward goal behaviors, utilizing the brain potential provided by the combination of habit loops to protect ourselves and world. We believe that you, the reader, are now poised with the skills needed to bring together humanity in shared behavior change. You are a key voice with the knowledge and skills needed to direct individual humans across the globe towards new habits that create a better future for all.

This text has focused on ways to optimize individual health-related habits. We have demonstrated the adverse and beneficial consequences of maladaptive and adaptive behaviors generated by the brain's five prefrontal habit loops using common individual challenges as examples. Throughout this book, you have learned ways to develop and maintain new habits and modify or stop old ones. As health professionals and health-oriented individuals, your understanding and application of the best practice recommendations embodied in this text in your work and lives can help optimize health and wellbeing for individuals. As we touched on in Chapter 7 using the example of health care system-level goals, these same skills and principles can also help reshape behaviors towards collective goals and benefits.

In sum, the health and survival of our species and the environments we live in depend on our collective habits and their global impact. As health experts armed with knowledge of how to change habit behaviors, you have the power to not only optimize health and wellbeing of individuals, but also develop and promote solutions and achieve benefits that arise from sharing and caring for each other. The habit loops of our brain help us guide behavior and optimize our brain potential. With your new knowledge of how to influence the habit loops of your and other's brains, you can take behavior change to the next level, optimizing behaviors and health choices for whole communities, and thereby enhancing the survival and well-being of the whole of humanity.

References Cited

Abler B, Walter H, Erk S, Kammerer H, Spitzer M. Prediction error as a linear function of reward probability is coded in human nucleus accumbens. Neuroimage. 2006; 31(2):790-5.

Abumaria N, Rygula R, Havemann-Reinecke U, Rüther E, Bodemer W, Roos C, Flügge G. Identification of genes regulated by chronic social stress in the rat dorsal raphe nucleus. Cell Mol Neurobiol. 2006; 26(2):145-62.

Adams WK, Sussman JL, Kaur S, D'souza AM, Kieffer TJ, Winstanley CA. Long-term, calorie-restricted intake of a high-fat diet in rats reduces impulse control and ventral striatal D2 receptor signaling: two markers of addiction vulnerability. Eur J Neurosci. 2015; 42(12):3095-3104.

Adolphs R. Looking at other people: mechanisms for social perception revealed in subjects with focal amygdala damage. Novartis Found Symp. 2007; 278:146-59.

Agency for Health Care Research and Quality. "Culture of Safety". Updated on Sept 7, 2019. Available at: https://psnet.ahrq.gov/primer/culture-safety .

Aharon I, Etcoff N, Ariely D, Chabris CF, O'Connor E, Breiter HC. Beautiful faces have variable reward value: fMRI and behavioral evidence. Neuron. 2001; 32(3):537-51.

Ahluwalia SC, Giannitrapani KF, Dobscha SK, Cromer R, Lorenz KA. "It Encourages Them to Complain": A Qualitative Study of the Unintended Consequences of Assessing Patient-Reported Pain. J Pain. 2018;19(5):562-568.

Ainslie G, Monterosso J. Building blocks of self-control: Increased tolerance for delay with bundled rewards. Journal of the Experimental Analysis of Behavior. 2003; 79 (1): 37-48.

Ainslie GW. Impulse control in pigeons. J Exp Anal Behav. 1974; 21(3):485-9.

Ajazi EM, Dasgupta N, Marshall SW, Monaco J, Howard AG, Preisser JS, Schwartz TA. Revisiting the X:BOT Naltrexone Clinical Trial Using a Comprehensive Survival Analysis. J Addict Med. 2022;16(4):440-446.

Alexander GE, DeLong MR, Strick PL. Parallel organization of functionally segregated circuits linking basal ganglia and cortex. Ann Rev Neurosci. 1986; 9(1), 357-381.

Allen SM, Shah AC, Nezu AM, Nezu CM, Ciambrone D, Hogan J, Mor V. A problem-solving approach to stress reduction among younger women with breast carcinoma: a randomized controlled trial. Cancer. 2002; 94(12):3089-100.

Allport G, Vernon, PE, Lindzey G. Study of values: a scale for measuring the dominant interests in personality (3rd edition). Boston: Houghton Mifflin, 1970.

Alonso M, Petit AC, Lledo PM. The impact of adult neurogenesis on affective functions: of mice and men. Mol Psychiatry. 2024; Epub ahead of print. PMID: 38499657.

Anic GM, Titus-Ernstoff L, Newcomb PA, Trentham-Dietz A, Egan KM. Sleep duration and obesity in a population-based study. Sleep Med. 2010; 11(5):447-51.

American Psychiatric Association. Learn about the Collaborative Care Model. Available at: https://www.psychiatry.org/psychiatrists/practice/professional-interests/integrated-care/learn. Accessed on May 28, 2023.

Andrews G, Basu A, Cuijpers P, Craske MG, McEvoy P, English CL, Newby JM. Computer therapy for the anxiety and depression disorders is effective, acceptable and practical health care: An updated meta-analysis. J Anxiety Disord. 2018; 55:70-78.

Antony MM, Swinson RP. Shyness & social anxiety workbook. Oakland: New Harbinger Publications, Inc., 2008.

Arora S, Thornton K, Komaromy M, Kalishman S, Katzman J, Duhigg D. Demonopolizing medical knowledge. Acad Med. 2014 ; 89(1):30-2.

Arora S, Thornton K, Murata G, Deming P, Kalishman S, Dion D, Parish B, Burke T, Pak W, Dunkelberg J, Kistin M, Brown J, Jenkusky S, Komaromy M, Qualls C. Outcomes of treatment for hepatitis C virus infection by primary care providers. N Engl J Med. 2011; 364(23):2199-207.

Ashburner JM, Horn DM, O'Keefe SM, Zai AH, Chang Y, Wagle NW, Atlas SJ. Chronic disease outcomes from primary care population health program implementation. Am J Manag Care. 2017; 23(12):728-735.

Ashe ML, Wilson SJ. A brief review of choice bundling: A strategy to reduce delay discounting and bolster self-control. Addict Behav Rep. 2020;11: 100262.

Baker DW. The Joint. Commission's Pain Standards: Origins and Evolution. Oakbrook Terrace, IL: The Joint Commission, 2017, available at: https://www.jointcommission.org/-/media/tjc/documents/resources/pain-management/pain_std_history_web_version_05122017pdf

Ballard ME, Mandelkern MA, Monterosso JR, Hsu E, Robertson CL, Ishibashi K, Dean AC, London ED. Low Dopamine D2/D3 Receptor Availability is Associated with Steep Discounting of Delayed Rewards in Methamphetamine Dependence. Int J Neuropsychopharmacol. 2015;18(7): pyu119.

Balldin J, Berglund KJ, Berggren U, Wennberg P, Fahlke C. TAQ1A1 Allele of the DRD2 Gene Region Contribute to Shorter Survival Time in Alcohol Dependent Individuals When Controlling for the Influence of Age and Gender. A Follow-up Study of 18 Years. Alcohol. 2018; 53(3):216-220.

Banasr M, Duman RS. Regulation of neurogenesis and gliogenesis by stress and antidepressant treatment. CNS Neurol Disord Drug Targets. 2007; 6(5):311-20.

Bandura A. Self-efficacy: the exercise of control. W.H. Freeman and Company: United States, 1997.

Baran SE, Campbell AM, Kleen JK, Foltz CH, Wright RL, Diamond DM, Conrad CD. Combination of high fat diet and chronic stress retracts hippocampal dendrites. Neuroreport. 2005; 16(1):39-43.

Barbey AK, Koenigs M, Grafman J. Dorsolateral prefrontal contributions to human working memory. Cortex. 2013; 49(5):1195-205.

Barbieri L, Boggian I, Falloon I, Lamonaca D; Centro Diurno 5 (CD5) collaborators. Problem-solving skills for cognitive rehabilitation among persons with chronic psychotic disorders in Italy. Psychiatr Serv. 2006; 57(2):172-4.

Bardo MT. Neuropharmacological mechanisms of drug reward: beyond dopamine in the nucleus accumbens. Crit Rev Neurobiol. 1998; 12(1-2):37-67.

Barlow RL, Gorges M, Wearn A, Niessen HG, Kassubek, Dalley JW, Pekcec A. Ventral Striatal D2/3 Receptor Availability Is Associated with Impulsive Choice Behavior As Well As Limbic Corticostriatal Connectivity. Int J Neuropsychopharmacol. 2018; 21(7):705-715.

Barnhill JL, Roth IJ, Faurot KR, Honvoh GD, Lynch CE, Thompson KL, Gaylord SA. Cultural Transformation in Healthcare: How Well Does the Veterans Health Administration Vision for Whole Person Care Fit the Needs of Patients at an Academic Rehabilitation Center? Glob Adv Health Med. 2022; 11:2164957X221082994.

Barnett JA, Gibson DL. Separating the Empirical Wheat From the Pseudoscientific Chaff: A Critical Review of the Literature Surrounding Glyphosate, Dysbiosis and Wheat-Sensitivity. Front Microbiol. 2020; 11:556729.

Barry RL, Byun NE, Williams JM, Siuta MA, Tantawy MN, Speed NK, Saunders C, Galli A, Niswender KD, Avison MJ. Brief exposure to obesogenic diet disrupts brain dopamine networks. PLoS One. 2018; 13(4):e0191299.

Barry CN, Abraham KM, Weaver KR, Bowersox NW. Innovating team-based outpatient mental health care in the Veterans Health Administration: Staff-perceived benefits and challenges to pilot implementation of the Behavioral Health Interdisciplinary Program (BHIP). Psychol Serv. 2016;13(2):148-155.

Bauer MS, Miller CJ, Kim B, Lew R, Stolzmann K, Sullivan J, Riendeau R, Pitcock J, Williamson A, Connolly S, Elwy AR, Weaver K. Effectiveness of Implementing a Collaborative Chronic Care Model for Clinician Teams on Patient Outcomes and Health

Status in Mental Health: A Randomized Clinical Trial. JAMA Netw Open. 2019; 2(3): e190230.

Bault N, di Pellegrino G, Puppi M, Opolczynski G, Monti A, Braghittoni D, Thibaut F, Rustichini A, Coricelli G. Dissociation between Private and Social Counterfactual Value Signals Following Ventromedial Prefrontal Cortex Damage. J Cogn Neurosci. 2019; 31(5): 639-656.

Bechara A, Tranel D, Damasio H. Characterization of the decision-making deficit of patients with ventromedial prefrontal cortex lesions. Brain. 2000; 123(Pt 11):2189-202.

Beck AT. Cognitive therapy and the emotional disorders. New York: Penguin Books, 1976.

Benazon NR, Moore GJ, Rosenberg DR. Neurochemical analyses in pediatric obsessive-compulsive disorder in patients treated with cognitive-behavioral therapy. J Am Acad Child Adolesc Psychiatry. 2003; 42(11):1279-85.

Benedetti F. Placebo effects: understanding the mechanisms in health and disease. New York: Oxford University Press, 2021.

Blakeslee S, Blakeslee M. The body has a mind of its own: how body maps in your brain help you do (almost) everything better. New York: Random House, 2007.

Boles JM, Maccarone D, Brown B, Archer A, Trotter MG, Friedman NMG, Chittams J, Mazzone L, Ballinghoff J, Burchill CN, Cacchione PZ. Nurse, Provider, and Emergency Department Technician: Perceptions and Experiences of Violence and Aggression in the Emergency Department. J Emerg Nurs. 2022; S0099-1767(22)00180-5.

Bolster L, Rourke L. The Effect of Restricting Residents' Duty Hours on Patient Safety, Resident Well-Being, and Resident Education: An Updated Systematic Review. J Grad Med Educ. 2015; 7(3):349-63.

Boysen PG 2nd. Just culture: a foundation for balanced accountability and patient safety. Ochsner J. 2013; 13(3):400-6.

Brady KT, Killeen TK, Brewerton T, Lucerini S. Comorbidity of psychiatric disorders and posttraumatic stress disorder. J Clin Psychiatry. 2000; 61 Suppl 7:22-32.

Brake WG, Zhang TY, Diorio J, Meaney MJ, Gratton A. Influence of early postnatal rearing conditions on mesocorticolimbic dopamine and behavioural responses to psychostimulants and stressors in adult rats. Eur J Neurosci. 2004; 19(7):1863-74.

Braun K, Lange E, Metzger M, Poeggel G. Maternal separation followed by early social deprivation affects the development of monoaminergic fiber systems in the medial prefrontal cortex of Octodon degus. Neuroscience. 2000; 95(1):309-18.

Bray S, O'Doherty J. Neural coding of reward-prediction error signals during classical conditioning with attractive faces. J Neurophysiol. 2007; 97(4):3036-45.

Bremner JD, Elzinga B, Schmahl C, Vermetten E. Structural and functional plasticity of the human brain in posttraumatic stress disorder. Prog Brain Res. 2008; 167:171-86.

Brunner EJ, Chandola T, Marmot MG. Prospective effect of job strain on general and central obesity in the Whitehall II Study. Am J Epidemiol. 2007; 165(7):828-37.

Bryan CJ, Mintz J, Clemans TA, Leeson B, Burch TS, Williams SR, Maney E, Rudd MD. Effect of crisis response planning vs. contracts for safety on suicide risk in U.S. Army Soldiers: A randomized clinical trial. J Affect Disord. 2017; 212:64-72.

Bryant RA, Felmingham K, Kemp A, Das P, Hughes G, Peduto A, Williams L. Amygdala and ventral anterior cingulate activation predicts treatment response to cognitive behaviour therapy for post-traumatic stress disorder. Psychol Med. 2008; 38(4):555-61.

Buckworth J, Sears L. Increasing and maintaining physical activity in clinical populations. In: Best practices in the behavioral management of chronic disease: volume 2 other medical disorders. Trafton JA, Gordon WP (eds.), Los Altos: Institute for Brain Potential, 2008.

Buljac-Samardžić M, Dekker-van Doorn CM, Maynard MT. What Do We Really Know About Crew Resource Management in Healthcare?: An Umbrella Review on Crew Resource Management and Its Effectiveness. J Patient Saf. 2021; 17(8):e929-e958.

Bulley A, Gullo MJ. The influence of episodic foresight on delay discounting and demand for alcohol. Addict Behav. 2017; 66:1-6.

Burgess PW, Scott SK, Frith CD. The role of the rostral frontal cortex (area 10) in prospective memory: a lateral versus medial dissociation. Neuropsychologia. 2003; 41(8): 906-18.

Burns D. The feeling good handbook. New York: William Morrow and Company, Inc., 1989.

Burton CR, Williams L, Bucknall T, Fisher D, Hall B, Harris G, Jones P, Makin M, Mcbride A, Meacock R, Parkinson J, Rycroft-Malone J, Waring J. Theory and practical guidance for effective de-implementation of practices across health and care services: a realist synthesis. Health Services and Delivery Research. 2021; 9(2).

Butler RN, Forette F, Greengross BS. Maintaining cognitive health in an ageing society. J R Soc Health. 2004; 124(3):119-21.

Cain SW, Filtness AJ, Phillips CL, Anderson C. Enhanced preference for high-fat foods following a simulated night shift. Scand J Work Environ Health. 2015;41(3):288-93.

Carlsson SV, Clauss C, Benfante N, Manasia M, Sollazzo T, Lynch J, Frank J, Quadri S, Lin X, Vickers AJ, Ehdaie B. Shared Medical Appointments for Prostate Cancer Active

Surveillance Follow-Up Visits. Urol Pract. 2021; 8(5):541-545.

Castrén E, Rantamäki T. The role of BDNF and its receptors in depression and antidepressant drug action: Reactivation of developmental plasticity. Dev Neurobiol. 2010; 70(5):289-97.

Catalan MJ, Honda M, Weeks RA, Cohen LG, Hallett M. The functional neuroanatomy of simple and complex sequential finger movements: a PET study. Brain: A Journal of Neurology. 1998; 121(2): 253-264.

Champagne F, Meaney MJ. Like mother, like daughter: evidence for non-genomic transmission of parental behavior and stress responsivity. Prog Brain Res. 2001; 133:287-302.

Chambers L, Seidler K, Barrow M. Circadian misalignment in obesity: The role for time-restricted feeding. Clin Nutr ESPEN. 2023; 57:430-447.

Chapados C, Petrides, M. Impairment only on the fluency subtest of the Frontal Assessment Bettery after prefrontal lesions. Brain. 2013; 136(Pt 10): 2966-78.

Chaput JP, Tremblay A. Sleeping habits predict the magnitude of fat loss in adults exposed to moderate caloric restriction. Obes Facts. 2012;5(4):561-6.

Chinman M, Gellad WF, McCarthy S, Gordon AJ, Rogal S, Mor MK, Hausmann LRM. Protocol for evaluating the nationwide implementation of the VA Stratification Tool for Opioid Risk Management (STORM). Implement Sci. 2019; 14(1):5.

CDC. Data Brief 427: Mortality in the United States, 2020. Available at: https://www.cdc.gov/nchs/data/databriefs/db427-tables.pdf#4. Accessed on April 28, 2024.

Chard, P. Wellness programs don't make workplace stressors go away. Milwaukee journal sentinel. 2018. Available at: https://www.jsonline.com/story/life/green-sheet/advice/philip-chard/2018/05/10/wellness-workplace-stress/585881002/

Chein JM, Schneider W. Neuroimaging studies of practice-related change: fMRI and meta-analytic evidence of a domain-general control network for learning. Cognitive Brain Res. 2005; 25(3): 607-623.

Chen Y, Mark G, Ali S. Promoting Positive Affect through Smartphone Photography. Psychol Well Being. 2016; 6:8.

Chernoff RA, Davison GC. An evaluation of a brief HIV/AIDS prevention intervention for college students using normative feedback and goal setting. AIDS Educ Prev. 2005; 17(2):91-104.

Chester DS, DeWall CN. The pleasure of revenge: retaliatory aggression arises from a neural imbalance toward reward. Soc Cog Affect Neurosci. 2016; 11(7):1173-82.

Chiou WB, Wu WH. Episodic Future Thinking Involving the Nonsmoking Self Can Induce Lower Discounting and Cigarette Consumption. J Stud Alcohol Drugs. 2017; 78(1):106-112.

Christakis NA, Fowler JH. The spread of obesity in a large social network over 32 years. N Engl J Med. 2007; 357(4):370-9.

Christakis NA, Fowler JH. The collective dynamics of smoking in a large social network. N Engl J Med. 2008; 358(21): 2249-58.

Christiansen BA, Smith DT, Roehling PV, Goldman MS. Using alcohol expectancies to predict adolescent drinking behavior after one year. J Consult Clini Psychol 1989; 57(1): 93-99.

Christiansen BA, Goldman MS. Alcohol-related expectancies versus demographic/background variables in the prediction of adolescent drinking. J Consult Clin Pschol 1983; 51: 249-257.

Christianson JP, Paul ED, Irani M, Thompson BM, Kubala KH, Yirmiya R, Watkins LR, Maier SF. The role of prior stressor controllability and the dorsal raphé nucleus in sucrose preference and social exploration. Behav Brain Res. 2008; 193(1):87-93.

Cinko C, Thrasher A, Sawyer C, Kramer K, West S, Harris E. Using the Project ECHO Model to Increase Pediatric Primary Care Provider Confidence to Independently Treat Adolescent Depression. Acad Psychiatry. 2023: 47(4): 360-367.

Clark C, Cole J, Winter C, Williams K, Grammer G. A Review of Transcranial Magnetic Stimulation as a Treatment for Post-Traumatic Stress Disorder. Curr Psychiatry Rep. 2015;17(10):83.

Cohen DA. Neurophysiological pathways to obesity: below awareness and beyond individual control. Diabetes. 2008; 57(7):1768-73.

Coles NA, Larsen JT, Lench HC. A meta-analysis of the facial feedback literature: Effects of facial feedback on emotional experience are small and variable. Psychol Bull. 2019; 145(6):610-651.

Colloca L, Benedetti F. Placebo analgesia induced by social observational learning. Pain. 2009; 144(1-2):28-34.

Colman RJ, Anderson RM, Johnson SC, Kastman EK, Kosmatka KJ, Beasley TM, Allison DB, Cruzen C, Simmons HA, Kemnitz JW, Weindruch R. Caloric restriction delays disease onset and mortality in rhesus monkeys. Science. 2009; 325(5937): 201-4.

Comalli PE Jr, Wapner S, Werner H. Interference effects of Stroop color-word test in childhood, adulthood, and aging. J Genet Psychol. 1962; 100:47-53.

Comings DE, Blum K. Reward deficiency syndrome: genetic aspects of behavioral disorders. Prog Brain Res. 2000; 126:325-41.

Cooper MA, McIntyre KE, Huhman KL. Activation of 5-HT1A autoreceptors in the dorsal raphe nucleus reduces the behavioral consequences of social defeat. Psychoneuroendocrinology. 2008; 33(9):1236-47.

Costa G. The impact of shift and night work on health. Applied Ergonomics. 1996; 27(1): 9-16.

Côté S, Bouchard S. Documenting the efficacy of virtual reality exposure with psychophysiological and information processing measures. Appl Psychophysiol Biofeedback. 2005; 30(3):217-32.

Crandall CJ, Danz M, Trung Dung H, Baxi SM, Rubenstein LV, Thompson G, Al-Ibrahim H, Larkin J, Motala A, Akinniranye G, Hempel S. Peer-to-Peer Support Interventions for Health Care Providers: A Series of Literature Reviews. 2022, RAND. Available at: https://www.rand.org/content/dam/rand/pubs/research_reports/RRA400/RRA428-2/RAND_RRA428-2.pdf, accessed on Nov. 12, 2023.

Crum AJ, Phillips DJ, Goyer JP, Akinola M, Higgins ET. Transforming Water: Social Influence Moderates Psychological, Physiological, and Functional Response to a Placebo Product. PLoS One. 2016; 11(11):e0167121.

Culpin I, Stapinski L, Budanur Miles O, Araya R, Joinson C. Exposure to socioeconomic adversity in early life and risk of depression at 18 years: The mediating role of locus of control J Affect Disord. 2015; 183: 269–278.

Cummings JL, Mega JS. Neuropsychiatry and behavioral neuroscience. New York: Oxford University Press, 2003.

Czéh B, Müller-Keuker JI, Rygula R, Abumaria N, Hiemke C, Domenici E, Fuchs E. Chronic social stress inhibits cell proliferation in the adult medial prefrontal cortex: hemispheric asymmetry and reversal by fluoxetine treatment. Neuropsychopharmacology. 2007; 32(7):1490-503.

Daley A. Exercise and depression: a review of reviews. J Clin Psychol Med Settings. 2008; 15(2):140-7.

Damasio A. Descartes' error: emotion, reason, and the human brain. New York: G.P. Putnam's Sons, 1994.

Damasio AR, Tranel D, Damasio H. Individuals with sociopathic behavior caused by frontal damage fail to respond autonomically to social stimuli. Behav Brain Res. 1990; 41(2):81-94.

Daniel TO, Said M, Stanton CM, Epstein LH. Episodic future thinking reduces delay discounting and energy intake in children. Eat Behav. 2015; 18:20-4.

Daniels JK, Anadria D. Experiencing and Witnessing Patient Violence - an Occupational Risk for Outpatient Therapists? Psychiatr Q. 2019; 90(3):533-541.

Darkes J, Goldman MS. Expectancy challenge and drinking reduction: experimental evidence for a mediational process. J Consult Clin Psychol. 1993; 61(2):344-53.

Darkes J, Goldman MS. Expectancy challenge and drinking reduction: process and structure in the alcohol expectancy network. Exp Clin Psychopharmacol. 1998; 6:64-76.

Darnall BD, Roy A, Chen AL, Ziadni MS, Keane RT, You DS, Slater K, Poupore-King H, Mackey I, Kao MC, Cook KF, Lorig K, Zhang D, Hong J, Tian L, Mackey SC. Comparison of a Single-Session Pain Management Skills Intervention With a Single-Session Health Education Intervention and 8 Sessions of Cognitive Behavioral Therapy in Adults With Chronic Low Back Pain: A Randomized Clinical Trial. JAMA Netw Open. 2021; 4(8):e2113401.

Dassen FCM, Jansen A, Nederkoorn C, Houben K. Focus on the future: Episodic future thinking reduces discount rate and snacking. Appetite. 2016; 96:327-332.

Davis C, Carter JC. Compulsive overeating as an addiction disorder. A review of theory and evidence. Appetite. 2009; 53(1):1-8.

DeBusk RF, Miller NH, Superko HR, Dennis CA, Thomas RJ, Lew HT, Berger WE 3rd, Heller RS, Rompf J, Gee D, Kraemer HC, Bandura A, Ghandour G, Clark M, Shah RV, Fisher L, Taylor CB. A case-management system for coronary risk factor modification after acute myocardial infarction. Ann Intern Med. 1994; 120(9):721-9.

Defrin R, Ginzburg K, Solomon Z, Polad E, Bloch M, Govezensky M, Schreiber S. Quantitative testing of pain perception in subjects with PTSD-implications for the mechanism of the coexistence between PTSD and chronic pain. Pain. 2008; 138(2):450-9.

Dekker S. Just culture: balancing safety and accountability. London: CRC Press; 2016.

De Martino B, Camerer CF, Adolphs R. Amygdala damage eliminates monetary loss aversion. Proc Natl Acad Sci U S A. 2010; 107(8):3788-92.

de Quervain DJ, Fischbacher U, Treyer V, Schellhammer M, Schnyder U, Buck A, Fehr E. The neural basis of altruistic punishment. Science. 2004; 305(5688):1246-7.

Del Arco A, Mora F. Prefrontal cortex-nucleus accumbens interaction: in vivo modulation by dopamine and glutamate in the prefrontal cortex. Pharmacol Biochem Behav. 2008; 90(2):226-35.

Delsignore A, Schnyder U. Control expectancies as predictors of psychotherapy outcome: a systematic review. Br J Clin Psychol. 2007; 46(Pt 4):467-83.

Denneson LM, Purcell N, McGrath SL, Abadjian LR, Becker WC, Seal KH. Integration of Health Coaches in a Whole Health Team Model of Chronic Pain Care: A Qualitative Study. J Gen Intern Med. 2023; 38(16):3574-3580.

Diliberti N, Bordi PL, Conklin MT, Roe LS, Rolls BJ. Increased portion size leads to increased energy intake in a restaurant meal. Obes Res. 2004; 12(3):562-8.

Dilk MN, Bond GR. Meta-analytic evaluation of skills training research for individuals with severe mental illness. J Consult Clin Psychol. 1996; 64(6):1337-1346.

Dominey PF, Inui T. Cortico-striatal function in sentence comprehension: insights from neurophysiology and modeling. Cortex. 2009; 45(8):1012-8.

Dong Y, Green T, Saal D, Marie H, Neve R, Nestler EJ, Malenka RC. CREB modulates excitability of nucleus accumbens neurons. Nat Neurosci. 2006; 9(4):475-7.

Dreisoerner A, Junker NM, Schlotz W, Heimrich J, Bloemeke S, Ditzen B, van Dick R. Self-soothing touch and being hugged reduce cortisol responses to stress: A randomized controlled trial on stress, physical touch, and social identity. Compr Psychoneuroendocrinol. 2021; 8:100091.

du Boisgueheneuc F, Levy R, Volle E, Seassau M, Duffau H, Kinkingnehun S, Samson Y, Zhang S, Dubois B. Functions of the left superior frontal gyrus in humans: a lesion study. Brain. 2006;129(Pt 12):3315-28.

Dugdale DC, Epstein R, Pantilat SZ. Time and the patient-physician relationship. J Gen Intern Med. 1999;14 Suppl 1:S34-40.

Edelman D, Gierisch JM, McDuffie JR, Oddone E, Williams JW Jr. Shared medical appointments for patients with diabetes mellitus: a systematic review. J Gen Intern Med. 2015; 30(1):99-106.

Efron G, Wootton BM. Remote cognitive behavioral therapy for panic disorder: A meta-analysis. J Anxiety Disord. 2021; 79:102385.

Eisenberg D, Quinn BC. Estimating the effect of smoking cessation on weight gain: an instrumental variable approach. Health Serv Res. 2006; 41(6):2255-66.

Embry DD, Flannery DJ, Vazsonyi AT, Powell KE, Atha H. Peacebuilders: a theoretically driven, school-based model for early violence prevention. Am J Prev Med. 1996; 12(5 Suppl):91-100.

Evans JA, Davidson AJ. Health consequences of circadian disruption in humans and animal models. Prog Mol Biol Transl Sci. 2013;119:283-323.

Eyberg SM, Boggs SR, Algina J. Parent-child interaction therapy: a psychosocial model for the treatment of young children with conduct problem behavior and their families. Psychopharmacol Bull. 1995; 31(1):83-91.

Fales CL, Barch DM, Rundle MM, Mintun MA, Mathews J, Snyder AZ, Sheline YI. Antidepressant treatment normalizes hypoactivity in dorsolateral prefrontal cortex during emotional interference processing in major depression. J Affect Disord. 2009;112(1-3):206-11.

Féart C, Samieri C, Rondeau V, Amieva H, Portet F, Dartigues JF, Scarmeas N, Barberger-Gateau P. Adherence to a Mediterranean diet, cognitive decline, and risk of dementia. JAMA. 2009; 302(6):638-48.

Fellows LK, Farah MJ. The role of ventromedial prefrontal cortex in decision making: judgment under uncertainty or judgment per se? Cereb Cortex. 2007;17(11):2669-74.

Feredoes E, Heinen K, Weiskopf N, Ruff C, Driver J. Causal evidence for frontal involvement in memory target maintenance by posterior brain areas during distracter interference of visual working memory. Proc Natl Acad Sci U S A. 2011; 108(42):17510-5.

Fillit HM, Butler RN, O'Connell AW, Albert MS, Birren JE, Cotman CW, Greenough WT, Gold PE, Kramer AF, Kuller LH, Perls TT, Sahagan BG, Tully T. Achieving and maintaining cognitive vitality with aging. Mayo Clin Proc. 2002; 77(7):681-96.

Fissler P, Kolassa IT, Schrader C. Educational games for brain health: revealing their unexplored potential through a neurocognitive approach. Front Psychol. 2015; 6:1056.

Flannery DJ, Vazsonyi AT, Liau AK, Guo S, Powell KE, Atha H, Vesterdal W, Embry D. Initial behavior outcomes for the peacebuilders universal school-based violence prevention program. Dev Psychol. 2003; 39(2):292-308.

Flor H, Lutzenberger W, Knost B. Spouse presence alters brain response to pain. Society for Neuroscience abstracts, 2002, Orlando, FL.

Fond G, Fernandes S, Lucas G, Greenberg N, Boyer L. Depression in healthcare workers: Results from the nationwide AMADEUS survey. Int J Nurs Stud. 2022; 135:104328.

Forbes, CE, Grafman, J. The role of the human prefrontal cortex in social cognition and moral judgment. Ann Rev Neurosci. 2010; 33: 299-324.

Fountaine AR, Iyar MM, Lutes LD. Examining the Utility of a Telehealth Warm Handoff in Integrated Primary Care for Improving Patient Engagement in Mental Health Treatment: Randomized Video Vignette Study. JMIR Form Res. 2023; 7:e40274.

Fowler JH, Christakis NA. Dynamic spread of happiness in a large social network: longitudinal analysis over 20 years in the Framingham Heart Study. BMJ. 2008; 337: a2338.

Francis DD, Kuhar MJ. Frequency of maternal licking and grooming correlates negatively with vulnerability to cocaine and alcohol use in rats. Pharmacol Biochem Behav. 2008; 90(3):497-500.

Franco G. The impact of productivity standards on psychotherapy. Front Psychol. 2023; 14:1229628.

Francis DD, Diorio J, Plotsky PM, Meaney MJ. Environmental enrichment reverses the effects of maternal separation on stress reactivity. J Neurosci. 2002; 22(18):7840-3.

Freeman LR, Haley-Zitlin V, Rosenberger DS, Granholm AC. Damaging effects of a high-fat diet to the brain and cognition: a review of proposed mechanisms. Nutr Neurosci. 2014;17(6):241-51.

French SA, Story M, Jeffery RW. Environmental influences on eating and physical activity. Ann Rev Public Health. 2001; 22: 309-35.

Friedberg MW, Chen PG, Simmons M, Sherry T, Mendel P, Raaen L, Ryan J, Orr P, Vargo C, Carlasare L, Botts C, Blake K. Effects of Health Care Payment Models on Physician Practice in the United States: Follow-Up Study. Rand Health Q. 2020; 9(1):1.

Froeliger B, Mathew AR, McConnell PA, Eichberg C, Saladin ME, Carpenter MJ, Garland EL. Restructuring Reward Mechanisms in Nicotine Addiction: A Pilot fMRI Study of Mindfulness-Oriented Recovery Enhancement for Cigarette Smokers. Evid Based Complement Alternat Med. 2017; 2017:7018014.

Fullana MA, Cardoner N, Alonso P, Subira M, Lopez-Sola C, Puiol J, Segalas C, Real E, Bossa M, Zacur E, Martinez-Zalacain I, Bulbena A, Menchon JM, Olmos S, Soriano-Mas C. Brain regions related to fear extinction in obsessive-compulsive disorder and its relation to exposure therapy outcome: a morphometric study. Psychol Med. 2014;44(4): 845-56.

Fuster, J. The prefrontal cortex (4th edition). Academic Press, 2008.

Gadagkar V, Puzerey PA, Chen R, Baird-Daniel E, Farhang AR, Goldberg JH. Dopamine neurons encode performance error in singing birds. Science. 2016; 354: 1278-1282.

Gallardo-Gómez D, Del Pozo-Cruz J, Noetel M, Álvarez-Barbosa F, Alfonso-Rosa RM, Del Pozo Cruz B. Optimal dose and type of exercise to improve cognitive function in older adults: A systematic review and Bayesian model-based network meta-analysis of RCTs. Ageing Res Rev. 2022; 76:101591.

Gander P, Purnell H, Garden A, Woodward A. Work patterns and fatigue-related risk among junior doctors. Occup Environ Med. 2007; 64(11):733-8.

Gangwisch JE, Heymsfield SB, Boden-Albala B, Buijs RM, Kreier F, Pickering TG, Rundle AG, Zammit GK, Malaspina D. Sleep duration as a risk factor for diabetes incidence in a large U.S. sample. Sleep. 2007; 30(12):1667-73.

Gardner KL, Thrivikraman KV, Lightman SL, Plotsky PM, Lowry CA. Early life experience alters behavior during social defeat: focus on serotonergic systems. Neuroscience. 2005; 136(1):181-91.

Garland EL. Restructuring reward processing with Mindfulness-Oriented Recovery Enhancement: novel therapeutic mechanisms to remediate hedonic dysregulation in addiction, stress, and pain. Ann N Y Acad Sci. 2016; 1373(1):25-37.

Garland EL, Fix ST, Hudak JP, Bernat EM, Nakamura Y, Hanley AW, Donaldson GW, Marchand WR, Froeliger B. Mindfulness-Oriented Recovery Enhancement remediates anhedonia in chronic opioid use by enhancing neurophysiological responses during savoring of natural rewards. Psychol Med. 2023; 53(5):2085-2094.

Gatz JD, Gingold DB, Lemkin DL, Wilkerson RG. Association of Resident Shift Length with Procedural Complications. J Emerg Med. 2021; 61(2):189-197.

George SZ, Zeppieri G Jr, Cere AL, Cere MR, Borut MS, Hodges MJ, Reed DM, Valencia C, Robinson ME. A randomized trial of behavioral physical therapy interventions for acute and sub-acute low back pain (NCT00373867). Pain. 2008; 140(1):145-57.

Genis-Mendoza AD, Lopez-Narvaez ML, Tovilla-Zarate CA, Sarmiento E, Chavez A, Martinez-Magaña JJ, et al. Association between polymorphisms of the DRD2 and ANKK1 genes and suicide attempt: A preliminary case-control study in a Mexican population. Neuropsychobiology. 2017;76(4):193–198.

Gerontakos S, Leach M, Steel A, Wardle J. Feasibility and efficacy of implementing group visits for women's health conditions: a systematic review. BMC Health Serv Res. 2023; 23(1):549.

Gilbert P. Introducing compassion-focused therapy. Adv Psychiatr Treat 2009; 15: 199–208.

Gilbert P. The origins and nature of compassion focused therapy. Brit J Clin Psychol. 2014; 53(1): 6–41.

Gitterman A, Schulman L (eds.). Mutual aid groups, vulnerable and resilient populations, and the life cycle. New York: Columbia University Press, 2005.

Goehler L. Food for Thought: Changing How We Feel By Changing How We Eat. Los Altos: Institute for Brain Potential, 2022.

Goldstein, RZ, Alia-Klein, N, Cottone, LA, Volkow, ND. The orbitofrontal cortex in drug addiction (pp. 481-522). In: Zald, DH, Rauch, SL (eds.). The orbitofrontal cortex. New York: Oxford University Press, 2006.

Gómez-Martínez C, Babio N, Júlvez J, Nishi SK, Fernández-Aranda F, Martínez-González MÁ, Cuenca-Royo A, Fernández R, Jiménez-Murcia S, de la Torre R, Pintó X, Bloemendaal M, Fitó M, Corella D, Arias A, Salas-Salvadó J. Impulsivity is longitudinally associated with healthy and unhealthy dietary patterns in individuals with overweight or obesity and metabolic syndrome within the framework of the PREDIMED-Plus trial. Int J Behav Nutr Phys Act. 2022; 19(1):101.

Gondré-Lewis MC, Bassey R, Blum K. Pre-clinical models of reward deficiency syndrome: A behavioral octopus. Neurosci Biobehav Rev. 2020; 115:164-188.

Gosselin N, Peretz I, Johnsen E, Adolphs R. Amygdala damage impairs emotion recognition from music. Neuropsychologia. 2007; 45(2):236-44.

Grabiel AM. Habits, rituals, and the evaluative brain. Ann Rev Neurosci. 2008; 31: 359-87.

Grace AA, Floresco SB, Goto Y, Lodge DJ. Regulation of firing of dopaminergic neurons and control of goal-directed behaviors. Trends Neurosci. 2007; 30(5):220-7.

Grol R, Mokkink H, Smits A, van Eijk J, Beek M, Mesker P, Mesker-Niesten J. Work satisfaction of general practitioners and the quality of patient care. Fam Pract. 1985; 2(3):128-35.

Gu X, Lohrenz T, Salas R, Baldwin PR, Soltani A, Kirk U, Cinciripini PM, Montague PR. Belief about nicotine selectively modulates value and reward prediction error signals in smokers. Proc Natl Acad Sci U S A. 2015;112(8):2539-44.

Haber SN. Corticostriatal circuitry. Dialog Clinical Neurosci. 2016;18(1):7-21.

Hagemann N, Strauss B, Busch D. The complex problem-solving competence of team coaches. Psychol Sport Exercise. 2008; 9(3): 301-317.

Hambrick EP, Williams JL, Hardt MM, Collins JO, Punt SE, Rincon Caicedo M, Zhang EA, Maras M, Lopez Mader L, Stiles R, Nelson EL. Disseminating early interventions for disaster mental health response using the ECHO model. J Community Psychol. 2023; 51(5):2213-2228.

Hampton AN, Adolphs R, Tyszka MJ, O'Doherty JP. Contributions of the amygdala to reward expectancy and choice signals in human prefrontal cortex. Neuron. 2007; 55(4): 545-55.

Harris AH, Bowe T, Hagedorn H, Nevedal A, Finlay AK, Gidwani R, Rosen C, Kay C, Christopher M. Multifaceted academic detailing program to increase pharmacotherapy for alcohol use disorder: interrupted time series evaluation of effectiveness. Addict Sci Clin Pract. 2016;11(1):15.

Hart AS, Rutledge RB, Glimcher PW, Phillips PE. Phasic dopamine release in the rat nucleus accumbens symmetrically encodes a reward prediction error term. J Neurosci. 2014; 34(3):698-704.

Hasan F, Tu YK, Lin CM, Chuang LP, Jeng C, Yuliana LT, Chen TJ, Chiu HY. Comparative efficacy of exercise regimens on sleep quality in older adults: A systematic review and network meta-analysis. Sleep Med Rev. 2022; 65:101673.

Hasan S, Alhaj H, Hassoulas A. The Efficacy and Therapeutic Alliance of Augmented Reality Exposure Therapy in Treating Adults with Phobic Disorders: Systematic Review. JMIR Ment Health. 2023;10: e51318.

Hatchett GT, Coaston SC. Surviving fee-for-service and productivity standards. J Mental Health Couns. 2018; 40: 199–210.

Hayes SC, Strosahl KD, Wilson KG. Acceptance and commitment therapy: an experiential approach to behavior change. New York: Guilford Press, 1999.

Helmeke C, Ovtscharoff W Jr, Poeggel G, Braun K. Imbalance of immunohistochemically characterized interneuron populations in the adolescent and adult rodent medial prefrontal cortex after repeated exposure to neonatal separation stress. Neurosci. 2008; 152(1):18-28.

Hester R, Garavan H. Executive dysfunction in cocaine addiction: evidence for discordant frontal, cingulate, and cerebellar activity. J Neurosci. 2004; 24(49):11017-22.

Higgins ST, Petry NM. Contingency management. Incentives for sobriety. Alcohol Res Health. 1999; 23(2): 122-7.

Hofmann SG, Asnaani A, Vonk IJ, Sawyer AT, Fang A. The Efficacy of Cognitive Behavioral Therapy: A Review of Meta-analyses. Cognit Ther Res. 2012; 36(5):427-440.

Hofmann SG, Gómez AF. Mindfulness-Based Interventions for Anxiety and Depression. Psychiatr Clin North Am. 2017;40(4):739-749.

Hofmeyr A, Ainslie G, Charlton R, Ross D. The relationship between addiction and reward bundling: An experiment comparing smokers and non-smokers. Addiction. 2010. 106 (2): 402-409.

Hollon SD, Steward MO, Strunk D. Enduring effects for cognitive behavioral therapy in the treatment of depression and anxiety. Ann Rev Psychol. 2006; 57: 285-315.

Holmes CJ, Kim-Spoon J. Adolescents' Religiousness and Substance Use Are Linked via Afterlife Beliefs and Future Orientation. J Early Adolesc. 2017;37(8):1054-1077.

Holt TA, Thorogood M, Griffiths F. Changing clinical practice through patient specific reminders available at the time of the clinical encounter: systematic review and meta-analysis. J Gen Intern Med. 2012; 27(8):974-84.

Hölzl R, Kleinböhl D, Huse E. Implicit operant learning of pain sensitization. Pain. 2005; 115(1-2):12-20.

Hornak J, O'Doherty J, Bramham J, Rolls ET, Morris RG, Bullock PR, Polkey CE. Reward-related reversal learning after surgical excisions in orbito-frontal or dorsolateral prefrontal cortex in humans. J Cogn Neurosci. 2004;16(3):463-78.

Howe LC, Leibowitz KA, Crum AJ. When Your Doctor "Gets It" and "Gets You": The Critical Role of Competence and Warmth in the Patient-Provider Interaction. Front Psychiatry. 2019; 10:475.

Howe RJ, Poulin LM, Federman DG. The Personal Health Inventory: Current Use, Perceived Barriers, and Benefits. Fed Pract. 2017; 34(5):23-26.

Huizenga HM, Crone EA, Jansen BJ. Decision-making in healthy children, adolescents and adults explained by the use of increasingly complex proportional reasoning rules. Dev Sci. 2007; 10(6): 814-25.

Hull JG, Bond CF Jr. Social and behavioral consequences of alcohol consumption and expectancy: a meta-analysis. Psychol Bull. 1986; 99(3):347-60.

Humphreys K. Circles of recovery. New York: Cambridge University Press, 2004.

Humphreys K, Barreto NB, Alessi SM, Carroll KM, Crits-Christoph P, Donovan DM, Kelly JF, Schottenfeld RS, Timko C, Wagner TH. Impact of 12 step mutual help groups on drug use disorder patients across six clinical trials. Drug Alcohol Depend. 2020; 215:108213.

Huot RL, Gonzalez ME, Ladd CO, Thrivikraman KV, Plotsky PM. Foster litters prevent hypothalamic-pituitary-adrenal axis sensitization mediated by neonatal maternal separation. Psychoneuroendocrinol. 2004; 29(2):279-89.

Hurley KM, Black MM, Papas MA, Caulfield LE. Maternal symptoms of stress, depression, and anxiety are related to nonresponsive feeding styles in a statewide sample of WIC participants. J Nutr. 2008; 138(4):799-805.

Iacoboni M. Imitation, empathy, and mirror neurons. Annu Rev Psychol. 2009; 60:653-70.

Insel TR. Is social attachment an addictive disorder? Physiol. Behav. 2003; 79, 351–357.

Ipser J, Seedat S, Stein DJ. Pharmacotherapy for post-traumatic stress disorder - a systematic review and meta-analysis. S Afr Med J. 2006; 96(10):1088-96.

Ipser JC, Wilson D, Akindipe TO, Sager C, Stein DJ. Pharmacotherapy for anxiety and comorbid alcohol use disorders. Cochrane Database Syst Review. 2015; 20(1): CD007505.

Iyasere CA, Wing J, Martel JN, Healy MG, Park YS, Finn KM. Effect of Increased Interprofessional Familiarity on Team Performance, Communication, and Psychological Safety on Inpatient Medical Teams: A Randomized Clinical Trial. JAMA Intern Med. 2022; 182(11):1190-1198.

Jason LA, O'Donnell WT Jr. Behavioral interventions to reduce youth exposure to unhealthful media. In: Best practices in the behavioral management of chronic disease: volume 3 from preconception to adolescence, Trafton JA, Gordon WP (eds.), Los Altos: Institute for Brain Potential, 2008.

Jia L, Meng Q, Scott A, Yuan B, Zhang L. Payment methods for healthcare providers working in outpatient healthcare settings. Cochrane Database Syst Rev. 2021; 1(1):CD011865.

Joen H, Lee SH. From Neurons to Social Beings: Short Review of the Mirror Neuron System Research and Its Socio-Psychological and Psychiatric Implications. Clin Psychopharmacol Neurosci. 2018; 16(1): 18–31.

Johnson PM, Kenny PJ. Dopamine D2 receptors in addiction-like reward dysfunction and compulsive eating in obese rats. Nat Neurosci. 2010; 13:635–641.

Jollant F, Lawrence NS, Olie E, O'Daly O, Malafosse A, Courtet P, Phillips ML. Decreased activation of lateral orbitofrontal cortex during risky choices under uncertainty is associated with disadvantageous decision-making and suicidal behavior. NeuroImage. 2010; 51: 1275–1281.

Jolliffe CD, Nicholas MK. Verbally reinforcing pain reports: an experimental test of the operant model of chronic pain. Pain. 2004; 107(1-2):167-75.

Jones K, Daley D, Hutchings J, Bywater T, Eames C. Efficacy of the Incredible Years Programme as an early intervention for children with conduct problems and ADHD: long-term follow-up. Child Care Health Dev. 2008; 34(3):380-90.

Jones K, Daley D, Hutchings J, Bywater T, Eames C. Efficacy of the Incredible Years Basic parent training programme as an early intervention for children with conduct problems and ADHD. Child Care Health Dev. 2007; 33(6):749-56.

Kalivas PW, Volkow N. The neural basis of addiction: a pathology of motivation and choice. Am J Psychiatry. 2005;162(8):1403-13.

Kawamoto K, Houlihan CA, Balas EA, Lobach DF. Improving clinical practice using clinical decision support systems: a systematic review of trials to identify features critical to success. BMJ. 2005; 330(7494):765.

Kazdin AE, Siegel TC, Bass D. Cognitive problem-solving skills training and parent management training in the treatment of antisocial behavior in children. J Consult Clin Psychol. 1992; 60(5):733-47.

Kedzior KK, Reitz SK, Azorina V, Loo C. Durability of the antidepressant effect of the high-frequency repetitive transcranial magnetic stimulation (rTMS) In the absence of maintenance treatment in major depression: A systematic review and meta-analysis of 16 double-blind, randomized, sham-controlled trials. Depress Anxiety. 2015; 32(3):193-203.

Keeler JF, Pretsell DO, Robbins TW. Functional implications of dopamine D1 vs. D2 receptors: A 'prepare and select' model of the striatal direct vs. indirect pathways. Neurosci. 2014; 282: 156 – 175.

Kelleher J, Zola S, Cui X, Chen S, Gerber C, Parker MW, Davis C, Law S, Golden M, Vaughan CP. Personalized Visual Mapping Assistive Technology to Improve Functional Ability in Persons With Dementia: Feasibility Cohort Study. JMIR Aging. 2021; 4(4): e28165.

Kelly JF, Humphreys K, Ferri M. Alcoholics Anonymous and other 12-step programs for alcohol use disorder. Cochrane Database Syst Rev. 2020; 3(3):CD012880.

Keltikangas-Järvinen L, Pulkki-Råback L, Elovainio M, Raitakari OT, Viikari J, Lehtimäki T. DRD2 C32806T modifies the effect of child-rearing environment on adulthood novelty seeking. Am J Med Genet B Neuropsychiatr Genet. 2009; 150B(3):389-94.

Kennedy SH, Konarski JZ, Segal ZV, Lau MA, Bieling PJ, McIntyre RS, Mayberg HS. Differences in brain glucose metabolism between responders to CBT and venlafaxine in a 16-week randomized controlled trial. Am J Psychiatry. 2007; 164(5):778-88.

Kenny PJ, Voren G, Johnson PM. Dopamine D2 receptors and striatopallidal transmission in addiction and obesity. Curr Opin Neurobiol. 2013; 23(4):535-8.

Kerr DL, McLaren DG, Mathy RM, Nitschke JB. Controllability modulates the anticipatory response in the human ventromedial prefrontal cortex. Front Psychol. 2012 14;3:557.

Kessler RM, Hutson PH, Herman BK, Potenza MN. The Neurobiological basis of binge-eating disorder. Neurosci Biobehav Rev. 2016; 63: 223-38.

Khoury Z, Maloyan M, Conroy K, Epee-Bounya A. Improving delivery of preventative care services using population management strategies. BMJ Open Qual. 2022; 11(2):e001695.

Kiehl KA. A cognitive neuroscience perspective on psychopathy: evidence for paralimbic system dysfunction. Psychiatr Res. 2006;142(2-3):107-28.

Kiehl KA, Anderson NE, Aharoni E, Maurer JM, Harenski KA, Rao V, Claus ED, Harenski C, Koenigs M, Decety J, Kosson D, Wager TD, Calhoun VD, Steele VR. Age of gray matters: Neuroprediction of recidivism. Neuroimage Clin. 2018; 19:813-823.

Killgore WD, Balkin TJ, Wesensten NJ. Impaired decision making following 49 h of sleep deprivation. J Sleep Res. 2006; 15(1):7-13.

Killgore WD, Lipizzi EL, Kamimori GH, Balkin TJ. Caffeine effects on risky decision making after 75 hours of sleep deprivation. Aviat Space Environ Med. 2007;78(10):957-62.

Kim E, Lee D, Do K, Kim J. Interaction Effects of DRD2 Genetic Polymorphism and Interpersonal Stress on Problematic Gaming in College Students. Genes (Basel). 2022; 13(3):449.

Kimbrel NA, Ashley-Koch AE, Qin XJ, Lindquist JH, Garrett ME, Dennis MF, Hair LP, Huffman JE, Jacobson DA, Madduri RK, Trafton JA, Coon H, Docherty AR, Kang J, Mullins N, Ruderfer DM; VA Million Veteran Program (MVP); MVP Suicide Exemplar Workgroup; International Suicide Genetics Consortium; Harvey PD, McMahon BH, Oslin DW, Hauser ER, Hauser MA, Beckham JC. A genome-wide association study of suicide attempts in the million veterans program identifies evidence of pan-ancestry and ancestry-specific risk loci. Mol Psychiatry. 2022; 27(4):2264-2272.

Kirby LG, Pan YZ, Freeman-Daniels E, Rani S, Nunan JD, Akanwa A, Beck SG. Cellular effects of swim stress in the dorsal raphe nucleus. Psychoneuroendocrinology. 2007; 32(6):712-23.

Kirgios EL, Mandel GH, Park Y, Milkman KL, Gromet DM, Kay JS, Duckworth AL. Teaching temptation bundling to boost exercise: A field experiment. Organizational Behavior and Human Decision Processes. 2020; 161: 20-35.

Kirsh SR, Aron DC, Johnson KD, Santurri LE, Stevenson LD, Jones KR, Jagosh J. A realist review of shared medical appointments: How, for whom, and under what circumstances do they work? BMC Health Serv Res. 2017; 17(1):113.

Kjellgren A, Bood SA, Axelsson K, Norlander T, Saatcioglu F. Wellness through a comprehensive yogic breathing program - a controlled pilot trial. BMC Complement Altern Med. 2007; 7:43.

Knowlden AP, Ottati M, McCallum M, Allegrante JP. The relationship between sleep quantity, sleep quality and weight loss in adults: A scoping review. Clin Obes. 2023: e12634.

Knutson B, Rick S, Wimmer GE, Prelec D, Loewenstein G. Neural predictors of purchases. Neuron. 2007; 53(1):147-56.

Knutson KL, Van Cauter E. Associations between sleep loss and increased risk of obesity and diabetes. Ann N Y Acad Sci. 2008; 1129:287-304.

Kopelovich SL, Blank J, McCain C, Hughes M, Strachan E. Applying the Project ECHO Model to Support Implementation and Sustainment of Cognitive Behavioral Therapy for Psychosis. J Contin Educ Health Prof. 2023; 10.1097/CEH.0000000000000511.

Koran LM, Bullock KD, Hartston HJ, Elliott MA, D'Andrea V. Citalopram treatment of compulsive shopping: an open-label study. J Clin Psychiatry. 2002; 63(8):704-8.

Koyama T, McHaffie JG, Laurienti PJ, Coghill RC. The subjective experience of pain: where expectations become reality. Proc Natl Acad Sci U S A. 2005; 102(36):12950-5.

Kraft TL, Pressman SD. Grin and bear it: the influence of manipulated facial expression on the stress response. Psychol Sci. 2012; 23(11):1372-8.

Kringelbach, ML. The hedonic brain: a functional neuroanatomy of human pleasure. In: Kringelbach, ML, Berridge, KC. Pleasures of the brain. New York: Oxford University Press, 2010.

Kroenke K, Theobald D, Wu J, Norton K, Morrison G, Carpenter J, Tu W. Effect of Telecare Management on Pain and Depression in Patients with Cancer: A Randomized Trial. JAMA. 2010; 304(2): 163–171.

Kroeze W, Oenema A, Dagnelie PC, Brug J. Examining the minimal required elements of a computer-tailored intervention aimed at dietary fat reduction: results of a randomized controlled dismantling study. Health Educ Res. 2008; 23(5):880-91.

Krug EG, Brener ND, Dahlberg LL, Ryan GW, Powell KE. The impact of an elementary school-based violence prevention program on visits to the school nurse. Am J Prev Med. 1997; 13(6):459-63.

Krug I, Treasure J, Anderluh M, Bellodi L, Cellini E, di Bernardo M, Granero R, Karwautz A, Nacmias B, Penelo E, Ricca V, Sorbi S, Tchanturia K, Wagner G, Collier D, Fernández-Aranda F. Present and lifetime comorbidity of tobacco, alcohol and drug use in eating disorders: a European multicenter study. Drug Alcohol Depend. 2008; 97(1-2):169-79.

Kruger J, Blanck HM, Gillespie C. Dietary and physical activity behaviors among adults successful at weight loss maintenance. Int J Behav Nutr Phys Act. 2006; 3:17.

Kumari V, Peters ER, Fannon D, Antonova E, Premkumar P, Anilkumar AP, Williams SC, Kuipers E. . Biol Psychiatry. 2009;66(6):594-602.

Kunzler AM, Helmreich I, Chmitorz A, König J, Binder H, Wessa M, Lieb K. Psychological interventions to foster resilience in healthcare professionals. Cochrane Database Syst Rev. 2020; 7(7):CD012527.

Lally P, van Jaarsveld CHM, Potts HWW, Wardle J. How are habits formed: modelling habit formation in the real world. Eur J Social Psychol. 2010; 46(6):998-1009.

Larsson B, Fossum S, Clifford G, Drugli MB, Handegård BH, Mørch WT. Treatment of oppositional defiant and conduct problems in young Norwegian children: results of a randomized controlled trial. Eur Child Adolesc Psychiatry. 2009; 18(1):42-52.

Lau-Barraco C, Dunn ME. Evaluation of a single-session expectancy challenge intervention to reduce alcohol use among college students. Psychol Addict Behav. 2008; 22(2):168-75.

Lee JY, Kim JM, Kim JW, Cho J, Lee WY, Kim HJ, Jeon BS. Association between the dose of dopaminergic medication and the behavioral disturbances in Parkinson disease. Parkinsonism Relat Disord. 2010; 16(3):202-7.

Leeuw M, Goossens ME, van Breukelen GJ, de Jong JR, Heuts PH, Smeets RJ, Köke AJ, Vlaeyen JW. Exposure in vivo versus operant graded activity in chronic low back pain patients: results of a randomized controlled trial. Pain. 2008; 138(1):192-207.

Leung LB, Rose D, Rubenstein LV, Guo R, Dresselhaus TR, Stockdale S. Does Mental Health Care Integration Affect Primary Care Clinician Burnout? Results from a Longitudinal Veterans Affairs Survey. J Gen Intern Med. 2020; 35(12):3620-3626.

Levine JA, Lanningham-Foster LM, McCrady SK, Krizan AC, Olson LR, Kane PH, Jensen MD, Clark MM. Interindividual variation in posture allocation: possible role in human obesity. Science. 2005; 307(5709):584-6.

Lewis ET, Cucciare MA, Trafton JA. What do patients do with unused opioid medications? Clin J Pain. 2014; 30(8):654-62.

Liberzon I, Britton JC, Phan KL. Neural correlates of traumatic recall in posttraumatic stress disorder. Stress. 2003; 6(3):151-6.

Liberman RP, Eckman TA, Marder SR. Training in social problem-solving among persons with schizophrenia. Psychiatric Services. 2001; 52:31–33.

Lillis J, Hayes SC, Bunting K and Masuda A. Teaching acceptance and mindfulness to improve the lives of the obese: a preliminary test of a theoretical model. Annals of Behavioral Medicine. 2009; 37(1): 58-69.

Lin W, Li N, Yang L, Zhang Y. The efficacy of digital cognitive behavioral therapy for insomnia and depression: a systematic review and meta-analysis of randomized controlled trials. PeerJ. 2023;11:e16137.

Lin Y, Saper R, Patil SJ. Long COVID Shared Medical Appointments: Lifestyle and Mind-Body Medicine With Peer Support. Ann Fam Med. 2022; 20(4):383.

Linden DE. How psychotherapy changes the brain--the contribution of functional neuroimaging. Mol Psychiatry. 2006; 11(6):528-38.

Linehan MM. *Cognitive Behavioral Therapy of Borderline Personality Disorder*. New York, NY: Guilford Press; 1993.

Linzer M, Jin JO, Shah P, Stillman M, Brown R, Poplau S, Nankivil N, Cappelucci K, Sinsky CA. Trends in Clinician Burnout With Associated Mitigating and Aggravating Factors During the COVID-19 Pandemic. JAMA Health Forum. 2022; 3(11):e224163.

Lockley SW, Barger LK, Ayas NT, Rothschild JM, Czeisler CA, Landrigan CP; Harvard Work Hours, Health and Safety Group. Effects of health care provider work hours and sleep deprivation on safety and performance. Jt Comm J Qual Patient Saf. 2007; 33(11 Suppl):7-18.

Lu MA, O'Toole J, Shneyderman M, Brockman S, Cumpsty-Fowler C, Dang D, Herzke C, Rand CS, Sateia HF, Van Dyke E, Eakin MN, Daugherty Biddison EL. "Where You Feel Like a Family Instead of Co-workers": a Mixed Methods Study on Care Teams and Burnout. J Gen Intern Med. 2023; 38(2):341-350.

Magee L, Hale L. Longitudinal associations between sleep duration and subsequent weight gain: a systematic review. Sleep Med Rev. 2012;16(3):231-41.

Maier SF. Behavioral control blunts reactions to contemporaneous and future adverse events: medial prefrontal cortex plasticity and a corticostriatal network. Neurobiol Stress. 2015;1:12-22.

Malejko K, Abler B, Plener PL, Straub J. Neural Correlates of Psychotherapeutic Treatment of Post-traumatic Stress Disorder: A Systematic Literature Review. Front Psychiatry. 2017; 8: 85.

Mandyam CD, Wee S, Eisch AJ, Richardson HN, Koob GF. Methamphetamine self-administration and voluntary exercise have opposing effects on medial prefrontal cortex gliogenesis. J Neurosci. 2007; 27(42):11442-50.

Mangory KY, Ali LY, Rø KI, Tyssen R. Effect of burnout among physicians on observed adverse patient outcomes: a literature review. BMC Health Serv Res. 2021; 21(1):369.

Mansouri FA, Tanaka K, Buckley MJ. Conflict-induced behavioural adjustment: a clue to the executive functions of the prefrontal cortex. Nature Reviews Neuroscience 2009; 10:141-152.

Marcus CL, Loughlin GM. Effect of sleep deprivation on driving safety in housestaff. Sleep. 1996; 19(10):763-6.

Marmot MG, Shipley MJ, Rose G. Inequalities in death--specific explanations of a general pattern? Lancet. 1984; 1(8384):1003-6.

Marosits MJ. Improving financial and patient outcomes: the future of demand management. Healthc Financ Manage. 1997; 51(8):43-4.

Marshall NS, Glozier N, Grunstein RR. Is sleep duration related to obesity? A critical review of the epidemiological evidence. Sleep Med Rev. 2008; 12(4):289-98.

Marshall V, Jewett-Tennant J, Shell-Boyd J, Stevenson L, Hearns R, Gee J, Schaub K, LaForest S, Taveira TH, Cohen L, Parent M, Dev S, Barrette A, Oliver K, Wu WC, Ball SL. Healthcare providers experiences with shared medical appointments for heart failure. PLoS One. 2022; 17(2):e0263498.

Martell BA, O'Connor PG, Kerns RD, Becker WC, Morales KH, Kosten TR, Fiellin DA. Systematic review: opioid treatment for chronic back pain: prevalence, efficacy, and association with addiction. Ann Intern Med. 2007; 146(2):116-27.

Martín-Sánchez E, Furukawa TA, Taylor J, Martin JL. Systematic review and meta-analysis of cannabis treatment for chronic pain. Pain Med. 2009; 10(8):1353-68.

Martikainen IK, Nuechterline EB, Pecina M, Love TM, Cummiford CM, Green CR, Stohler CS, Zubieta JK. Chronic Back Pain Is Associated with Alterations in Dopamine Neurotransmission in the Ventral Striatum. J Neurosci. 2015 Jul 8;35(27):9957-65.

Matsumoto M, Smith JC. Progressive muscle relaxation, breathing exercises, and ABC relaxation theory. J Clin Psychol. 2001; 57(12):1551-7.

Mayberg, HS. Targeted electrode-based modulation of neural circuits for depression. J. Clin Invest. 2009; 119 (4) 717-725.

Mayberg HS, Lozano AM, Voon V, McNeely HE, Seminowicz D, Hamani C, Schwalb JM, Kennedy SH. Deep brain stimulation for treatment-resistant depression. Neuron. 2005; 45(5):651-60.

McCrady B, Stout R, Noel N. Effectiveness of three types of spouse-involved alcohol treatment: outcomes 18 months after treatment. Br J Addict. 1991; 86(11):1415-1424.

McEwen BS. Stress and hippocampal plasticity. Annu Rev Neurosci. 1999; 22:105-22.

McGinnis JM, Foege WH. Actual causes of death in the United States. JAMA. 1993; 270(18):2207-12.

McGuire MT, Wing RR, Klem ML, Seagle HM, Hill JO. Long-term maintenance of weight loss: do people who lose weight through various weight loss methods use different behaviors to maintain their weight? Int J Obes Relat Metab Disord. 1998; 22(6):572-7.

McKellar JM. Increasing Self-Efficacy for Health Behavior Change: A Review of Self-Management Interventions. In: Trafton J, Gordon W (eds.), Best Practices in the Behavioral Management of Chronic Disease, Volume I: Neuropsychiatric Disorders. Los Altos: Institute for Brain Potential, 2010.

McLean N, Griffin S, Toney K, Hardeman W. Family involvement in weight control, weight maintenance and weight-loss interventions: a systematic review of randomised trials. Int J Obes Relat Metab Disord. 2003; 27(9):987-1005.

Meier MH, Caspi A, Ambler A, Harrington H, Houts R, Keefe RS, McDonald K, Ward A, Poulton R, Moffitt TE. Persistent cannabis users show neuropsychological decline from childhood to midlife. Proc Natl Acad Sci U S A. 2012;109(40): E2657-64.

Melgar-Locatelli S, de Ceglia M, Mañas-Padilla MC, Rodriguez-Pérez C, Castilla-Ortega E, Castro-Zavala A, Rivera P. Nutrition and adult neurogenesis in the hippocampus: Does what you eat help you remember? Front Neurosci. 2023;17:1147269.

Meloni EG, Reedy CL, Cohen BM, Carlezon WA Jr. Activation of raphe efferents to the medial prefrontal cortex by corticotropin-releasing factor: correlation with anxiety-like behavior. Biol Psychiatry. 2008;63(9):832-9.

Michaels CC, Holtzman SG. Early postnatal stress alters place conditioning to both mu- and kappa-opioid agonists. J Pharmacol Exp Ther. 2008; 325(1):313-8.

Midboe AM, Wu J, Erhardt T, Carmichael JM, Bounthavong M, Christopher MLD, Gale RC. Academic Detailing to Improve Opioid Safety: Implementation Lessons from a Qualitative Evaluation. Pain Med. 2018; 19(suppl_1):S46-S53.

Millder BL, Cummings JL (eds). The human frontal lobes: functions and disorders (2nd edition). New York: Guilford Press, 2007.

Miller WR, Rollnick S. Motivational Interviewing: Preparing people for change (2nd edition). New York: Guilford Press, 2002.

Miller CJ, Griffith KN, Stolzmann K, Kim B, Connolly SL, Bauer MS. An Economic Analysis of the Implementation of Team-based Collaborative Care in Outpatient General Mental Health Clinics. Med Care. 2020; 58(10):874-880.

Miller MA. Time for bed: diet, sleep and obesity in children and adults. Proc Nutr Soc. 2023: 1-8.

Minegishi T, Frakt AB, Garrido MM, Gellad WF, Hausmann LRM, Lewis ET, Pizer SD, Trafton JA, Oliva EM. Randomized program evaluation of the Veterans Health Administration Stratification Tool for Opioid Risk Mitigation (STORM): A research and clinical operations partnership to examine effectiveness. Subst Abus. 2019; 40(1):14-19.

Mladenovic Djordjevic A, Perovic M, Tesic V, Tanic N, Rakic L, Ruzdijic S, Kanazir S. Long-term dietary restriction modulates the level of presynaptic proteins in the cortex and hippocampus of the aging rat. Neurochem Int. 2010; 56(2):250-5.

Mokdad AH, Marks JS, Stroup DF, Gerberding JL. Actual causes of death in the United States, 2000. JAMA 2004; 291(10): 1238-1245.

Moffett MC, Vicentic A, Kozel M, Plotsky P, Francis DD, Kuhar MJ. Maternal separation alters drug intake patterns in adulthood in rats. Biochem Pharmacol. 2007; 73(3):321-30.

Monterosso J, Ainslie G. The behavioral economics of will in recovery from addiction. Drug Alcohol Depend. 2007; 90 Suppl 1:S100-11.

Moreira MT, Smith LA, Foxcroft D. Social norms interventions to reduce alcohol misuse in university or college students. Cochrane Database Syst Rev. 2009; (3):CD006748.

Morgan D, Grant KA, Gage HD, Mach RH, Kaplan JR, Prioleau O, Nader SH, Buchheimer N, Ehrenkaufer RL, Nader MA. Social dominance in monkeys: dopamine D2 receptors and cocaine self-administration. Nat Neurosci. 2002; 5(2):169-74.

Morgenthaler T, Kramer M, Alessi C, Friedman L, Boehlecke B, Brown T, Coleman J, Kapur V, Lee-Chiong T, Owens J, Pancer J, Swick T; American Academy of Sleep Medicine. Practice parameters for the psychological and behavioral treatment of insomnia: an update. An American Academy of Sleep Medicine report. Sleep. 2006; 29(11):1415-9.

Morres ID, Hatzigeorgiadis A, Stathi A, Comoutos N, Arpin-Cribbie C, Krommidas C, Theodorakis Y. Aerobic exercise for adult patients with major depressive disorder in mental health services: A systematic review and meta-analysis. Depress Anxiety. 2019; 36(1):39-53.

Müller-Vahl KR, Kaufmann J, Grosskreutz J, Dengler R, Emrich HM, Peschel T, O'Doherty, JP, Dolan, RJ. The role of human orbitofrontal cortex in reward prediction and behavioral choice: insights from neuroimaging (pp. 265-283). In: Zald, DH, Rauch, SL (eds.). The orbitofrontal cortex. New York: Oxford University Press, 2006.

Murray JS, Clifford J, Larson S, Lee JK, Sculli GL. Implementing Just Culture to Improve Patient Safety. Mil Med. 2023; 188(7-8): 1596-1599.

Naehrig D, Schokman A, Hughes JK, Epstein R, Hickie IB, Glozier N. Effect of interventions for the well-being, satisfaction and flourishing of general practitioners-a systematic review. BMJ Open. 2021; 11(8):e046599.

Neprash HT, Barnett ML. Association of Primary Care Clinic Appointment Time with Opioid Prescribing. JAMA Netw Open. 2019; 2(8):e1910373.

Nash J. 24 Best Self-Soothing Techniques and Strategies for Adults. 2022; Available at: https://positivepsychology.com/self-soothing/, accessed on Oct 9, 2023.

National Institute of Health and the friends of the National Library of Medicine. PTSD: A Growing Epidemic. NIH Medline Plus. 2009; 4(1):10-14.

Ng HJH, Kansal A, Abdul Naseer JF, Hing WC, Goh CJM, Poh H, D'souza JLA, Lim EL, Tan G. Optimizing Best Practice Advisory alerts in electronic medical records with a multi-pronged strategy at a tertiary care hospital in Singapore. JAMIA Open. 2023; 6(3): ooad056.

NHS. "A just culture guide". 2023; Accessed on July 30, 2023; available at: https://www.england.nhs.uk/patient-safety/a-just-culture-guide/.

Nigam JA, Barker RM, Cunningham TR, Swanson NG, Chosewood LC. Vital Signs: Health Worker–Perceived Working Conditions and Symptoms of Poor Mental Health — Quality of Worklife Survey, United States, 2018–2022. MMWR Morb Mortal Wkly Rep 2023; 72:1197–1205.

Nilsson U. Soothing music can increase oxytocin levels during bed rest after open-heart surgery: a randomised control trial. J Clin Nurs. 2009;18(15):2153-61.

Nixon RD, Sweeney L, Erickson DB, Touyz SW. Parent-child interaction therapy: one- and two-year follow-up of standard and abbreviated treatments for oppositional preschoolers. J Abnorm Child Psychol. 2004; 32(3):263-71.

Nixon RD, Sweeney L, Erickson DB, Touyz SW. Parent-child interaction therapy: a comparison of standard and abbreviated treatments for oppositional defiant preschoolers. J Consult Clin Psychol. 2003; 71(2):251-60.

Olson AK, Eadie BD, Ernst C, Christie BR. Environmental enrichment and voluntary exercise massively increase neurogenesis in the adult hippocampus via dissociable pathways. Hippocampus. 2006; 16(3): 250-60.

Occupational Safety and Health Administration. Preventing Workplace Violence: A Road Map for Healthcare Facilities. U.S. Department of Labor. 2015; Accessed on January 3, 2024; Available at: https://www.osha.gov/sites/default/files/OSHA3827.pdf.

Occupational Safety and Health Administration. Guidelines for Preventing Workplace Violence for Healthcare and Social Service Workers. U.S. Department of Labor report: OSHA 3128-06R 2016. 2016; Accessed on January 3, 2024; Available at: https://www.osha.gov/sites/default/files/publications/osha3148.pdf

O'dea A, O'Connor P, Keogh I. A meta-analysis of the effectiveness of crew resource management training in acute care domains. Postgrad Med J. 2014; 90:699–708.

O'Donnell S, Oluyomi Daniel T, Epstein LH. Does goal relevant episodic future thinking amplify the effect on delay discounting? Conscious Cogn. 2017; 51:10-16.

O'Farrell TJ. Behavioral couples therapy for alcohol and drug use. Psychiatric Times, 1999: XVI (4), available at: http://www.psychosocial.com/addiction/bct.html.

O'Farrell TJ, Cutter HSG, Choquette KA. Behavioral marital therapy for male alcoholics: marital and drinking adjustment during the two years after treatment. Behavior Therapy. 1992; 23:529-549.

Oomen CA, Bekinschtein P, Kent BA, Saksida LM, Bussey TJ. Oomen CA, Bekinschtein P, Kent BA, Saksida LM, Bussey TJ. Adult hippocampal neurogenesis and its role in cognition. Wiley Interdiscip Rev Cogn Sci. 2014; 5(5):573-87.

Osorio RS, Gumb T, Pirraglia E, Varga AW, Lu SE, Lim J, Wohlleber ME, Ducca EL, Koushyk V, Glodzik L, Mosconi L, Avappa I, Rapoport DM, de Leon MJ. Alzheimer's Disease Neuroimaging Initiative. Sleep-disordered breathing advances cognitive decline in the elderly. Neurology. 2015; 84(19):1964-71.

Page N, Baysari MT, Westbrook JI. A systematic review of the effectiveness of interruptive medication prescribing alerts in hospital CPOE systems to change prescriber behavior and improve patient safety. Int J Med Inform. 2017; 105:22-30.

Paladini CA, Roeper J. Generating bursts (and pauses) in the dopamine midbrain neurons. Neuroscience. 2014; 282C:109-121.

Papadakis A, Pfoh ER, Hu B, Liu X, Rothberg MB, Misra-Hebert AD. Shared Medical Appointments and Prediabetes: The Power of the Group. Ann Fam Med. 2021; 19(3):258-261.

Park B, Gold SB, Bazemore A, Liaw W. How Evolving United States Payment Models Influence Primary Care and Its Impact on the Quadruple Aim. J Am Board Fam Med. 2018; 31(4):588-604.

Park CL, Gaffey AE. Relationships between psychosocial factors and health behavior change in cancer survivors: an integrative review. Ann Behav Med. 2007; 34(2):115-34.

Park DC, Reuter-Lorenz P. The adaptive brain: aging and neurocognitive scaffolding. Annu Rev Psychol. 2009; 60:173-96.

Parker MW, Davis C, White K, Johnson D, Golden M, Zola S. Reduced care burden and improved quality of life in African American family caregivers: Positive impact of personalized assistive technology. Technology and Health Care. 2022; 30(2):379-87.

Parsons AC, Shraim M, Inglis J, Aveyard P, Hajek P. Interventions for preventing weight gain after smoking cessation. Cochrane Database Syst Rev. 2009; (1):CD006219.

Patel SR, Hu FB. Short sleep duration and weight gain: a systematic review. Obesity. 2008; 16(3):643-53.

Pawlow LA, Jones GE. The impact of abbreviated progressive muscle relaxation on salivary cortisol. Biol Psychol. 2002; 60(1):1-16.

Pawlow LA, O'Neil PM, Malcolm RJ. Night eating syndrome: effects of brief relaxation training on stress, mood, hunger, and eating patterns. Int J Obes Relat Metab Disord. 2003; 27(8):970-8.

Pearcy CP, Anderson RA, Egan SJ, Rees CS. A systematic review and meta-analysis of self-help therapeutic interventions for obsessive-compulsive disorder: Is therapeutic contact key to overall improvement? J Behav Ther Exp Psychiatry. 2016; 51:74-83.

Perkonigg A, Owashi T, Stein MB, Kirschbaum C, Wittchen HU. Posttraumatic stress disorder and obesity: evidence for a risk association. Am J Prev Med. 2009; 36(1):1-8.

Petry NM. A comprehensive guide to the application of contingency management procedures in clinical settings. Drug Alcohol Depend. 2000; 58(1-2):9-25.

Porto PR, Oliveira L, Mari J, Volchan E, Figueira I, Ventura P. Does cognitive behavioral therapy change the brain? A systematic review of neuroimaging in anxiety disorders. J Neuropsychiatry Clin Neurosci. 2009; 21(2):114-25.

Pressman SD, Acevedo AM, Hammond KV, Kraft-Feil TL. Smile (or grimace) through the pain? The effects of experimentally manipulated facial expressions on needle-injection responses. Emotion. 2021; 21(6):1188-1203.

Qaseem A, Kansagara D, Forciea MA, Cooke M, Denberg TD; Clinical Guidelines Committee of the American College of Physicians. Management of Chronic Insomnia Disorder in Adults: A Clinical Practice Guideline From the American College of Physicians. Ann Intern Med. 2016;165(2):125-33.

Ragan AP, Aikens GB, Bounthavong M, Brittain K, Mirk A. Academic Detailing to Reduce Sedative-Hypnotic Prescribing in Older Veterans. J Pharm Pract. 2021; 34(2):287-294.

Rathert C, Williams ES, Linhart H. Evidence for the Quadruple Aim: A Systematic Review of the Literature on Physician Burnout and Patient Outcomes. Med Care. 2018; 56(12):976-984.

Ravussin E, Lillioja S, Anderson TE, Christin L, Bogardus C. Determinants of 24-hour energy expenditure in man. Methods and results using a respiratory chamber. J Clin Invest. 1986; 78(6):1568-78.

Read D, Van Leeuwen B. Predicting hunger: the effects of appetite and delay on choice. Organizational behavior and human decision processes. 1998: 76(2): 189-205.

Reindersma T, Sülz S, Ahaus K, Fabbricotti I. The Effect of Network-Level Payment Models on Care Network Performance: A Scoping Review of the Empirical Literature. Int J Integr Care. 2022; 22(2):3.

Reed DA, Fletcher KE, Arora VM. (2010) Systematic Review: Association of Shift Length, Protected Sleep Time and Night Float with Patient Care, Resident's Health and Education. Ann Int Med, 153(12): 829-842.

Redish AD. Addiction as a computational process gone awry. Science. 2004; 306(5703): 1944-7.

Regier PS, Redish AD. Contingency Management and Deliberative Decision-Making Processes. Front Psychiatry. 2015; 6: 76.

Regnier SD, Traxler HK, Devoto A, DeFulio A. A Systematic Review of Treatment Maintenance Strategies in Token Economies: Implications for Contingency Management. Perspect Behav Sci. 2022;45(4):819-861.

Reis HT, Rusbult CE (eds). Close relationships. New York: Psychology Press, 2004.

Rod NH, Dissing AS, Clark A, Gerds TA, Lund R. Overnight smartphone use: A new public health challenge? A novel study design based on high-resolution smartphone data. PLoS One. 2018; 13(10): e0204811.

Rodriguez PF, Aron AR, Poldrack RA. Ventral-striatal/nucleus-accumbens sensitivity to prediction errors during classification learning. Hum Brain Mapp. 2006; 27(4):306-13.

Rodziewicz TL, Houseman B, Hipskind JE. Medical Error Reduction and Prevention. 2023. In: StatPearls [Internet]. Treasure Island (FL): StatPearls Publishing; 2023 Jan.

Roesch MR, Olson CR. Neuronal activity related to reward value and motivation in primate frontal cortex. Science. 2004; 304(5668):307-10.

Rolle CE, Pedersen ML, Johnson N, Amemori KI, Ironside M, Graybiel AM, Pizzagalli DA, Etkin A. The Role of the Dorsal-Lateral Prefrontal Cortex in Reward Sensitivity During Approach-Avoidance Conflict. Cereb Cortex. 2022; 32(6):1269-1285.

Rolls BJ, Morris EL, Roe LS. Portion size of food affects energy intake in normal-weight and overweight men and women. Am J Clin Nutr. 2002; 76(6):1207-13.

Roman E, Nylander I. The impact of emotional stress early in life on adult voluntary ethanol intake-results of maternal separation in rats. Stress. 2005; 8(3):157-74.

Romano JM, Turner JA, Jensen MP, Friedman LS, Bulcroft RA, Hops H, Wright SF. Chronic pain patient-spouse behavioral interactions predict patient disability. Pain. 1995; 63(3):353-60.

Rominger A, Cumming P, Xiong G, Koller G, Boning G, Wulff M, Zwergal A, Forster S, Reilhac A, Munk O, Soyka M, Wangler B, Bartenstein P, la Fougere C, Pogarell O. [18F]Fallypride PET measurement of striatal and extrastriatal dopamine D2/3 receptor availability in recently abstinent alcoholics. Addict Biol. 2012; 17(2): 490-503.

Rosenblum LA, Coplan JD, Freidman S, Bassoff T, Gorman JM, Andrews MW. Adverse early experiences affect noradrenergic and serotonergic functioning in adult primates. Biol Psycho. 1994; 35: 221-227.

Ross A, Thomas S. The health benefits of yoga and exercise: a review of comparison studies. J Altern Complement Med. 2010; 16(1): 3-12.

Rotge JY, Guehl D, Dilharreguy B, Tignol J, Bioulac B, Allard M, Burbaud P, Aouizerate B. Meta-analysis of brain volume changes in obsessive-compulsive disorder. Biol Psychiatry. 2009; Jan 1;65(1):75-83.

Rozeske RR, Der-Avakian A, Bland ST, Beckley JT, Watkins LR, Maier SF. The medial prefrontal cortex regulates the differential expression of morphine-conditioned place preference following a single exposure to controllable or uncontrollable stress. Neuropsychopharmacology. 2009; 34(4):834-43.

Rubak S, Sandbaek A, Lauritzen T, Christensen B. Motivational interviewing: a systematic review and meta-analysis. Br J Gen Pract. 2005; 55(513):305-12.

Ruderman MA, Byers AL, Bauer MS, Stolzmann K, Miller CJ, Connolly SL, Kim B. One-Year All-Cause Mortality and Delivery of the Collaborative Chronic Care Model in General Mental Health Clinics. Psychiatr Serv. 2023; appips20220428.

Rung JM, Peck S, Hinnenkamp J, Preston E, Madden GJ. Changing Delay Discounting and Impulsive Choice: Implications for Addictions, Prevention, and Human Health. Perspect Behav Sci. 2019; 42(3):397-417.

Ryder AL, Azcarate PM, Cohen BE. PTSD and Physical Health. Curr Psychiatry Rep. 2018; 20(12):116.

Saint-Exupery A. The Little Prince. Gaillimard, 1943.

Saling LL, Phillips JG. Automatic behaviour: efficient not mindless. Brain Res Bull. 2007; 73(1-3):1-20.

Sapolsky RM. Why zebras don't get ulcers (3rd edition). New York: Henry Holt and Company, 2004.

Sapolsky RM. Glucocorticoids, stress, and their adverse neurological effects: relevance to aging. Exp Gerontol. 1999; 34(6):721-32.

Satyal MK, Basso JC, Wilding H, Athamneh LN, Bickel WK. Examining neurobehavioral differences that support success in recovery from alcohol and other substance use disorders. J Subst Use Addict Treat. 2023; 148:209007.

Saxena, S. Neurobiology and treatment of compulsive hoarding. CNS Spectrum. 2008; 13(9)14: 29-36.

Scarmeas N, Luchsinger JA, Schupf N, Brickman AM, Cosentino S, Tang MX, Stern Y. Physical activity, diet, and risk of Alzheimer disease. JAMA. 2009; 302(6):627-37.

Schienle A, Schäfer A, Hermann A, Rohrmann S, Vaitl D. Symptom provocation and reduction in patients suffering from spider phobia: an fMRI study on exposure therapy. Eur Arch Psychiatry Clin Neurosci. 2007; 257(8):486-93.

Schmidt EM, Wright D, Cherkasova E, Harris AHS, Trafton J. Evaluating and Improving Engagement in Care After High-Intensity Stays for Mental or Substance Use Disorders. Psychiatr Serv. 2022; 73(1):18-25.

Schnider A. Orbitofrontal reality filtering. Front Behav Neurosci. 2013; 10;7:67.

Schneider W, Chein JM. Controlled & automatic processing: behavior, theory, and biological mechanisms, Cognitive Science: A Multidisciplinary Journal. 2003; 27:3,525-559.

Schuch FB, Vancampfort D, Richards J, Rosenbaum S, Ward PB, Stubbs B. Exercise as a treatment for depression: A meta-analysis adjusting for publication bias. J Psychiatr Res. 2016; 77: 42-51.

Schultz W. Predictive reward signal of dopamine neurons. J Neurophysiol. 1998; 80(1):1-27.

Schultz W. Potential vulnerabilities of neuronal reward, risk, and decision mechanisms to addictive drugs. Neuron. 2011;69(4):603-17.

Schutte-Rodin S; Broch L; Buysse D; Dorsey C; Sateia M. Clinical guideline for the evaluation and management of chronic insomnia in adults. J Clin Sleep Med 2008; 4(5): 487-504.

Scott DJ, Stohler CS, Egnatuk CM, Wang H, Koeppe RA, Zubieta JK. Individual differences in reward responding explain placebo-induced expectations and effects. Neuron. 2007; 55(2):325-36.

Seid AA, Mohammed AA, Hasen AA. Progressive muscle relaxation exercises in patients with COVID-19: Systematic review and meta-analysis. Medicine (Baltimore). 2023; 102(14):e33464.

Seminowicz DA, Mayberg HS, McIntosh AR, Goldapple K, Kennedy S, Segal Z, Rafi-Tari S. Limbic-frontal circuitry in major depression: A path modeling metanalysis. Neuroimage. 2004; 22(1):409-18.

Sephien A, Reljic T, Jordan J, Prida X, Kumar A. Resident duty hours and resident and patient outcomes: Systematic review and meta-analysis. Med Educ. 2023; 57(3):221-232.

Serafine KM, O'Dell LE, Zorrilla EP. Converging vulnerability factors for compulsive food and drug use. Neuropharmacology. 2021; 196:108556.

Shanafelt TD, Hasan O, Dyrbye LN, Sinsky C, Satele D, Sloan J, West CP. Changes in burnout and satisfaction with work-life balance in physicians and the general US working population between 2011 and 2014. Mayo Clin Proc 2015; 90: 1600–13.

Shiri R, Nikunlaakso R, Laitinen J. Effectiveness of Workplace Interventions to Improve Health and Well-Being of Health and Social Service Workers: A Narrative Review of Randomised Controlled Trials. Healthcare. 2023; 11(12):1792.

Shibuya K, Ji X, Pfoh ER, Milinovich A, Weng W, Bauman J, Ganguly R, Misra-Hebert AD, Hobbs TM, Kattan MW, Pantalone KM, Ramasamy A, Burguera B. Association between shared medical appointments and weight loss outcomes and anti-obesity medication use in patients with obesity. Obes Sci Pract. 2020; 6(3):247-254.

Shin LM, Wright CI, Cannistraro PA, Wedig MM, McMullin K, Martis B, Macklin ML, Lasko NB, Cavanagh SR, Krangel TS, Orr SP, Pitman RK, Whalen PJ, Rauch SL. A functional magnetic resonance imaging study of amygdala and medial prefrontal cortex responses to overtly presented fearful faces in posttraumatic stress disorder. Arch Gen Psychiatry. 2005; 62(3):273-81.

Shipherd JC, Keyes M, Jovanovic T, Ready DJ, Baltzell D, Worley V, Gordon-Brown V, Hayslett C, Duncan E. Veterans seeking treatment for posttraumatic stress disorder: what about comorbid chronic pain? J Rehabil Res Dev. 2007; 44(2):153-66.

Shonkoff JP, Boyce WT, McEwen BS. Neuroscience, molecular biology, and the childhood roots of health disparities: building a new framework for health promotion and disease prevention. JAMA. 2009; 301(21):2252-9.

Siegle GJ, Carter CS, Thase ME. Use of FMRI to predict recovery from unipolar depression with cognitive behavior therapy. Am J Psychiatry. 2006; 163(4):735-8.

Simon L, Steinmetz L, Feige B, Benz F, Spiegelhalder K, Baumeister H. Comparative efficacy of onsite, digital, and other settings for cognitive behavioral therapy for insomnia: a systematic review and network meta-analysis. Sci Rep. 2023; 13(1):1929.

Small DM, Zatorre RJ, Dagher A, Evans AC, Jones-Gotman M. Changes in brain activity related to eating chocolate: from pleasure to aversion. Brain. 2001; 124(9): 1720-1733.

Smith-Coggins R, Howard SK, Mac DT, Wang C, Kwan S, Rosekind MR, Sowb Y, Balise R, Levis J, Gaba DM. Improving alertness and performance in emergency department physicians and nurses: the use of planned naps. Ann Emerg Med. 2006; 48(5):596-604.

Sobstyl M, Kupryjaniuk A, Prokopienko M, Rylski M. Subcallosal Cingulate Cortex Deep Brain Stimulation for Treatment-Resistant Depression: A Systematic Review. Front Neurol. 2022; 13:780481.

Sokol R, Albanese M, Albanese C, Coste G, Grossman E, Morrill D, Roll D, Sobieszczyk A, Schuman-Olivier Z. Implementing group visits for opioid use disorder: A case series. Subst Abus. 2020; 41(2):174-180.

Sorbi MJ, Peters ML, Kruise DA, Maas CJ, Kerssens JJ, Verhaak PF, Bensing JM. Electronic momentary assessment in chronic pain I: psychological pain responses as predictors of pain intensity. Clin J Pain. 2006; 22(1):55-66.

Sorrell JT, Trafton JA, McKellar, JD. Integrated management of pain. Unpublished workbook: VA Palo Alto, 2005.

Spikmans FJ, Brug J, Doven MM, Kruizenga HM, Hofsteenge GH, van Bokhorst-van der Schueren MA. Why do diabetic patients not attend appointments with their dietitian? J Hum Nutr Diet. 2003; 16(3):151-8.

Sripada RK, Grau PP, Porath BR, Burgess J, Van T, Kim HM, Boden MT, Zivin K. Role of Institutional Support for Evidence-Based Psychotherapy in Satisfaction and Burnout Among Veterans Affairs Therapists. Psychiatr Serv. 2024: 75(3): 206-213.

Stanley B, Brown GK, Brenner LA, Galfalvy HC, Currier GW, Knox KL, Chaudhury SR, Bush AL, Green KL. Comparison of the Safety Planning Intervention With Follow-up vs Usual Care of Suicidal Patients Treated in the Emergency Department. JAMA Psychiatry. 2018; 75(9):894-900.

Steele CC, Pirkle JRA, Kirkpatrick K. Diet-induced impulsivity: Effects of a high-fat and a high-sugar diet on impulsive choice in rats. PLoS One. 2017; 12(6):e0180510.

Stein JS, Wilson AG, Koffarnus MN, Daniel TO, Epstein LH, Bickel WK. Unstuck in time: episodic future thinking reduces delay discounting and cigarette smoking. Psychopharmacology (Berl). 2016; 233(21-22):3771-3778.

Stein JS, Smits RR, Johnson PS, Liston KJ, Madden GL. Effects of reward bundling on male rats' preferences for larger-later food rewards. J Exper Analysis Behavior. 2013; 99 (2): 150-158.

Stitzer M, Petry N. Contingency management for treatment of substance abuse. Annu Rev Clin Psychol. 2006; 2:411-34.

Strombotne KL, Legler A, Minegishi T, Trafton JA, Oliva EM, Lewis ET, Sohoni P, Garrido MM, Pizer SD, Frakt AB. Effect of a Predictive Analytics-Targeted Program in Patients on Opioids: a Stepped-Wedge Cluster Randomized Controlled Trial. J Gen Intern Med. 2023; 38(2):375-381.

Stubbs B, Vancampfort D, Rosenbaum S, Firth J, Cosco T, Veronese N, Salum GA, Schuch FB. An examination of the anxiolytic effects of exercise for people with anxiety and stress-related disorders: A meta-analysis. Psychiatry Res. 2017; 249:102-108.

Stulz N, Lutz W, Kopta SM, Minami T, Saunders SM. Dose-effect relationship in routine outpatient psychotherapy: does treatment duration matter? J Couns Psychol. 2013 Oct;60(4):593-600.

Stroop, JR. Studies of interference in serial verbal reactions. J Exper Psychol. 1935; 18: 643-662.

Suda A, Kawanishi C, Kishida I, Sato R, Yamada T, Nakagawa M,et al. Dopamine D2 receptor gene polymorphisms are associated with suicide attempt in the Japanese population. Neuropsychobiology. 2009; 59(2):130–134.

Sutton RT, Pincock D, Baumgart DC, Sadowski DC, Fedorak RN, Kroeker KI. An overview of clinical decision support systems: benefits, risks, and strategies for success. NPJ Digit Med. 2020; 3:17.

Taber KH, Hurley RA, Yudofsky. Diagnosis and treatment of neuropsychiatric disorders. Ann Rev of Med. 2010; 61:121-133.

Taha SA, Fields HL. Inhibitions of nucleus accumbens neurons encode a gating signal for reward-directed behavior. J Neurosci. 2006; 26(1):217-22.

Tam EK, De Arrigunaga S, Shah M, Kefella H, Soriano S, Rowe S. Patient and Clinician Satisfaction With Shared Medical Appointments for Glaucoma. Semin Ophthalmol. 2022; 37(1):17-22.

Taylor JJ, Borckardt JJ, Canterberry M, Li X, Hanlon CA, Brown TR, George MS. Naloxone-reversible modulation of pain circuitry by left prefrontal rTMS. Neuropsychopharmacology. 2013; 38(7): 1189-1197.

Temiz G, Sébille SB, Francois C, Bardinet E, Karachi C. The anatomo-functional organization of the hyperdirect cortical pathway to the subthalamic area using in vivo structural connectivity imaging in humans. Brain Structure and Function. 2020; 225: 551-565.

The ASAM National Practice Guideline for the Treatment of Opioid Use Disorder: 2020 Focused Update. J Addict Med. 2020; 14(2S Suppl 1):1-91.

Thomas R, Zimmer-Gembeck MJ. Behavioral outcomes of Parent-Child Interaction Therapy and Triple P-Positive Parenting Program: a review and meta-analysis. J Abnorm Child Psychol. 2007; 35(3):475-95.

Thompson PM, Hayashi KM, Simon SL, Geaga JA, Hong MS, Sui Y, Lee JY, Toga AW, Ling W, London ED. Structural abnormalities in the brains of human subjects who use methamphetamine. J Neurosci. 2004; 24(26):6028-36.

Timko C, DeBenedetti A. A randomized controlled trial of intensive referral to 12-step self-help groups: one-year outcomes. Drug Alcohol Depend. 2007; 90(2-3):270-9.

Tobler PN, Fiorillo CD, Schultz W. Adaptive coding of reward value by dopamine neurons. Science. 2005; 307(5715):1642-5.

Tomosugi N, Koshino Y. Gentle, Massage-like, Head Stroking Provokes Salivary Oxytocin Release. Altern Ther Health Med. 2023; 29(5):188-191.

Torrens M, Fonseca F, Mateu G, Farre M. Efficacy of antidepressants in substance use disorders with and without comorbid depression. A systematic review and meta-analysis. Drug Alcohol Depend. 2005; 78(1): 1-22.

Trafton JA, Gifford EV. Behavioral reactivity and addiction: the adaptation of behavioral response to reward opportunities. J Neuropsychiatry Clin Neurosci. 2008; 20(1):23-35.

Trafton JA, Gordon W (eds.). Best practices in the behavioral management of chronic disease: volume 1 neuropsychiatric disorders. Los Altos: Institute for Brain Potential. 2008a.

Trafton JA, Gordon W (eds). Best practices in the behavioral management of chronic disease: volume 2 other medical disorders. Los Altos: Institute for Brain Potential, 2008b.

Trafton J, Martins S, Michel M, Lewis E, Wang D, Combs A, Scates N, Tu S, Goldstein MK. Evaluation of the acceptability and usability of a decision support system to encourage safe and effective use of opioid therapy for chronic, noncancer pain by primary care providers. Pain Med. 2010; 11(4):575-85.

Trafton JA, Sorrell JT, Holodniy M, Pierson H, Link P, Combs A, Israelski D. Outcomes associated with a cognitive-behavioral chronic pain management program implemented in three public HIV primary care clinics. J Behav Health Serv Res. 2012; 39(2):158-73.

Tranel D, Gullickson G, Koch M, Adolphs R. Altered experience of emotion following bilateral amygdala damage. Cogn Neuropsychiatry. 2006; 11(3):219-32.

Truby H, Baic S, deLooy A, Fox KR, Livingstone MB, Logan CM, Macdonald IA, Morgan LM, Taylor MA, Millward DJ. Randomised controlled trial of four commercial weight loss programmes in the UK: initial findings from the BBC "diet trials". BMJ. 2006; 332(7553):1309-14.

Tsuchida A, Doll BB, Fellows LK. Beyond reversal: a critical role for human orbitofrontal cortex in flexible learning from probabilistic feedback. J Neuroscience. 2010; 30(50): 16868-16875.

Turner JK, Athamneh LN, Basso JC, Bickel WK. The phenotype of recovery V: Does delay discounting predict the perceived risk of relapse among individuals in recovery from alcohol and drug use disorders. Alcohol Clin Exp Res. 2021; 45(5):1100-1108.

Ulman, MT. Is Broca's area part of a basal ganglia thalamocortical circuit? Cortex. 2006; 42(4):480-5.

Umilta MA, Kohler E, Gallese V, Fogassi L, Fadiga L. I know what you are doing. A neurophysiological study. Neuron. 2001; 31: 155-65.

Uvnäs-Moberg K, Handlin L, Petersson M. Self-soothing behaviors with particular reference to oxytocin release induced by non-noxious sensory stimulation. Front Psychol. 2015; 5:1529.

Internal Revenue Service. Clean Vehicle Tax Credits. Available at: https://www.irs.gov/clean-vehicle-tax-credits. Accessed on April 28, 2024.

U.S. Department of Veterans Affairs. "VHA National Center for Patient Safety: VA's Approach to Patient Safety." 2023; Accessed on July 30, 2023. Available at: https://www.patientsafety.va.gov/about/approach.asp.

van Baarle E, Hartman L, Rooijakkers S, Wallenburg I, Weenink JW, Bal R, Widdershoven G. Fostering a just culture in healthcare organizations: experiences in practice. BMC Health Serv Res. 2022; 22(1):1035.

van der Elst W, van Boxtel MP, van Breukelen GJ, Jolles J. The Stroop color-word test: influence of age, sex, and education; and normative data for a large sample across the adult age range. Assessment. 2006; 13(1):62-79.

van der Heijden AA, Hu FB, Rimm EB, van Dam RM. A prospective study of breakfast consumption and weight gain among U.S. men. Obesity (Silver Spring). 2007; 15(10): 2463-9.

Vander Wal JS, Maraldo TM, Vercellone AC, Gagne DA. Education, progressive muscle relaxation therapy, and exercise for the treatment of night eating syndrome. A pilot study. Appetite. 2015; 89:136-44.

van Honk J, Hermans EJ, Putman P, Montagne B, Schutter DJ. Defective somatic markers in sub-clinical psychopathy. Neuroreport. 2002; 13(8):1025-7.

van Peppen L, Faber TJE, Erasmus V, Dankbaar MEW. Teamwork Training With a Multiplayer Game in Health Care: Content Analysis of the Teamwork Principles Applied. JMIR Serious Games. 2022; 10(4): e38009.

Vance DE, Moore BS, Farr KF, Struzick T. Prefrontal and anterior cingulate cortex abnormalities in Tourette Syndrome: evidence from voxel-based morphometry and magnetization transfer imaging. BMC Neurosci. 2009;10:47.

Venkatraman V, Chuah YM, Huettel SA, Chee MW. Sleep deprivation elevates expectation of gains and attenuates response to losses following risky decisions. Sleep. 2007; 30(5):603-9.

Vidal J, Soldevilla JM. Effect of compassion-focused therapy on self-criticism and self-soothing: A meta-analysis. Br J Clin Psychol. 2023; 62(1):70-81.

Vieweg WV, Julius DA, Bates J, Quinn JF 3rd, Fernandez A, Hasnain M, Pandurangi AK. Posttraumatic stress disorder as a risk factor for obesity among male military veterans. Acta Psychiatr Scand. 2007; 116(6):483-7.

Vitay J, Hamker FH. Timing and expectation of reward: a neuro-computational model of the afferents to the ventral tegmental area. Front Neurorobot. 2014; 8:4.

Vlaeyen JW, de Jong J, Geilen M, Heuts PH, van Breukelen G. Graded exposure in vivo in the treatment of pain-related fear: a replicated single-case experimental design in four patients with chronic low back pain. Behav Res Ther. 2001; 39(2):151-66.

Vlaeyen JWS, Linton SJ. Fear-avoidance and its consequences in chronic musculoskeletal pain: a state of the art. Pain. 2000; 85(3):317-332.

Volpp KG, John LK, Troxel AB, Norton L, Fassbender J, Loewenstein G. Financial incentive-based approaches for weight loss: a randomized trial. JAMA. 2008; 300(22): 2631-7.

Wadsworth KH, Archibald TG, Payne AE, Cleary AK, Haney BL, Hoverman AS. Shared medical appointments and patient-centered experience: a mixed-methods systematic review. BMC Fam Pract. 2019; 20(1):97.

Wager TD, Rilling JK, Smith EE, Sokolik A, Casey KL, Davidson RJ, Kosslyn SM, Rose RM, Cohen JD. Placebo-induced changes in FMRI in the anticipation and experience of pain. Science. 2004; 303(5661):1162-7.

Walch JM, Rabin BS, Day R, Williams JN, Choi K, Kang JD. The effect of sunlight on postoperative analgesic medication use: a prospective study of patients undergoing spinal surgery. Psychosomatic Med. 2005; 67: 156-163.

Wall-Haas CL, Kulbok P, Kirchgessner J, Rovnyak V. Shared medical appointments: facilitating care for children with asthma and their caregivers. J Pediatr Health Care. 2012; 26(1):37-44.

Walker R, Ramasamy V, Sturgiss E, Dunbar J, Boyle J. Shared medical appointments for weight loss: a systematic review. Fam Pract. 2022; 39(4):710-724.

Wagas A, Akhtar P, Afzaal TA, Meraj H, Naveed S. Social support interventions for young healthcare professionals: In- sight analyses based on a mixed-methods systematic review & meta-analysis. Wellcome's 2020 Workplace Mental Health Commission report. Available at: https://cms.wellcome.org/sites/default/files/2021-05/social-support-interventions-healthcare-workers-wellcome-workplace-mental-health.pdf .

Wang Y, Yang L, Lin G, Huang B, Sheng X, Wang L, Chen L, Qiu X, Wu X, Lin R. The efficacy of progressive muscle relaxation training on cancer-related fatigue and quality of life in patients with cancer: A systematic review and meta-analysis of randomized controlled studies. Int J Nurs Stud. 2024;152:104694.

Wansink B, van Ittersum K. Portion size me: downsizing our consumption norms. J Am Diet Assoc. 2007; 107(7):1103-6.

Webber KH, Tate DF, Michael Bowling J. A randomized comparison of two motivationally enhanced Internet behavioral weight loss programs. Behav Res Ther. 2008; 46(9):1090-5.

Webster-Stratton C, Jamila Reid M, Stoolmiller M. Preventing conduct problems and improving school readiness: evaluation of the Incredible Years Teacher and Child Training Programs in high-risk schools. J Child Psychol Psychiatry. 2008; 49(5):471-88.

Weinberg A, Kotov R, Proudfit GH. Neural indicators of error processing in generalized anxiety disorder, obsessive-compulsive disorder, and major depressive disorder. J Abnorm

Psychol. 2015;124(1):172-85.

Weintraub D. Dopamine and impulse control disorders in Parkinson's disease. Ann Neurol. 2008; 64 Suppl 2:S93-100.

West CP, Dyrbye LN, Shanafelt TD. Physician burnout: contributors, consequences and solutions. J Intern Med. 2018; 283(6):516-529.

West DS, DiLillo V, Bursac Z, Gore SA, Greene PG. Motivational interviewing improves weight loss in women with type 2 diabetes. Diabetes Care. 2007; 30(5):1081-7.

White B, Sanders SH. The influence on patients' pain intensity ratings of antecedent reinforcement of pain talk or well talk. J Behav Ther Exp Psychiatry. 1986; 17(3):155-9.

Wikipedia. Employer transportation benefits in the United States. Available at: http://en.wikipedia.org/wiki/Employer_transportation_benefits_in_the_United_States. Accessed 2/19/24.

Wise RA, Bozarth MA. Brain mechanisms of drug reward and euphoria. Psychiatr Med. 1985; 3(4):445-60.

Woods MP, Asmundson GJ. Evaluating the efficacy of graded in vivo exposure for the treatment of fear in patients with chronic back pain: a randomized controlled clinical trial. Pain. 2008; 136(3): 271-80.

Worbe Y, Gerardin E, Hartmann A, Valabrégue R, Chupin M, Tremblay L, Vidailhet M, Colliot O, Lehéricy S. Distinct structural changes underpin clinical phenotypes in patients with Gilles de la Tourette syndrome. Brain. 2010; 133(Pt 12):3649-60.

Wu AW. Medical error: the second victim. The doctor who makes the mistake needs help too. BMJ. 2000; 320(7237):726-7.

Zack M, Poulos CX. A D2 antagonist enhances the rewarding and priming effects of a gambling episode in pathological gamblers. Neuropsychopharmacology. 2007; 32(8): 1678-86.

Zalocusky KA, Ramakrishnan C, Lerner TN, Davidson TJ, Knutson B, Deisseroth K. Nucleus accumbens D2R cells signal prior outcomes and control risky decision-making. Nature. 2016; 531(7596):642-646.

Zeller D, Gross C, Bartsch A, Johansen-Berg H, Classen J. Ventral premotor cortex may be required for dynamic changes in the feeling of limb ownership: a lesion study. J Neurosci. 2011; 31(13):4852-7.

Zhang W, Cao Y, Wang M, Ji L, Chen L, Deater-Deckard K. The Dopamine D2 Receptor Polymorphism (DRD2 TaqIA) Interacts with Maternal Parenting in Predicting Early Adolescent Depressive Symptoms: Evidence of Differential Susceptibility and Age Differences. J Youth Adolesc. 2015; 44(7):1428-40.

Ziadni MS, Gonzalez-Castro L, Anderson S, Krishnamurthy P, Darnall BD. Efficacy of a Single-Session "Empowered Relief" Zoom-Delivered Group Intervention for Chronic Pain: Randomized Controlled Trial Conducted During the COVID-19 Pandemic. J Med Internet Res. 2021; 23(9):e29672.

Use this page to list how you can benefit from applying the 5 brain challenges:

Made in the USA
Las Vegas, NV
03 October 2024

96224632R00210